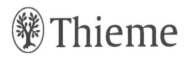

The Art of Refractive Cataract Surgery

For Residents, Fellows, and Beginners

Fuxiang Zhang, MD
Medical Director
Department of Ophthalmology
Downriver Supervision Center
Henry Ford Health System
Taylor, Michigan, USA

Alan Sugar, MD
Professor
Department of Ophthalmology and Visual Sciences
W.K. Kellogg Eye Center
University of Michigan Medical School
Ann Arbor, Michigan, USA

Lisa Brothers Arbisser, MD
Co-founder and Ophthalmologist Emerita
Eye Surgeons Associates PC
Iowa and Illinois Quad Cities;
Adjunct Professor
John A. Moran Eye Center
University of Utah
Salt Lake City, Utah, USA

185 illustrations

Thieme
New York • Stuttgart • Delhi • Rio de Janeiro

Library of Congress Cataloging-in-Publication Data
is available with the publisher.

Important note: Medicine is an ever-changing science undergoing continual development. Research and clinical experience are continually expanding our knowledge, in particular our knowledge of proper treatment and drug therapy. Insofar as this book mentions any dosage or application, readers may rest assured that the authors, editors, and publishers have made every effort to ensure that such references are in accordance with **the state of knowledge at the time of production of the book.**

Nevertheless, this does not involve, imply, or express any guarantee or responsibility on the part of the publishers in respect to any dosage instructions and forms of applications stated in the book. **Every user is requested to examine carefully** the manufacturers' leaflets accompanying each drug and to check, if necessary in consultation with a physician or specialist, whether the dosage schedules mentioned therein or the contraindications stated by the manufacturers differ from the statements made in the present book. Such examination is particularly important with drugs that are either rarely used or have been newly released on the market. Every dosage schedule or every form of application used is entirely at the user's own risk and responsibility. The authors and publishers request every user to report to the publishers any discrepancies or inaccuracies noticed. If errors in this work are found after publication, errata will be posted at www.thieme.com on the product description page.

Some of the product names, patents, and registered designs referred to in this book are in fact registered trademarks or proprietary names even though specific reference to this fact is not always made in the text. Therefore, the appearance of a name without designation as proprietary is not to be construed as a representation by the publisher that it is in the public domain.

Thieme addresses people of all gender identities equally. We encourage our authors to use gender neutral or gender-equal expressions wherever the context allows.

Thieme Medical Publishers, Inc.
333 Seventh Avenue, 18th Floor,
New York, NY 10001, USA
www.thieme.com
+1 800 782 3488,
customerservice@thieme.com

Cover design: © Thieme

Cover image source: Composed by Thieme using following image:
3D Eye Anatomy © PIC4U/stock.adobe.com

Typesetting by Thomson Digital, India

Printed in USA by King Printing Company, Inc.   5 4 3 2 1

ISBN 978-1-68420-257-7

Also available as an e-book:
eISBN (PDF): 978-1-68420-258-4
eISBN (epub): 978-1-63853-709-0

This book is dedicated to W.K. Kellogg Eye Center, University of Michigan, with sincere gratitude for the residency training I received from 1994 to 1997.

Fuxiang Zhang, MD

Contents

Contents

Videos

Video 23.4   Enlargement of CCC after ReStor lens. This video shows the tangential cut with a pair of scissors to make a tag that can be grasped and torn in a spiral fashion to enlarge a continuous circular capsulorhexis once the IOL is in position forming a template for perfect sizing.

Video 23.5   CCC runout; complication prevention. Close observation reveals an unintended direction of the tear within a millimeter. OVD is placed peripherally over the area of the tear to deepen the chamber and change the downhill direction for return to the proper vector and completion.

Video 23.6   Continuous rhexis or bust for crystalens. This shows the efforts without regard to time to complete a CCC at all costs including the use of Trypan Blue dye to visualize and reduce elasticity of the capsule to retrieve a continuous outcome.

Video 23.7   Intumescent cataract surgery. This video demonstrates the use of adaptive OVD to maintain the flat shape of a lens with extreme intralenticular pressure and the method of moving emerging lens milk peripherally for visualization with dispersive OVD eliminating the risk of Argentinian flag tears. It also demonstrates the chop technique for a dense lens, leaving a clean bag for optimal outcome.

Video 23.8   Central dimple down technique for FLACS. This surgery, courtesy of Professor H. Burkhard Dick, demonstrates the use of the OVD cannula to press down directly on the femtolaser anterior flap to safely prevent any tags from resulting in radial tears of the CCC.

Video 23.9   Pearls for stable chamber. Prevention of reverse pupillary block in a high myope is demonstrated along with the use of irrigation through the sideport while removing the phaco and I/A handpieces from the CCI to prevent anterior chamber collapse and CCI irrigation for immediate closure after OVD removal, all to maintain a stable anterior chamber for quiet eyes and best outcome.

Video 23.10   Iris prolapse with posterior pressure. Many pearls are demonstrated for the high-pressure eye's management at every step of the cataract procedure, from preventing full and repeated iris prolapse to chamber maintenance even during incision closure.

Video 23.11   5+ Brunescent with circumferential disassembly vertical chop technique. This voiced over video of a very dense lens is disassembled with minimal CDE showing the steps and explaining the principles of Circumferential Disassembly with Cross Action Vertical chop technique at the iris plane or below. A clear cornea is evident at completion.

Video 23.12   Vitrectomy lessons to avoid traction. This shows the value of amputation of anterior-posterior vitreous connection rather than sweeping and the one port pars plana technique for anterior vitrectomy as well as the safe implantation of a 3-piece IOL with optic capture.

Video 23.13   Posterior optic capture after primary posterior capsulorhexis. This video shows the technique of primary posterior capsulorhexis with posterior optic capture into Berger's space during the author's early learning curve.

Foreword

Cataract surgery is a modern-day miracle. According to Market Scope, since 1995, over 500 million cataract surgeries with intraocular lens implantation have been performed on 300 million patients worldwide. About 60,000 cataract surgeries are performed every day in the world and close to 20,000 per working day in the USA. The growing elderly population is driving a 3% plus increase per year in the USA cataract surgery volume, which means surgeons in training today will perform twice as much cataract surgery per year as today's cataract surgeon in 24 years. The American baby boom generation is very demanding regarding the vision they desire after cataract surgery for their active lifestyles. Today's patients with cataract want to be able to see after cataract surgery like they did in their 30s, and every year patient expectations increase. To achieve our patient's goals, ophthalmic surgeons must not only restore clear vision, but also enhance vision through the treatment of pre-existing refractive errors and thereby reducing dependence on glasses or contact lenses.

Although cataract surgery has always impacted our patients' refractive status, it is only in the past two decades that the tools required to provide patients with clear seamless vision from far to near without optical correction had become possible. The goal of refractive cataract surgery is to not only restore clear vision but also enhance visual performance. Today's refractive cataract surgeon must treat the patient's base refractive error, correct pre-existing astigmatism, reduce the handicap of presbyopia, obtain the patient's desired postoperative target refraction, and reduce higher-order aberrations and corneal irregularities. The knowledge and skills required are significant. They include a broad base of understanding, a good communication skill, and access to advanced diagnostics, devices, and drugs, complemented by surgical excellence.

In their book *The Art of Refractive Cataract Surgery: For Residents, Fellows, and Beginners*, master refractive cataract surgeons Fuxiang Zhang, MD; Alan Sugar, MD; Lisa Brothers Arbisser, MD; and a carefully selected team of outstanding colleagues share their broad experience with the reader. This is a book written by veteran educators for the refractive cataract surgeon in training, but many surgeons in active practice today will also benefit.

Richard L. Lindstrom, MD
Senior Lecturer and Foundation Trustee
University of Minnesota;
Visiting Professor
University of California Irvine Gavin Herbert Eye Institute;
Founder and Surgeon Emeritus
Minnesota Eye Consultants/Unifeye Vision Partners
Bloomington, Minnesota, USA

Preface

Everyone develops cataracts if they live long enough. Presbyopia is also an integral part of human aging. The estimated number of presbyopes worldwide was 1.4 billion in 2020.[1] Although topical medications for presbyopia are currently under investigation, the main nonsurgical management of presbyopia remains spectacle correction. The most practical permanent solution for the dysfunctional lens in presbyopia, however, is undeniably refractive cataract surgery (RCS).

The annual estimated volume of US cataract surgery is 3.6 million cases.[2] In our clinical survey in 2016 (Fuxiang Zhang), 50% of cataract patients sought partial relief from spectacles (readers only) and about 25% desired total spectacle independence. We believe RCS is clearly a growing trend. The public has come to expect it. Loosely defined, RCS has been practiced by Alan Sugar and Lisa Brothers Arbisser since the days of intracapsular surgery with timed selective suture removal. A leap forward was taken when astigmatism became manageable in a reasonably predictable manner with corneal incisions, refined by toric implants and femtosecond laser incisions. Presbyopia correcting lenses began with the Array lens in 1997[3] and has progressed to ever more sophisticated ways of providing a range of lenses for spectacle independent vision. Upcharging medicare patients for the refractive component of cataract surgery has forever changed the playing field.

In 2013, the American Society of Cataract and Refractive Surgery (ASCRS) sent a survey to 2,279 residents, fellows, young practicing physicians (practicing for 5 years or less), and program directors of 118 ACGME accredited ophthalmology programs throughout the United States. The study showed that 52% had not performed corneal relaxing incisions and 60% had no experience in implanting toric intraocular lenses (IOLs); 78% had not implanted a presbyopia-correcting IOL.[4] The 2018 ASCRS survey showed modest improvement. More than two-thirds of the surveyed residents and about one-third of surveyed fellows and young professionals had not done any limbal relaxing incisions (LRIs) or inserted presbyopia-correcting IOLs. Approximately two-thirds of fellows and young professionals did not feel competent to manage unhappy presbyopia-correcting IOL patients.[5] Training programs for future surgeons vary widely in providing advanced procedures and techniques likely needed immediately following residency both to be competitive and, especially, to deliver the best care with a full range of patient options.

As no perfect solution for presbyopia exists yet and technology continues to evolve, many seasoned surgeons are hesitant to provide presbyopia solutions. However, we can be successful in fulfilling the needs of the vast majority of our patients who at least deserve to hear about the available options. The 2018 ASCRS survey indicated that more than 30% of respondents did not even feel sufficiently trained to integrate toric IOLs into their practices. Among American respondents, this number increased to 39%, which may reflect this major gap in residency training.[6]

There are a few wonderful books on the topic of RCS and premium IOLs, but this book is specifically written for residents, fellows, and beginners who wish to engage in and improve their RCS skills. The triggers to write this book were the questions from our own residents as well as from attendees of the annual American Academy of Ophthalmology (AAO) when I (Fuxiang Zhang) was responsible for the Breakfast with the Experts sessions on Pseudophakic Monovision/Refractive Cataract Surgery. Our impression was that commercially available books were excellent for those with moderate experience in RCS, but may not be optimal for true beginners, as they assume a pre-existing fund of knowledge.

Most medical textbooks are at least 1 year behind when printed with regard to advanced technology and even medical theory. This book is no exception. This book does not introduce the most advanced technology, but instead helps beginners become familiar with and master the fundamentals in the process of incorporating RCS and its principles into practice. Therefore, we hope that it is timeless. We aim to cover the basics, with the experience of seasoned practitioners added, where and how to start limbal relaxing incisions, toric IOLs, IOL monovision, multifocal/accommodating/EDOF/trifocal IOLs, intraoperative aberrometers such as ORA, IOL formulas, femtosecond laser-assisted cataract surgery, and more. For each premium IOL, we start with criteria for candidate selection. Understanding who are the best candidates for one's first few cases (and whom to avoid) is a critical first step. This book encourages surgeons to ford the challenging river of learning curves with clearly defined basic and fundamental knowledge and its application. We hope that this book helps beginners enjoy home run success as they engage in RCS. This book uniquely focuses its chapters on our residents' and junior colleagues' questions and has been refined by their feedback. Enjoy!

Fuxiang Zhang, MD
Alan Sugar, MD
Lisa Brothers Arbisser, MD

References

1. Holden BA, Fricke TR, Ho SM, et al. Global vision impairment due to uncorrected presbyopia. Arch Ophthalmol 2008;126(12):1731–1739
2. Werner L. Aerosol generation: the safety of phacoemulsification in the pandemic era. J Cataract Refract Surg 2020;46(9):1215–1216
3. Allergan AMO Array multifocal IOL roll-out slated for end of October. Medtech Insight. Published September 15, 1997. Accessed July 17, 2021. https://medtech.pharmaintelligence.informa.com/MT008736/Allergan-AMO-Array-multifocal-IOL-rollout-slated-for-end-of-October
4. Yeu E, Reeves SW, Wang L, Randleman JB; ASCRS Young Physicians and Residents Clinical Committee. Resident surgical experience with lens and corneal refractive surgery: a survey of the ASCRS young physicians and residents membership. J Cataract Refract Surg 2013;39(2):279–284
5. ASCRS Clinical Survey results highlight key issues for young physicians. EyeWorld (suppl). 2019:16–18
6. ASCRS Clinical Survey 2018. EyeWorld (suppl). Published November 20, 2018. Accessed July 30, 2021. https://supplements.eyeworld.org/eyeworld-supplements/december-2018-clinical-survey

About the Authors

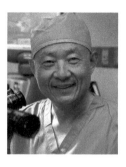

Fuxiang Zhang, MD

Dr. Fuxiang Zhang started to use multifocal intraocular lenses (MFIOL) in the same year that he graduated from his ophthalmology residency at the W. K. Kellogg Eye Center, University of Michigan in 1997 when the Array IOL had just been approved by the FDA. He did not wait to use the first Star Toric IOL in 1998 when it was just approved by FDA. He has performed cataract surgery using all of the premium IOLs approved in the US and has been actively involved in American Society of Cataract and Refractive Surgery (ASCRS) and American Academy of Ophthalmology (AAO) refractive cataract surgery teaching and lecturing. He has published influential peer-reviewed papers as the first author in prestigious journals in the field of refractive cataract surgery, including the debate on IOL monovision vs MFIOL, conventional monovision vs. crossed monovision, limitations of ORA for post radial keratotomy (RK) patients, etc. He has also been invited by numerous national and international conferences as a keynote speaker. Together with Alan Sugar and Graham Barrett, his first ophthalmologic book, *Pseudophakic Monovision: A Clinic Guide*, was published in 2018. Besides refractive cataract surgery, Dr. Zhang has been actively involved in other ophthalmic innovation projects, among which the Zhang Ring Test (Precision Vision, Woodstock, Illinois) has been used to promote early diagnosis of retinal detachment. A few new sulcus IOL and Toric IOL designs are illustrated in this current book.

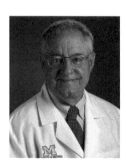

Alan Sugar, MD

Dr. Alan Sugar is Professor of Ophthalmology and Visual Sciences at the W. K. Kellogg Eye Center at the University of Michigan. A graduate of the University of Michigan Medical School, he was an ophthalmology resident at Washington University in St Louis and a Cornea Fellow at the University of Florida. He has been on the faculty at Michigan since 1979. His interest has been in corneal and cataract surgery. He served as editor-in-chief of Cornea, the journal of the Cornea Society. He is also interested in clinical research ethics and serves as a chair of the Institutional Review Board of the University of Michigan Medical School.

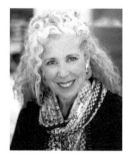

Lisa Brother Arbisser, MD

Dr. Lisa Brothers Arbisser, a recognized leader in cataract and anterior segment surgery, co-founded Eye Surgeons Associates, PC: An 8-office, 22-doctors, 180-employees integrated Iowa, Illinois practice. Graduating with honors from Princeton University, she received her MD (AOA) from the University of Texas Health Science Center at Houston and NIH fellowship in neurobiology and retina before completing ophthalmology residency and associate fellowship in anterior segment surgery at the University of Iowa. She is adjunct professor at the University of Utah Moran Eye Center, a frequent-visiting professor and invited speaker, an author of textbook chapters, and former writer/editor of Focal Points. She surgical coaches privately since retiring from direct patient care after 30 years in practice. Numerous awards include two AAO Secretariat awards and two ASCRS peer-voted Golden Apple Awards for surgical teaching. She has performed satellite surgery in the US and abroad. She served on the AAO online news and education network (ONE) for over a decade as well on numerous editorial boards. She is a former president of the American College of Eye Surgeons and served as education director on the board of Women in Ophthalmology. She was voted among the top 50 opinion leaders by Cataract and Refractive Surgery Today and was one of the earliest female KOL's for industry in cataract surgery. The American Women's Medical Association recognized her as an Iowa Living Legend, and she's been honored as a lifetime member of the Iowa Volunteer Hall of Fame. She is a third-generation professional woman, wife and mother of 4, and grandmother of 4.

Acknowledgments

First and foremost, our wholehearted gratitude to our patients who trust us with their precious vision. Special thanks to the patients of all of this book's contributors. Their willingness to participate in our research projects has made our learning possible.

Sir Isaac Newton said, "If I have seen further than others, it is by standing upon the shoulders of giants." It has been my great gratitude to work with such giants over the whole course of writing this book. I cannot thank them enough, my coauthors, Alan Sugar and Lisa Brothers Arbisser, for their knowledge, expertise and meticulous collaborative contributions, without which, this book would have been impossible.

This book is also the work of our chapter contributors who are among the top-notch refractive cataract surgeons and leaders in our profession. Needless to say, they spent much of their precious personal time in composing and editing their chapters. Without their great contributions, this book would not be able to provide a full spectrum of modern refractive cataract surgery. I extend my sincere appreciation to Richard Lindstrom, Robert Osher, Cynthia Matossian, Kendall Donaldson, Nandini Venkateswaran, Burkhard Dick, Ronald Gerste, and Samuel Masket (in the order of their chapters).

Paul Edwards, my department chair at Henry Ford Health System, deserves heartfelt thanks for his strong support for all of my research work. Collected questions and comments from our residents, young professional beginners and conference audiences were the original triggers and significant contributors for this book. Their practical questions and close feedback made possible the uniqueness of this book for teaching beginners. I want to thank them for their sincere interest and enthusiasm in the process of starting and engaging in refractive cataract surgery. Special thanks to our last two years' chief residents, Andrew Hou, Dan Brill, Kevin Leikert, and Anjali Badami for their special connections in providing real world feedbacks for the main chapters. I am grateful to all the invaluable encouragement and instructive advice from my colleagues, among those, special thanks to Bithika Kheterpal, Robert Levine and Salma Noorulla.

I would specially like to express my deep appreciation to Rebecca Lopez, my part-time research assistant. Her wisdom and skills were fully reflected in assisting me in searching and confirming literature, drawing pictures, and editing photos and videos. Without her high-quality work, this book will not be what it is.

Along with my coauthors, this is the second textbook on which I have worked with Thieme Medical Publishers. I am very thankful for their vision, trust and professional and reliable collaboration to assure that this project was completed seamlessly. Thieme is a great publisher to work with.

I am deeply humbled and sincerely grateful for the instructive advice and support from David Chang, Warren Hill, Kendall E. Donaldson, Uday Devgan, John Berdahl, Louis Nichamin, Howard Gimbel, Tim Page and many others. The information shared by them has been an invaluable part of this book.

Fuxiang Zhang, MD

Contributors

Lisa Brothers Arbisser, MD
Co-founder and Ophthalmologist Emerita
Eye Surgeons Associates PC
Iowa and Illinois Quad Cities;
Adjunct Professor
John A. Moran Eye Center
University of Utah
Salt Lake City, Utah, USA

H. Burkhard Dick, MD, PhD, FEBOS-CR
Professor, Chairman, and Ophthalmologist
Ophthalmology Clinic
Ruhr-University Bochum
Bochum, Germany

Kendall E. Donaldson, MD, MS
Professor of Clinical Ophthalmology
Medical Director
Bascom Palmer Eye Institute
Plantation, Florida, USA

Ronald D. Gerste, MD, PhD
Ophthalmologist
Ophthalmology Clinic
Ruhr-University Bochum
Bochum, Germany

Samuel Masket, MD
Clinical Professor of Ophthalmology
David Geffen School of Medicine
UCLA
Los Angeles, California, USA

Cynthia Matossian, MD, FACS
Adjunct Clinical Assistant Professor
Department of Ophthalmology
School of Medicine
Temple University
Philadelphia, Pennsylvania, USA

Robert H. Osher, MD
Professor of Ophthalmology
University of Cincinnati College of Medicine;
Medical Director Emeritus
Cincinnati Eye Institute;
Founder and Editor
Video Journal of Cataract, Refractive, &
    Glaucoma
Cincinnati, Ohio, USA

Alan Sugar, MD
Professor
Department of Ophthalmology and Visual
    Sciences
W.K. Kellogg Eye Center
University of Michigan Medical School
Ann Arbor, Michigan, USA

Nandini Venkateswaran, MD
Cataract Cornea and Refractive Surgeon
Clinical Instructor of Ophthalmology
Ophthalmology Massachusetts Eye and Ear
    Infirmary
Harvard Medical School
Waltham, Massachusetts, USA

Fuxiang Zhang, MD
Medical Director
Department of Ophthalmology
Downriver Supervision Center
Henry Ford Health System
Taylor, Michigan, USA

1 A Career of Refractive Cataract Surgery

Robert H. Osher

Abstract

Being a refractive cataract surgeon has been a personal mission that the author has pursued for over four decades. A variety of concepts, technologies, and techniques are reviewed in this chapter. The ophthalmologist who performs cataract surgery should be committed to accept the challenge of becoming a refractive cataract surgeon.

Keywords: refractive cataract surgery, emmetropia, uncorrected vision, astigmatic keratotomy, hyperopic clear lensectomy, slow motion phacoemulsification, toric lens alignment, extreme pseudophakic monovision for diplopia

1.1 Introduction

A significant portion of my ophthalmic career has been devoted to the pursuit of emmetropia. Clear vision unaided by spectacles has been a personal "Holy Grail" worth pursuing for more than four decades. As a result, I have had the opportunity to write chapters about the evolution of refractive cataract surgery in multiple books.[1,2,3,4] This chapter will review my personal experience and preferred philosophy.

1.2 The Early Days

After completing my residency at the renowned Bascom Palmer Eye Institute (BPEI) in Miami and additional Fellowships in Neuro-ophthalmology and Retina, I delayed the start of my career in Academia to spend a few months with my father, Morris Osher, MD, whose primary interest was in cataract surgery. Observing his meticulous procedure and the universal elation of his postoperative patients, I made a dramatic career change and decided to join Dad in private practice. Moreover, I was resolved to develop one of the first practices limited to referral cataract surgery.

In the early 1980s, about 99% of surgeons were using a large incision planned ECCE and either an anterior or posterior chamber PMMA IOL (poly methyl metha acrylate intraocular lens). Clifford Terry, MD, had just developed a surgical keratoscope and Richard Kratz, MD, introduced a scleral tunnel incision that was closed with a running suture to avoid the high astigmatism associated with many radial sutures. But only the spherical component of a pseudophakic equation was being discussed; the cylindrical component was ignored. Reducing preexisting astigmatism had never even been considered.

I was fortunate to have been the first resident at BPEI to perform phacoemulsification and was fully committed to smaller incision surgery. I was also interested in a new corneal operation, radial keratotomy (RK), developed in Russia by Dr. Svyatoslav Fyodorov, MD. I visited Albert Neumann, MD, one of the American RK pioneers, in Deland, Florida and was fascinated by the effect that corneal incisions had on the refractive error. I also visited Spencer Thornton, MD, in Nashville, Tennessee, who was placing incisions in the cornea to reduce natural (congenital) astigmatism. I also heard about a surgeon in North Carolina, George Tate, MD, who was placing corneal incisions to correct high astigmatism after penetrating keratoplasty. I flew to Pinehurst to observe his surgery during which time I suddenly had an amazing thought that struck with the force of tsunami: what if I combined corneal incisions with phacoemulsification to reduce preexisting astigmatism? I could not wait to get started.

At first, I used sharp fragments of a carbon shaving blade to make a 3-mm straight incision in the peripheral cornea to a depth of 600 micra perpendicular to the steepest meridian. The result was minimal until a second incision in the peripheral cornea was placed 180 degrees away. I studied the effect of varying the optical zones between a conservative 10 mm and an aggressive 6 mm. For high amounts of astigmatism, I even added a second pair of incisions, for example, using 6-mm and 8-mm optical zones. After designing a diamond micrometer knife with Metico, the depth was increased to 690 micra achieving a greater effect (▶ Fig. 1.1).

I sent the data on the first 128 patients to Clifford Terry, MD, and Spencer Thornton, MD. They confirmed that the operation was successful in reducing astigmatism and 76% of patients achieved an uncorrected vision of 20/40 or better. With a sense of exhilaration and an endorsement

Source: Osher RH. A Career of Refractive Cataract Surgery. In: Buratto L, Packard R. History of Refractive Surgery. Milano, Italy: Fabiano Gruppo Editoriale; 2020.

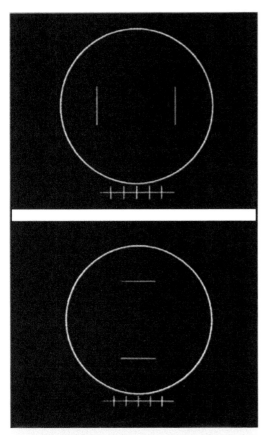

Fig. 1.1 Patterns of astigmatic keratotomy with phacoemulsification for reducing preexisting astigmatism in 1983.

from these leading astigmatism experts, I presented my study at the Cataract Congress in Houston, Texas, and at the AIOIS Meeting in 1984; the Annual Meeting of the United Kingdom Intraocular Implant Society in Guernsey, England in 1985; and the ASCRS Meeting in Los Angeles, California in 1986. The reception was cool and the reaction from colleagues was harsh. I was criticized, belittled, and even condemned. Fortunately, a few young, open-minded surgeons like Richard Lindstrom, MD, and Douglas Koch, MD, were excited about this new approach which they found worthy of further investigation. Despite the initial unpopularity of placing paired incisions in the virgin cornea, when combined with phacoemulsification, this operation represented the birth of refractive cataract surgery (▶ Fig. 1.2).[5]

1.3 Hyperopic Clear Lensectomy

Several years later, in about 1985, I had another opportunity to introduce a new refractive procedure. A chemist was referred with extreme hyperopia, a spherical equivalent of 11 D. He was unable to tolerate contact lenses and he detested his "Coke-bottle" thick glasses. At this time, there were still many aphakic patients with similar complaints which we were able to resolve by implanting a secondary IOL. But operating on a clear lens? I had read about an Italian surgeon, Dr. Franco Verzella, who reported removing the clear lens in high myopes, but the sight-threatening risk of a retinal detachment seemed to outweigh the benefits. However, this risk did not exist in high hyperopia, so I performed the first hyperopic clear lensectomy on this patient[6] (▶ Fig. 1.3). The phacoemulsification was routine, and the lens was placed into the capsular bag without difficulty. Even though the IOL power was undercorrected by several diopters, the patient was very happy. I expanded the study, presenting and publishing the results.[2,7,8,9]

Once again, the medical community was not supportive and there was a painful backlash of criticism for removing a clear lens from a "normal" eye. Over time, more refractive surgeons adopted this operation which remains a viable option to reduce high hyperopia today.

1.4 Slow Motion Phaco

In order for refractive cataract surgery to become embraced by ophthalmology, a number of technological advances were required to move the field forward. More accurate diagnostic equipment and improved IOL formulas were introduced. The hard PMMA IOL which required at least a 6-mm incision was replaced when California surgeon Thomas Mazzocco, MD, developed the "soft" foldable IOL which expedited the transition from planned extracapsular surgery to phacoemulsification. But there were still problems with the phaco machine.

In about 1984, I had been retained as a consultant by Cooper Vision, probably because of the success of the Osher-Fenzl IOL. This company manufactured the lion's share of the phaco machines which only offered the limited options of "maximum" and "minimum." I pleaded with management to develop a machine capable of

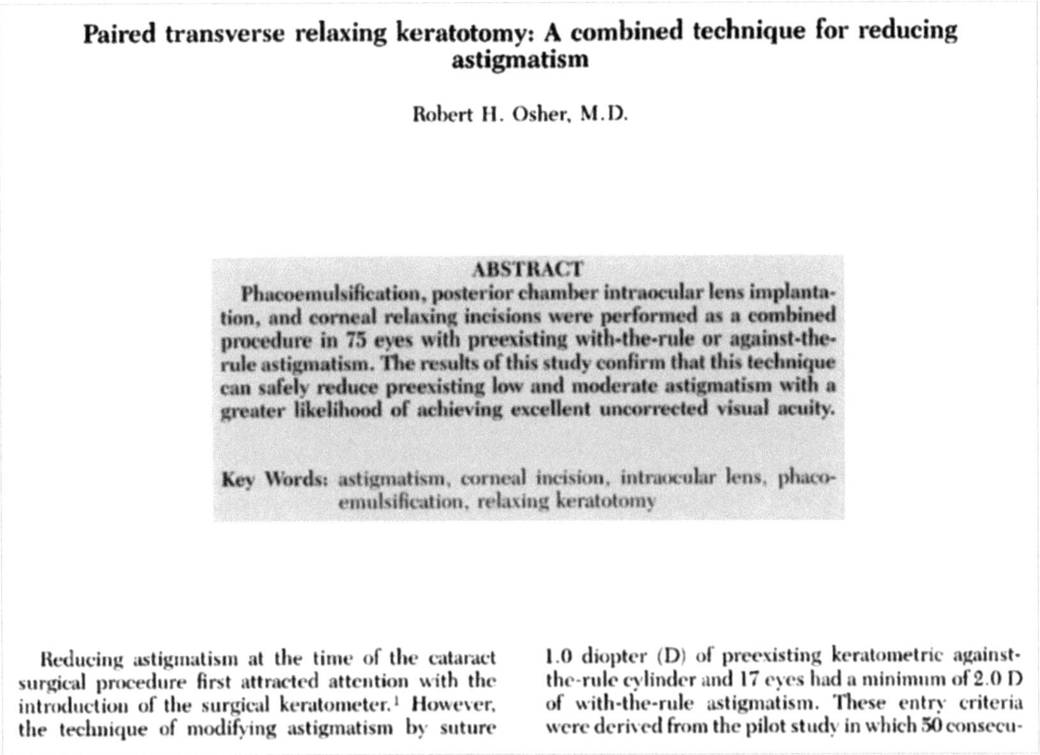

Paired transverse relaxing keratotomy: A combined technique for reducing astigmatism

Robert H. Osher, M.D.

ABSTRACT

Phacoemulsification, posterior chamber intraocular lens implantation, and corneal relaxing incisions were performed as a combined procedure in 75 eyes with preexisting with-the-rule or against-the-rule astigmatism. The results of this study confirm that this technique can safely reduce preexisting low and moderate astigmatism with a greater likelihood of achieving excellent uncorrected visual acuity.

Key Words: astigmatism, corneal incision, intraocular lens, phacoemulsification, relaxing keratotomy

Reducing astigmatism at the time of the cataract surgical procedure first attracted attention with the introduction of the surgical keratometer.[1] However, the technique of modifying astigmatism by suture 1.0 diopter (D) of preexisting keratometric against-the-rule cylinder and 17 eyes had a minimum of 2.0 D of with-the-rule astigmatism. These entry criteria were derived from the pilot study in which 50 consecu-

Fig. 1.2 The time was right for the birth of refractive cataract surgery.

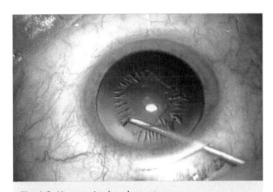

Fig. 1.3 Hyperopic clear lensectomy.

delivering infinite control of ultrasound power, aspiration rate, and vacuum. Because they showed no interest, I found a small Italian company, Optikon, who was intrigued by my idea of surgeon-controlled parameters. I identified another company, Jed Med in St. Louis, who was willing to develop a motorized IV pole for

surgeon-controlled infusion (▶ Fig. 1.4). Optikon introduced the Phacotron Gold, the first machine to incorporate features that would allow the surgeon to individualize the settings for different cataracts and situations. I named this new approach, Slow Motion Phaco (SMP), which received support from Dr. Charles Kelman himself (▶ Fig. 1.5). This was ironic because SMP eliminated Dr. Kelman's five contraindications to phacoemulsification: the loose lens, the brunescent lens, the small pupil, the shallow chamber, and the compromised cornea.[10,11] Surgeon-control of these parameters quickly became the standard of care and allowed the field of refractive cataract surgery to continue to evolve safely.

1.5 Early Uncorrected Vision: A New Standard

In 1986, I gave a presentation at the annual ASCRS Meeting in Los Angeles, California, that criticized the way we measure successful cataract surgery.

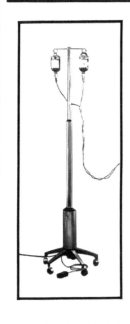
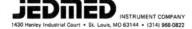

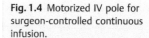

Fig. 1.4 Motorized IV pole for surgeon-controlled continuous infusion.

The standard was to determine if the patient attained a visual acuity 20/40 or better 6 weeks after surgery WITH glasses. I believed that this outdated and insensitive assessment would never allow us to precisely measure our results as refractive cataract surgeons. I argued that you could kick a cataract out with football cleats, and by 6 weeks, the eye had forgiven the sins of the surgeon, who with the help of glasses, qualified as a hero. How utterly absurd!

The title of the presentation was, "Early Uncorrected Vision: The New Gold Standard" which reported that 71% of patients achieved an unaided visual acuity of 20/40 or better on the first postoperative day. The "Early" was important because it reflected gentle surgery and intraoperative respect for the corneal endothelium. The "Uncorrected" vision indicated how well the surgeon had managed the spherical component of the pseudophakic refractive error by accurate biometry, keratometry, IOL selection, and IOL placement. It also indicated how well the surgeon had dealt with the astigmatic component, both preexisting and induced. I concluded that the refractive cataract surgeon must be willing to accept a more sensitive and demanding measurement of his or her outcomes. In 1993, the results improved to 91% of operated eyes obtaining an unaided vision of 20/40 or better.[12]

A 1994 guest editorial proclaimed, "The refractive cataract surgeon must be unafraid of stringent self-evaluation and must be willing to experience the discomfort that inevitably accompanies study, preparation, and change. I urge you to join this new and growing breed of surgeon. Accept this mission and you will enjoy the

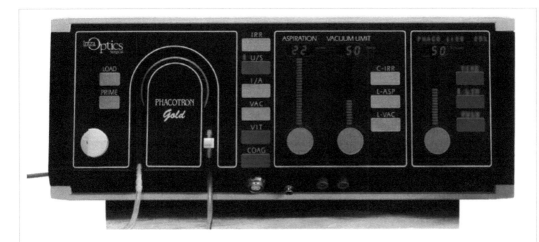

Dear Bob:

Thank you for responding to my request for an edited video of your surgical technique and accompanying commentary.

Your contribution regarding the technique of Slow Motion Phaco is highly important to phacoemulsification and I look forward to showing the videotape and crediting you for your achievement in this area.

With my thanks again and best wishes, I am

Sincerely yours,

Charles D. Kelman, M.D.

Fig. 1.5 Slow Motion Phaco with the surgeon-control features on the Phacotron Gold endorsed by Dr. Charles Kelman.

exhilaration of self-challenge for the remainder of your surgical career."[13] I published another peer-reviewed article in 2004 in which three fellows reviewed 100 consecutive cases showing that 49% of eyes attained an uncorrected vision of 20/20 or 20/25 on the first postoperative day which improved to 77% by 5 weeks.[14] Although it took years, more surgeons began reporting their visual results without glasses—the ultimate goal of refractive cataract surgery (▶ Fig. 1.6).

1.6 Emmetropia Trademark

With each passing year, my passion for attaining excellent uncorrected vision grew. I was convinced that refractive cataract surgery would eventually become embraced by industry, so I applied for and was granted trademarks for Mission Emmetropia, Target Emmetropia, and the Emmetropia Company (▶ Fig. 1.7). These trademarks were purchased by Clarity, a company committed to the development of intraoperative aberrometry. My initial enthusiasm for intraoperative refraction technology was tempered by mixed reports. However, I was encouraged to see new technology emerging from different sectors. For example, the preoperative sector was developing technology for measuring posterior corneal astigmatism and improved IOL formulas were being introduced. Intraoperative guidance was generating quite a bit

Early uncorrected visual acuity as a measurement of the visual outcomes of contemporary cataract surgery

Robert H. Osher, MD, Marcílio G. Barros, MD, Daniela M.V. Marques, MD, Frederico F. Marques, MD, James M. Osher, MS

Purpose: To determine the uncorrected visual acuity (UCVA) on the first postoperative day and the fifth week after routine slow-motion phacoemulsification with posterior chamber intraocular lens (IOL) implantation.

Setting: Cincinnati Eye Institute, Cincinnati, Ohio, USA.

Methods: This retrospective chart review performed by 3 research fellows analyzed the UCVA 1 day and 5 weeks postoperatively in 100 consecutive best-case scenario eyes of 99 patients who had routine slow-motion phacoemulsification with implantation of an AcrySof® single-piece IOL (Alcon). Reasons for UCVAs worse than 20/40 were sought. The stability of the visual result was analyzed.

Results: The UCVA was 20/40 or better in 98% of eyes at 1 day. Ninety-seven percent had a UCVA of at least 20/40 by 5 weeks, confirming stability of acuity. The percentage of patients with a UCVA of 20/20 or 20/25 increased from 49% at 1 day to 77% at 5 weeks.

Fig. 1.6 Article on Early Uncorrected Vision, the New Standard.

THE EMMETROPIA COMPANY
MISSION EMMETROPIA

Word Mark	THE **EMMETROPIA** COMPANY MISSION **EMMETROPIA**
Goods and Services	IC 010. US 026 039 044. G & S: Intraocular lenses
Standard Characters Claimed	
Mark Drawing Code	(4) STANDARD CHARACTER MARK
Serial Number	85491920
Filing Date	December 9, 2011
Current Basis	1B
Original Filing Basis	1B
Published for Opposition	June 19, 2012
Owner	(APPLICANT) Robert H. Osher INDIVIDUAL UNITED STATES 1945 CEI Drive Cincinnati OHIO 45242

Fig. 1.7 Trademarks for emmetropia applied for and granted.

of attention which will be discussed later in the chapter. Postoperative technology for modifying the IOL shape and refractive index was also being investigated. Although it remains impossible to predict which technology will ultimately prove best for helping the surgeon to hit the refractive target, it is certain that the percentage of eyes achieving the intended refractive target will continue to increase.

1.7 Toric Lens Alignment

Correcting astigmatism has always required accurate identification of the steepest corneal meridian. In the 1980s, I tried keratoscopy to facilitate placement of the paired corneal incisions. I designed the Osher Hyde Astigmatic Ruler, a series of astigmatic circles between 2 and 5 D that when placed above the cornea would both identify and quantitate the steep meridian. In the 1990s, when Kimiya Shimizu, MD, from Japan introduced the idea of a toric IOL, I knew that we were one step closer to achieving emmetropia in our cataract patients. After all, astigmatic keratotomy (AK) was not highly predictable because the incision depth had to be about 90% which was technically difficult to achieve by freehand. Moreover, there was variability in patient healing. While AK was an "Art," we believed that the toric lens would be more predictable as a "Science." Yet we were perplexed by the initial results until Douglas Koch, MD, discovered the missing link, posterior corneal astigmatism. What a difference this additional information made. Still, to achieve the best outcomes, it was necessary to identify and accurately mark the target meridian for precise toric lens alignment.

I thought it was absolutely crazy that we were using extraordinary technology to remove the cataract and sophisticated optics in the IOL. But the standard of care was to "guestimate" where the major and target meridia were located which were then marked with a $1.00 ink pen. Further compromising the task of accurate toric lens alignment was the fact that these ink blots would diffuse or even completely disappear. Every degree of inaccuracy resulted in about a 3% to 4% decrease in the amount of astigmatism reduction. There just had to be a better way!

I had an idea to use landmarks for orientation and discovered a small software company, Micron Imaging, in Memphis, Tennessee. They provided a high-definition camera which was installed on the slit lamp which allowed me to take a magnified picture of the anterior segment anatomy when the pupil was dilated. We created software which would overlay a protractor so every landmark would have a corresponding degree on a printed image (▶ Fig. 1.8). At first, I tried to use limbal vessels but quickly realized that Neo-Synephrine, topical antibiotics, and the presence of subconjunctival anesthetic would alter the appearance of these vessels in the operating room. So instead, I decided to use iris landmarks, like crypts, nevi, Brushfield spots, pigment, and unique stromal patterns which remained consistent in appearance from the initial dilated exam to the operating room. Unfortunately, a Mississippi flood bankrupted Micron Imaging, so I completed this work with Dr. Dominik Beck, the president of Haag-Streit USA, who introduced OTAS (Osher Toric Alignment System). Other companies like Eye Photo Systems and Tracey Technologies

developed variations of OTAS using landmarks to achieve accurate toric alignment (▶ Fig. 1.9). I called this method Iris Fingerprinting which was the subject of the 2009 ASCRS Innovator's Award Lecture.[15]

I even declared war on ink, developing Thermo-Dot with Beaver Visitec, International. After using a Mastel Osher Ring with fingerprinting, a tiny cautery mark was placed at the limbus to identify the target meridian (▶ Fig. 1.10). This eliminated ink diffusion or disappearance; prevented disorientation by loss of landmarks secondary to subconjunctival anesthetic, BSS, or hemorrhage; and could even be used to confirm the orientation of the toric lens on the day following surgery.

I was approached by other companies to work on sophisticated technology for toric IOL alignment utilizing the concept of registration. SMI in Germany developed a method to capture the preoperative image of the anterior segment and then register the live surgical image which was displayed in the interface within the microscope optics. This technology was sold to Alcon, who changed the name to Verion, and championed "guidance" for toric lens orientation. I also had the opportunity to work with Zeiss, who introduced the Callisto Markerless Z-Align System to interface with the Lumera microscope. The assault on astigmatism was heating up and bringing us one step closer to our goal of "nailing" the postoperative refractive target.

1.8 An IOL-Based Cure for Diplopia

An "out-of-the-box" refractive concept that I introduced was the unique approach to managing the cataract patient with stable diplopia. These were some of the most challenging patients, especially when the deviation was incomitant, preventing successful prism therapy. I had known for years that missing the diagnosis of a preexisting acquired tropia in a patient undergoing cataract surgery could have devastating consequences. I also knew that leaving any cataract patient with more than 3 D of aniseikonia could be disastrous, as the patient would be unable to fuse. But for the patient with acquired, stable diplopia, maybe by creating intentional extreme monovision, the inability to fuse might either reduce or eliminate preexisting diplopia.

I initiated a study enrolling a dozen cataract patients with longstanding, bothersome diplopia. They had a variety of diagnoses such as thyroid

Ophthalmology Times

All the Clinical News in Sight

www.ophthalmologytimes.com
MAY 15, 2009 ■ VOL. 34, NO. 10

Technique in development

'Iris fingerprinting' orients toric IOLs

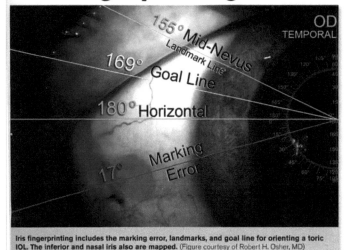

OD
TEMPORAL

155° Mid-Nevus
169° Goal Line
180° Horizontal
Marking Error
17°

Landmark Line

Iris fingerprinting includes the marking error, landmarks, and goal line for orienting a toric IOL. The inferior and nasal iris also are mapped. (Figure courtesy of Robert H. Osher, MD)

Technique helps surgeons address astigmatism and cataracts

By Ron Rajecki
Reviewed by Robert H. Osher, MD

Dr. Osher

San Francisco—Toric IOLs, precisely oriented in the eye via a new technique called "iris fingerprinting," represent a better way of performing astigmatic cataract surgery, according to **Robert H. Osher, MD**, who spoke during the annual meeting of the American Society of Cataract and Refractive Surgery.

"The treatment of astigmatism is absolutely an integral part of contemporary cataract surgery, and I'm amazed that more ophthalmologists are not embracing toric IOLs," said Dr. Osher, professor of ophthalmology, College of Medicine, University of Cincinnati, and medical director emeritus of the Cincinnati Eye Institute. "After all, no practitioner would do a refraction and ignore the

See **Technique** on page 26

Fig. 1.8 Iris fingerprinting using landmarks for toric intraocular lens (IOL) alignment in Ophthalmology Times 2009.

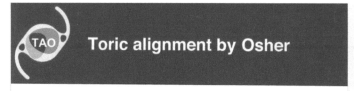

TAO
Toric alignment by Osher

Iris fingerprinting for intraoperative alignment of toric implants

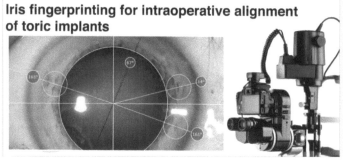

Fig. 1.9 Variations of toric alignment technology using landmarks for orientation.

eye disease, neurologic oculomotor palsies, unsuccessful strabismus surgery, etc., but they shared in common an unhappiness with prisms. Patients who were content with their prisms were not included in the study. The cardinal idea was to leave one eye emmetropic and the other eye with more than 3 D of residual myopia. Whenever

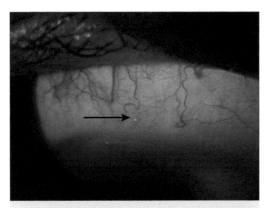

Fig. 1.10 ThermoDot system by BVI replaces ink with tiny cautery marks (*arrow*).

possible, I would offer a preview of extreme monovision using either trial lenses or contact lenses. I was surprised that the patient's choice of which eye to target for distance did not always respect ocular dominance. Informed consent was extensive and each patient was told that a lens exchange could be performed if he or she were unhappy with extreme monovision. Phacoemulsification was performed with implantation of an IOL placed into the capsular bag and associated astigmatism was always corrected using either AK or a toric IOL.

The results were dramatic! Every patient was thrilled to be able to enjoy uncorrected distance and near vision. All but two patients reported the elimination of their double vision. These two patients experienced less diplopia and said that their double vision was limited to intermediate distance. I learned that it was essential to create more than 3 D of aniseikonia and to underpromise the results. Eventually, I did encounter a patient outside of the original study who did request a lens exchange, but she was even unhappier when she had to again wear her prisms. Even though the peer-reviewed publication (▶ Fig. 1.11) generated

---

ARTICLE

Intentional extreme anisometropic pseudophakic monovision: New approach to the cataract patient with longstanding diplopia

Robert H. Osher, MD, Karl C. Golnik, MD, Graham Barrett, MD, Kimiya Shimizu, MD

PURPOSE: To determine whether extreme pseudophakic monovision can reduce or eliminate diplopia in patients with cataract and longstanding acquired strabismus.

SETTING: Department of Ophthalmology, University of Cincinnati, and the Cincinnati Eye Institute, Cincinnati, Ohio, USA.

DESIGN: Case series.

METHODS: Intentional extreme monovision was created in patients with stable diplopia having cataract surgery. Intraocular lens selection was targeted for emmetropia in 1 eye and at least 3.0 diopters of myopia in the fellow eye.

RESULTS: Twelve patients with stable diplopia attained excellent uncorrected distance and near vision with a marked reduction in or elimination of double vision.

Fig. 1.11 Controversial publication on treating diplopia using intentional extreme monovision, JCRS 2012.

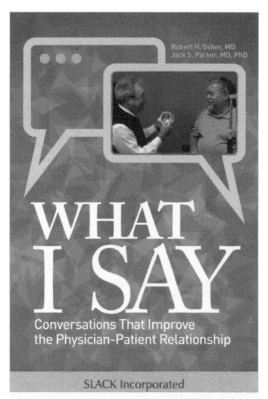

Fig. 1.12 Book entitled, *What I Say*, published by SLACK in 2019.

extreme controversy among the strabismus surgeons, the vast majority of patients were very pleased with this variant of refractive cataract surgery.[16]

1.9 What I Say

Jack Parker, MD, PhD, and I recently published a book entitled, *What I Say* in which we selected about 70 pre-, intra-, and postoperative situations which required important conversations with the patient (▶ Fig. 1.12). Although I have spent 40 years as a cataract surgeon trying to achieve emmetropia, I believe that we should always underpromise when discussing refractive outcomes with the patient. I always emphasize that a thin pair of glasses may be necessary to obtain the best possible vision after surgery, because we only have a limited number of IOL powers available, for example, +21, +22, +23, etc. I tell the patient that he or she may need a +21.68 to see perfect, but

we don't make this lens. Then I explain that we do our best to get close by selecting the nearest available IOL power. I also emphasize that every patient heals differently and if the eye heals with the IOL a fraction of a millimeter forwards or backwards, it may also change the requirement for glasses. Therefore, if I miss the refractive target, it is an expectation rather than a complication. Because I meld[17] (average) manual K, IOL Master K, LenStar K, Atlas topography K, iTrace K, Pentacam K; two axial lengths from the IOL Master and LenStar; and 8 formulas including the Barrett Universal and the Hill RBF, I expect to be within a 0.5 D of the intended target in 94% of patients undergoing routine cataract surgery.[18] Still, I would rather underpromise and subsequently enjoy a delighted patient whose expectations have been exceeded. This philosophy has proven to be a satisfying approach throughout my career.

In summary, I made a commitment in the early 1980s to become a refractive cataract surgeon, long before this term became popular. I have fulfilled the requirements of careful preparation, surgical innovation, and patient education in my attempt to achieve unaided vision and a happy patient. Not for one minute have I regretted this career-long mission.

References

[1] Osher RH. Evolution of refractive cataract surgery. In: Wallace III, RB, ed. Refractive cataract surgery and multifocal IOLs. SLACK Inc.; 2001:1–7

[2] Osher RH. Clear lensectomy. In: Fine IH, ed. Clear corneal lens surgery. SLACK Inc.; 1999:281–285

[3] Osher RH. American innovators: perspectives. In: Byron HM, Reshmi CS, Hirschman H, eds. Birth of the intraocular lens. 1st ed. Jaypee Brothers Medical Publishers (P) Ltd; 2008:134–137

[4] Osher RH. Combining astigmatism correction with cataract surgery: a personal crusade. In: Febbraro JL, Khan HN, Koch DD, eds. Surgical correction of astigmatism. Springer International Publishing AG; 2018:3–6

[5] Osher RH. Paired transverse relaxing keratotomy: a combined technique for reducing astigmatism. J Cataract Refract Surg. 1989; 15(1):32–37

[6] Osher RH. Controversies in cataract surgery. Audiovisual J Catar Implant Surg. 1989; 5(3)

[7] Osher RH. Discussant. Management of patients with high ametropia who seek refractive surgical correction. Eur J Implant Ref Surg. 1994; 6:298–299

[8] Osher RH. To the editor: clear lens extraction. J Cataract Refract Surg. 1994; 20(6):674

[9] Osher RH. Hyperopic lensectomy: an update. Paper presented at the American Academy of Ophthalmology Annual Meeting, San Francisco, CA; 1997

[10] Osher RH. Letter to the editor: slow motion phacoemulsification approach. J Cataract Refract Surg. 1993; 19(5):667

[11] Osher RH, Marques FF, Marques DMV, Osher JM. Slow-motion phacoemulsification technique. Tech Ophthalmol. 2003; 1(2):73–78

[12] Osher RH. Eur J Implant Refract Surg. 1993; 5:225–226

[13] Osher RH. Guest editorial. Ophthalmic Prac. 1994; 12:156–157

[14] Osher RH, Barros MG, Marques DM, Marques FF, Osher JM. Early uncorrected visual acuity as a measurement of the visual outcomes of contemporary cataract surgery. J Cataract Refract Surg. 2004; 30(9):1917–1920

[15] Osher RH. Iris fingerprinting: new method for improving accuracy in toric lens orientation. J Cataract Refract Surg. 2010; 36(2):351–352

[16] Osher RH, Golnik KC, Barrett G, Shimizu K. Intentional extreme anisometropic pseudophakic monovision: new approach to the cataract patient with longstanding diplopia. J Cataract Refract Surg. 2012; 38(8):1346–1351

[17] Browne AW, Osher RH. Optimizing precision in toric lens selection by combining keratometry techniques. J Refract Surg. 2014; 30(1):67–72

[18] Kim HJ, Stromberg K, Osher RH. Comparison of Barrett Universal II and Hill-RBF 2.0 formulas in patients undergoing routine cataract surgery. Highlights of Ophthalmology 2020; 48(6):26–30

2 Am I Ready to Become a Refractive Cataract Surgeon?–A Check-up List Before You Start

Fuxiang Zhang, Alan Sugar, and Lisa Brothers Arbisser

Abstract

This chapter briefly discusses some clinical pre-requisites before a resident or a beginner starts serious engagement in refractive cataract surgery (RCS). It does not mean that each and every item in the list must be fulfilled to prepare for RCS, but the surgeon should make a full self-evaluation and careful planning to maximize the chance of success. On the other end, it also means that not everyone should be a refractive cataract surgeon.

Keywords: refractive cataract surgery, readiness for refractive cataract surgery, prerequisite

2.1 Introduction

Loaded with all the ophthalmic knowledge and surgical skills you learned from your mentors during your 3 years of ophthalmology residency, you enter a new chapter of your career. If cataract surgery is the main surgical service you choose for your practice, you will have to decide whether to engage in refractive cataract surgery (RCS). Without the ability to meet patient's increasing expectations for relative spectacle independence, one's practice may be compromised in today's competitive environment.

We expect that more and more young ophthalmologists, as well as those who have not yet had a chance to integrate RCS into their current practice, will decide to initiate RCS. The next question will be "Am I ready?" This chapter will discuss 10 checklist-like topics. You do not have to be perfectly prepared for everything before your actual engagement, but these 10 items may help you to make your decision.

1. **Reasonable surgical skills with low complication rate:** Making all patients happy is a challenge, and often stressful. This may be amplified for RCS patients as the extra money they pay comes with added expectations. It does not make sense to initiate this premium service if you have not even achieved an acceptable outcome with your standard surgery. No one expects a young ophthalmic surgeon to have a surgical complication rate

only 10% of the national average, but young cataract surgeons should sharpen their surgical skills first, approaching the national average complication rate as a goal before starting premium services.

It is also very important to know how to fix problems intraoperatively. Complications happen to every surgeon. What makes a good surgeon stand out is not only a lower complication rate, but also the knowledge and the skill to appropriately fix problems intraoperatively and postoperatively. Until you feel comfortable on your operating room (OR) days, our advice is that you wait to start RCS. You need to be familiar with the use of different ophthalmic viscoelastic devices (OVD) for different situations, anterior vitrectomy, intraocular lens (IOL) repositioning, and IOL exchange, etc., independently without the luxury of having a supervisor.

For a cataract surgeon, it is absolutely necessary to know your phacoemulsification machine very well. Do not be shy about having the manufacturer's representative come to your OR for personal in-service tutorials. Pick a day when you do not have a fully packed schedule and have the expert technician observe all or most of your cases. After completion of all the cases, spend time to have a detailed discussion about the machine settings. It is even more important that you know how to make adjustments to the phaco machine for different settings in different situations because no phaco machine company's representative will be with you every single OR day.

No doubt there are many naturally gifted surgeons, but usually we all need continuous self-education to improve our skills. During my residency and first year of practice, I did not have access to a training simulator as do today's residents. I probably did hundreds of, if not thousands, simulated continuous curvilinear capsulorhexis (CCC) with my personal loupes and foil paper at home since that was the most challenging step for my cataract surgery at the time. I also religiously reviewed hundreds of my own routine surgical videos in my first postgraduate year. Watching my own videos helped me greatly in identifying subtle issues and improving my surgical skill.

2. **Proficiency with LRI and toric IOLs:** It is premature to start to insert extended depth of focus (EDOF), multifocal IOLs (MFIOLs), and trifocal IOLs before you feel comfortable with manual limbal relaxing incisions (LRI) and toric IOLs. We have watched some of our colleagues give up RCS permanently after a few attempts due to their inability to fix astigmatism. EDOF IOLs such as the Tecnis Symfony (Johnson & Johnson) are believed to be more forgiving in terms of residual astigmatism, but we would recommend that you approach it in the same way as you would an MFIOL and trifocal IOL. Do not rely on forgiveness to result in a happy patient. Our recommendation is to start by performing IOL monovision with manual LRI and/or a toric IOL. Pseudophakic monovision, especially mini-monovision and moderate monovision, provides great vision quality, and patients do not have to pay as much as for premium IOLs, so the expectation is tempered due to the lower cost. You will not have great clinical outcomes from IOL monovision if you do not know how to fix astigmatism with all modalities: realistic and informative preoperative consultation, reliable biometry, and solid surgical skills.

3. **Familiarity with modern IOL formulas and online calculators:** Accuracy and precision are the core of modern RCS. The IOL power and the axis of a toric IOL are calculated with IOL formulas. With this said, we know how critical it is to use the most accurate advanced IOL formulas. We did not understand the posterior corneal astigmatism until the much-appreciated study done by Douglas Koch and his colleagues in 2011. If you ignore these important factors, or if you are not familiar with the limitations of the most commonly used IOL formulas, you cannot expect to get satisfactory outcomes from RCS. Such peer-reviewed studies typically provide good guidelines.

4. **Familiarity with different IOL options:** There should be an ongoing accumulation of knowledge and experience, though not necessarily an absolute requisite. It will be very helpful if you already have a good grasp of the big picture at the very beginning. As we will discuss in Chapter 8, IOL monovision can be a starting point for RCS. However, IOL monovision is not and should not be the only option. In the spectrum of RCS, beginners should be knowledgeable about the existence of other options. What can we expect from Crystalens, EDOF, MFIOL, trifocals, and light adjustable lens? What are the pros and cons for each of them? What are the relative contraindications we should avoid?

5. **Reasonable basic consultation skill:** As suggested by the name of this book, The Art of Refractive Cataract Surgery, RCS is a combination of science and art. The purpose of RCS is to improve uncorrected near, intermediate distance, and far distance vision to make the patient happy. Unfortunately, happiness is a rather subjective psychological and mental state. You should never underestimate the importance of preoperative consultation and postoperative comprehensive management. These skills are enhanced by cumulative experience in practice.

A key component is to complete a thorough preoperative history and examination, on which to base a professional and honest consultation. The rationale for a thorough history and eye examination prior to decision-making is to reveal any hidden, but important, ocular comorbidities in order to educate patients about the possible limitations. This kind of observation and discussion does not help as much if it is done postoperatively without preoperative discussion. Focus on each individual preference, rather than the pure spectacle independence rate. Because we truly have no perfect option to restore vision to youthful perfection, the one thing we should never forget is the principle of "under promise and over deliver." Pursuing only a high rate of conversion to premium IOLs rather than patient satisfaction is not advisable or ethical.

6. **Passing your board examination:** The details of RCS are specific but general ophthalmic knowledge is critical to the safe diagnosis and treatment of every patient. We are not necessarily saying you should ignore RCS before you pass your ophthalmology board

exam, but it probably does not make much sense to spend lots of time and energy on this premium service at the time when you are still dealing with all the challenges of your board certification tests. Basically, you should at least feel pretty comfortable for the board test before you concentrate on RCS.

7. **A smoothly run office:** It is reasonable to say that there are three fundamental bases for a surgeon: home, office and OR. Each base should be appropriately sound and well run. Otherwise, it is hard to offer premium RCS as this will undoubtedly add more challenges and stress.

You must have a smoothly run office with a high patient satisfaction rate and relatively busy volume. Knowledge is the core of practice for a good physician. Continuous education and self-motivated learning will help us stay knowledgeable and competent.

Do not underestimate the importance of office appearance. The overall setting should be clean and neat. Patients should feel comfortable in your waiting room as well as in your examination lane. The appearance of your office is as vital as the appearance of your face, your hair, and your choice of clothing each morning at the time you leave your home. The same can be said for staff.

8. **Having enough office instruments:** The minimum diagnostic tools should include accurate biometry, immersion A-scan, corneal topography, and manual keratometry at the time when one starts RCS. A manual keratometer is not enough for astigmatism evaluation because it only measures a small central corneal zone. A corneal topographer is a must-have tool for RCS.

Today's environment is very different from decades ago. Patents did not have to pay out of pocket money for early premium lenses such as Array multifocal IOLs or Starr toric lenses at that time when we started our RCS decades ago. Once you have enough capital, the first tool to add or replace should be either an IOLMaster 700 (Zeiss) or a LenStar (Haag-Streit). These biometry devices can significantly improve refractive outcomes. Once sphere and cylinder are addressed, next is to consider minimization of higher order aberrations (HOA), such as spherical aberration, coma, and trefoil, etc.

9. **Quality of preoperative testing by technicians:** If the quality of preoperative tests is marginal, you will need to fix this problem before you start RCS. When we first started our practice, we personally performed all of the preoperative tests for several years. As our practice grew, we started to train our technicians. It is critical to pay special attention to the quality, reliability, and repeatability of the tests done by your assistants. Just as we concentrate on certain clinical subspecialties, it is also logical to train our technicians in the same way. Human errors do happen, but it is rare to have two people make the same mistake at the same time for a given patient. For this reason, we have always had two technicians do all preoperative tests for all RCS cases.

If you have a busy daily office schedule, it is advisable to have those fee-for-service patients come back another day for their preoperative tests. The quality may be compromised if it is done on the same day as the initial office visit during a busy clinic and when the pupils are dilated. Another option is to do the key biometry tests at the very beginning of the visit, prior to any eye drops and pupillary dilation.

Care must be taken to optimize the ocular surface prior to final measurements. Contact lens patients will need a period out of their lenses. This can be accomplished one eye at a time, bilaterally with changing temporary spectacles as required, or, if the patient cannot or will not go without contacts, they must understand this is a contraindication to RCS.

10. **Know one's limit:** If you feel comfortable with the above ten items, you are probably ready to start RCS and should not wait too long. It is not rare for surgeons to be reluctant to start new procedures. The longer they wait after residency, the more likely surgeons will be used to their beginning repertoire of procedures. Another issue is hesitation to initiate a new procedure when one becomes a "senior" surgeon. Actually, it is very acceptable for a senior surgeon to learn new skills from their juniors, but there are some surgeons who may be concerned with "losing face." Remember that the patient's needs should

always come first whether that means gaining new skills or referring to those who have mastered them.

In a 2018 American Society of Cataract and Refractive Surgery (ASCRS) survey,[1] more than 30% of respondents did not feel sufficiently trained to integrate toric IOLs into their practice. Among US respondents, this number surprisingly was 39%. In the same survey, 21% of respondents did not use presbyopia-correcting IOLs. However, almost half of them (21%) planned on using these types of lenses within the next 12 months.

It is a fact that RCS is not suitable for every surgeon and every patient. In today's challenging environment, making more than 90% of our patients happy is easier said than done. We do not want to give up this goal lightly due to obstacles, but if RCS always makes you lose sleep as a mental burden, it may be a wise decision to put it aside. If after sincere and carefully planned trials, you find yourself not suitable for RCS, there is no need to force yourself to make life unnecessarily stressful. Just as we often refer special cases to other experts who can perform certain procedures at a higher quality than in our own hands, referring these patients would actually be in the best interest of our patients.

Reference

[1] ASCRS Clinical Survey 2018. EyeWorld. Published November 20, 2018. Accessed April 15, 2020. http://supplements. eyeworld.org/eyeworld-supplements/december-2018-clinical-survey

3 Evaluating and Optimizing the Ocular Surface for Accurate Measurements

Cynthia Matossian

Abstract

A healthy ocular surface is essential to achieve the best visual outcomes in cataract surgery patients. Ocular surface disease has a significant impact on surgical planning, and hence, on surgical outcomes. As such, ocular surface disease must be identified and treated preoperatively. This requires eye care providers to actively look for and diagnose dry eye disease in cataract surgery candidates. The first step in diagnosis is asking questions about symptoms, followed by the application of objective point-of-care testing and a comprehensive slit lamp exam to identify signs. Educating patients of their preexisting disease is a critical step to achieve buy-in, especially if they are asymptomatic. Following diagnosis, presurgical treatment is essential to maximize postoperative outcomes and patient satisfaction. Treating ocular surface disease in the preoperative setting is different than maintenance chronic therapy, since the goal is rapid tear film homeostasis to enable reliable measurements for surgery. As such, preop treatment is often more aggressive if the patient desires surgery within a few weeks. Dry eye disease and meibomian gland dysfunction are complex, multifactorial processes. Therefore, in order to treat the underlying root cause, combination therapeutic approaches may be required. The end goal is to address ocular surface inflammation and meibomian gland dysfunction while restoring tear film health.

Keywords: cataract, dry eye, ocular surface, MGD, IOL, ocular surface disease, presurgical tear film stability

3.1 Introduction

As contemporary cataract surgeons, we correct refractive errors, including astigmatism, while providing our patients a broad range of vision from distance all the way to near. As such, the primary goal of a lens-based refractive surgeon is to provide the best possible surgical outcome, which is largely measured by patients in terms of visual acuity and comfort during surgery and in the immediate postoperative period. There are many variables that we endeavor to control, from lens selection and refractive targets to patient expectations. However, one of the most important considerations is ocular surface health. Fortunately, this is relatively easy to diagnose and treatment can almost always make a difference.

Ocular surface disease must be identified preoperatively. Presurgical treatment is essential to maximize postoperative outcomes and patient satisfaction. In order to maintain the achieved visual acuity, patients will be expected to take responsibility to maintain their tear health indefinitely after surgery.

3.2 Why Preoperative Treatment Is a Necessity

We put so much effort into optimizing biometry and personalizing A-constants, but this is all for naught if we don't also consider the impact of the tear film on presurgical measurements. We have known for quite some time that a healthy ocular surface is essential to achieve the best visual outcomes in cataract patients.[1] As such, it is incumbent on us to look for and diagnose dry eye disease in cataract surgery candidates. Indeed, an estimated 16 million adults in the United States have been diagnosed with dry eye and about 30 million adults in the United States report dry eye symptoms without a formal diagnosis.

Furthermore, a 2018 paper reported the overall prevalence of dry eye and ocular surface disease in cataract patients at about 80%.[2] Meibomian gland dysfunction (MGD) is another common culprit and is the most common underlying cause of dry eye.[3] Like any other chronic disease, MGD should be addressed upfront. It affects the ocular surface and the tear film interface, both of which play a key role in vision. Therefore, we need to treat MGD to provide the best possible vision for our patients.

In 2015, I published a paper with Dr. Alice Epitropoulos and colleagues showing that hyperosmolar tear film patients demonstrated significantly greater variability in average K readings and anterior corneal astigmatism, with the result that there was a higher probability of the

IOL power calculation being off by a diopter or more.[4] More recently, I conducted an unsponsored pilot study of 25 eyes to evaluate changes in topography, keratometry, and biometry in patients with MGD who were scheduled for cataract surgery.[5] In these 25 eyes that had a diagnosis of both a visually significant cataract and MGD, presurgical measurements were performed. I created an initial individualized surgical plan for each patient. Then, the patients underwent a thermal pulsation treatment with LipiFlow (Johnson & Johnson). We asked the patients to return in 6 weeks at which time we had the same technician repeat the topography, biometry, and keratometry using the same instruments. I recalculated each patient's IOL power and astigmatism management using their postthermal pulsation treatment data and compared the results to their prethermal pulsation treatment surgical plan. I found that 40% of the time I made a change in the surgical plan, either in the IOL power, or in the amount of astigmatism I had planned to correct. Interestingly, before the study, I hypothesized that the ocular surface issues would present as pseudoastigmatism, and that by stabilizing the tear film, I would find less astigmatism. Instead, I found that about 50% of eyes had higher amounts of astigmatism following thermal pulsation treatment, meaning that their dry ocular surface was actually masking the amount of astigmatism we had captured prior to treatment. In contrast, 25% of eyes showed less astigmatism following thermal pulsation treatment and the remaining 25% of eyes demonstrated no change pre- to posttreatment in the magnitude and axis of astigmatism.

The key takeaway here is that ocular surface disease has a significant impact on surgical planning and hence on surgical outcomes. Especially for patients who are paying out of pocket for a premium lens, we need to nail that refractive outcome; otherwise, we are going to have an unhappy patient who will gobble up an inordinate amount of chair time and publicly display their dissatisfaction by poor online reviews. Tuning up the surface to get more reliable information is essential, especially in the subset of patients seeking less dependence on spectacles.

But just how many of our patients require pretreatment? The Prospective Health Assessment of Cataract Patients' Ocular Surface (PHACO) study with Dr. William Trattler[6] and colleagues and a dry eye prevalence study with Dr. Preeya Gupta[2]

and colleagues both found that the majority of patients scheduled to undergo cataract surgery had signs of MGD. Specifically, the PHACO study found that 77% of patients being evaluated for cataract surgery had corneal staining, and 63% of patients had an unstable tear film (rapid tear breakup time).[6] With this in mind, I assume that every patient who comes into my office for a cataract consult has some level of MGD until proven otherwise.

3.3 Diagnostic Pearls

Very few patients who present for cataract evaluation call attention to a specific ocular surface disease complaint. Rather, most are unaware that they have preexisting dry eye disease, putting the responsibility to identify it squarely on our shoulders as refractive cataract surgeons. This is not surprising, since signs and symptoms of dry eye seldom correlate. That said, the first step in diagnosis is asking questions about symptoms. We begin with a short dry eye questionnaire such as the Standard Patient Evaluation of Eye Dryness (SPEED) or Symptom Assessment in Dry Eye (SANDE) option. There are many others from which a practice can select. Our technicians are also tasked to ask three very simple questions:

- How often do you use artificial tears? We don't ask if patients use tears; rather we ask how many times a day they use their artificial tears. This information tells me a lot about the level of discomfort the patient is experiencing.
- Does your vision change throughout the day?
- Do your eyes feel tired?

There are a number of diagnostics available when it comes to identifying dry eye. To organize these, the ASCRS Cornea Clinical Committee recently presented consensus guidelines on how to approach ocular surface disease in precataract patients.[7] It included a recommended ocular surface disease screening battery utilizing both a novel symptom questionnaire and an objective point-of-care testing for signs. In our practice, following the questionnaire, the technicians perform three tests: tear osmolarity, MMP-9, and meibomian gland imaging. This helps us identify a full range of ocular surface disease, from milder forms to Sjogren, for example. A multicenter study demonstrated that 85% of asymptomatic patients had an abnormal result in MMP-9, osmolarity, or both.[2]

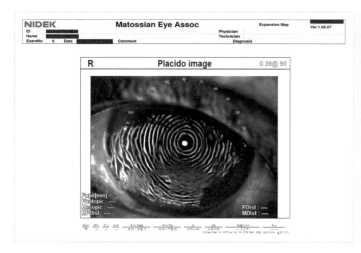

Fig. 3.1 A placido disc image taken with a Nidek OPD III with very warped mires representing an unstable tear film.

When I come into the exam room, I have all of this information in front of me. I proceed by using lissamine green to evaluate the lid margin, conjunctiva, and cornea, and fluorescein to further look at the cornea. Each dye tells me something different. I also examine the lid margins, the meibomian gland orifices, and press on them with my fingertip or a cotton swab to assess meibum quality and quantity. All of these steps don't even add a minute to my normal exam, yet they allow me to better grade the level of existing surface disease.

Since one of the main symptoms of dry eye is fluctuating vision, be on the lookout for that and distinguish it from cataract-induced blurry vision. Topography along with the black and white placido disc rings are other critical tools that can help identify irregular astigmatism, which can be a strong indicator of tear film instability in this population (▶ Fig. 3.1 and ▶ Fig. 3.2).

Finally, I review the gland images with my patients. The black and white meibography makes explaining the situation quite simple and is a powerful tool for patient education (▶ Fig. 3.3).

3.4 Treatment Options

Treating ocular surface disease in a preoperative cataract patient is a little different than maintenance chronic therapy, since the goal is rapid tear film homeostasis to enable reliable measurements for surgery. As such, preop treatment is often more aggressive if the patient desires surgery in a few weeks. Dry eye disease and MGD are complex,

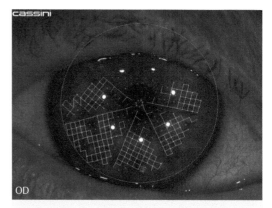

Fig. 3.2 Cassini surface qualifier imaging software demonstrates an unstable tear film, as evidenced by missing and irregular lines (broken pinecone appearance).

multifactorial processes. Therefore, in order to treat the underlying root cause, combination therapeutic approaches may be required. The end goal is to address ocular surface inflammation and MGD while regenerating the ocular surface epithelium and restoring the tear film. Depending on the cause of the disease and the patient's willingness to pay out of pocket, one or several of the following treatments may be considered:

- **Artificial tears:** Good quality artificial tears will rarely, singularly, create a healthy surface quickly enough, but are an important adjunct in the ocular surface restoration process. There is a wide variety of tear products, including tear

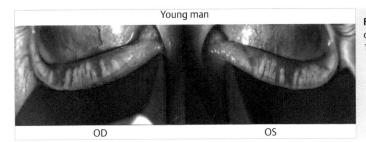

Young man

OD   OS

Fig. 3.3 LipiView image of a 42-year-old male IT worker who spends 10 + hours per day on his computer.

replacement, viscosity-enhancing, lipid-containing, gel-forming, ointments, and more. I always recommend preservative free tears preoperatively as they have the added benefit of getting patients acclimated to using drops, which is a practiced skill that will be needed postoperative.

- **Azithromycin:** Applied directly to the lid margins, topical azithromycin can be used preoperatively, particularly when MGD occurs in association with rosacea, since this therapy is believed to have an anti-inflammatory action in addition to properties that help control bacterial flora.[8]
- **Heated masks:** Warm compresses are a commonly used MGD treatment,[9,10,11] with several studies showing greater tear film stability and increased tear film lipid layer thickness following treatment in patients who have MGD.[12,13,14,15] This at-home remedy can be helpful in patients preparing for cataract surgery because the application of moist heat to the meibomian glands is thought to soften meibum viscosity, improve secretion, and, thus, increase tear lipid layer thickness.[14,16,17] There are many commercially available microwaveable masks, but it is important to look for one that offers consistent, moist heat at an appropriate temperature of approximately 42 to 43 °C that is sustainable for up to 8 minutes (Bruder Healthcare).
- **Hypochlorous acid:** Hypochlorous acid solution (Bruder Hygienic Eyelid Solution, Bruder Healthcare; Avenova, NovaBay Pharmaceuticals) may be helpful to decrease the bacterial load on the lid margin, particularly in patients who have MGD or ocular rosacea associated with blepharitis. As such, this can be a useful part of a preoperative prep kit. In one study, hypochlorous acid decreased the bacterial load by >90%.[18] This is an important consideration to minimize the risk of endophthalmitis, a rare yet

serious complication. Unlike antibiotics, hypochlorous acid also avoids contributing to resistance development by lid margin flora.

- **Immunomodulators:** The prescription of immunomodulating drugs such as cyclosporine ophthalmic emulsion 0.05% (Restasis, Allergan), lifitegrast ophthalmic solution 5% (Xiidra, Novartis), and, more recently, cyclosporine ophthalmic solution 0.09% (Cequa, Sun Pharma) formulated with nanomicelle technology can be used effectively in cataract candidates. Preservative-free compounded cyclosporine 0.1% ophthalmic emulsion in chondroitin sulfate (Klarity-C, ImprimisRx) is also available. Though not considered a short-term therapy option, these topical immunosuppressants can be initiated prior to surgery and are often continued postoperatively to maintain stable vision. Importantly, one needs to consider how quickly each of these therapies yields results in the presurgical setting, since most of these prescription drops may take anywhere from 2 to 12 weeks or longer to demonstrate improvement.
- **Intense pulsed light (IPL):** This drug-free, light-based treatment targets inflammation.[19,20,21] Specifically, it closes off abnormal blood vessels that perpetuate the inflammation, as the blood vessels leak proinflammatory mediators.[22,23]
- **Manual gland expression:** Due to the inherent discomfort of the procedure, gland expression may have limited utility as a stand-alone treatment without prior gland heating. However, it is both diagnostic and therapeutic in patients who have MGD.
- **Mechanical cleansing and exfoliation:** Removing excess bacteria, biofilm, and scurf from the lid margins is an essential part of ocular wellness. Therefore, microblepharoexfoliation (BlephEx, BlephEx) can be considered in some preoperative patients. This can be performed in the office by

the physician or by a trained technician. A milder, automated oscillating brush cleanser (NuLids, NuSight Medical) can be recommended as an adjunctive, home-based daily maintenance regimen for lid hygiene.

- **Mechanical warming and evacuation:** Several technologies exist in this category for patients who have MGD. Some devices offer the dual benefits of warming, along with nonmanual compression or pulsation to evacuate the meibomian glands (LipiFlow, Johnson & Johnson). Others can be used in an open-eye environment to facilitate the benefits of blinking during treatment (TearCare, Sight Sciences; iLux, Alcon). These latter options work well for patients with small interpalpebral fissures or those who are claustrophobic.

- **Neurostimulation:** Normal tear production can be stimulated via the lacrimal reflex by self-delivering mechanical vibrations to the external skin on the side of the nose for as little as 30 seconds per side (iTear, Olympic Ophthalmics). This has been shown to effectively improve both the signs and symptoms of dry eye disease.[8]

- **Oral omega supplements:** Omega-3 essential fatty acids (EFAs) and some Omega-6 EFAs are recognized to have a broad range of systemic anti-inflammatory effects, including inhibiting the production of several key proinflammatory cytokines and preventing T-lymphocyte proliferation processes.[8] As such, daily use may be beneficial in the months leading up to and following cataract surgery. Examples include PRN (Physician Recommended Nutriceuticals) and HydroEye (Science Based Health). Conversely, the National Eye Institute–sponsored DREAM study found that, among patients with dry eye disease, those who were randomly assigned to receive supplements containing 3000 mg of omega-3 fatty acids for 12 months did not have significantly better outcomes than those who were assigned to receive placebo.[24] In both groups, the regimen was five soft-gelatin capsules daily. Each active capsule contained 400 mg of EPA and 200 mg of docosahexaenoic acid (DHA), for a total daily dose of 2000 mg of EPA and 1000 mg of DHA.[24] Each placebo capsule contained 1000 mg of refined olive oil; each capsule was 68% oleic acid, 13% palmitic acid, and 11% linoleic acid.[24] The active and placebo capsules contained 3 mg

of vitamin E (alpha-tocopherol), as an antioxidant, as well as masking flavor and lemon flavor.[24] Symptoms and signs improved in patients who received the active supplement and in those who received placebo; there was no significant difference in improvement between the two groups.[24] The mean ocular surface disease index (OSDI) score decreased (improved) significantly, by approximately 13 points, in each group during follow-up, with greater improvement by 1.9 points (95% CI, −5.0 to 1.1; $p = 0.21$) in the active supplement group than in the placebo group. The authors noted that there was virtually no difference between the two groups in the improvement in four key signs of dry eye disease ($p \geq 0.25$ for all comparisons).[24]

- **Steroids:** A short course of low-dose steroids is a popular way to rapidly improve the tear film and reduce inflammation, especially in the presurgical setting. Both loteprednol etabonate ophthalmic drops (Lotemax, Bausch + Lomb; Inveltys, Kala Pharmaceuticals) and fluorometholone acetate ophthalmic suspension (Flarex, EyeVance/Santen) have been prescribed off label to treat dry eye disease. Also, used off-label, the allergy drug, loteprednol etabonate ophthalmic suspension 0.2% for seasonal allergic conjunctivitis (Alrex, Bausch + Lomb) is prescribed for milder dry eye disease. The newest addition to our armamentarium is the recently FDA-approved Loteprednol etabonate ophthalmic suspension 0.25% (Eysuvis, Kala Pharmaceuticals) for the short-term (up to 2 weeks) treatment of the signs and symptoms of dry eye disease including episodic flare-ups of dry eye disease. Some surgeons may choose to use this product to address presurgical ocular surface inflammation. A dexamethasone ophthalmic insert 0.4 mg (Dextenza, Ocular Therapeutix) was approved for the treatment of inflammation and pain following ophthalmic surgery. This intracanalicular insert, which also acts as a temporary plug, can be placed in the punctum preoperatively for continuous delivery of preservative-free dexamethasone to the ocular surface for up to 30 days. These dexamethasone inserts may be placed into the inferior punctum presurgically at the slit lamp within an office setting to optimize the ocular surface and improve surface inflammation.

- **Tea tree oil:** Tea tree oil is a useful short-term treatment for surgical candidates who present with Demodex infestation of their lashes. Blepharitis characterized by circular debris or collarettes at the base of the lashes may be an indication of Demodex infestation. This natural, essential oil exhibits antimicrobial, anti-inflammatory, antifungal, and antiviral properties,[25] and is toxic to Demodex.[8,26] There are several commercially available lid wipes with tea tree oil–soaked towelettes.
- **Tetracycline analogues:** Doxycycline and minocycline can be considered in MGD patients preparing for cataract surgery. Both oral agents have anti-inflammatory properties, with one study showing a significant reduction in matrix metalloproteinase, or MMP-9, a dry eye disease biomarker, in individuals who have rosacea following treatment with oral doxycycline.[27] It is important to advise patients that drug-induced photosensitivity may occur.

3.5 Closing

The responsibility to educate our patients that they have two distinct medical conditions: age-related lens opacification and ocular surface disease rests squarely on our shoulders, as eye care providers. I tell my patients, "You have two diseases. The cataract, I can 'cure' by removing it and it will never grow back. Whereas, dry eye is progressive, chronic and cannot be 'cured'. However, we can work together to find therapies to address this lifelong disease." The extra chair time on the front end of cataract surgery has an added benefit of reducing chair time postoperatively: First, by educating the patient about their ongoing ocular surface disease. If their condition flares up after surgery and their vision fluctuates a little or the quality of their vision changes, you can reference their preexisting diagnosis. This is an opportunity to remind them to continue using their prescribed regimen or have them restart their dry eye therapies if noncompliance has set in. Second, by tuning up the ocular surface preoperatively, you'll get closer to your refractive target and will likely have fewer IOL exchanges, photorefractive keratectomy (PRK), or laser-assisted in situ keratomileusis (LASIK) tune-ups. Overall, chair time postsurgery is minimized when you focus on the ocular surface on the front end.

When educating patients, try to make it as experiential as possible, with a lot of hands-on show and tell. For example, you might pull up the images of the meibomian glands on a large screen to better explain MGD to patients. The black and white "piano key" images readily convey the story. You might also ask patients to hold and look at the red line, an indicator of inflammation, in their MMP-9 test cartridges.

Importantly, if proper education is not provided to the patient preoperatively, patients may view postoperative dry eye as a surgical complication and they may likely blame the surgeon. For this reason, the more comprehensively we address dry eye before surgery, the less likely that the patient will attribute it to the surgery alone.

References

[1] Movahedan A, Djalilian AR. Cataract surgery in the face of ocular surface disease. Curr Opin Ophthalmol. 2012; 23(1): 68–72
[2] Gupta PK, Drinkwater OJ, VanDusen KW, Brissette AR, Starr CE. Prevalence of ocular surface dysfunction in patients presenting for cataract surgery evaluation. J Cataract Refract Surg. 2018; 44(9):1090–1096
[3] Nichols KK, Foulks GN, Bron AJ, et al. The international workshop on meibomian gland dysfunction: executive summary. Invest Ophthalmol Vis Sci. 2011; 52(4):1922–1929
[4] Epitropoulos AT, Matossian C, Berdy GJ, Malhotra RP, Potvin R. Effect of tear osmolarity on repeatability of keratometry for cataract surgery planning. J Cataract Refract Surg. 2015; 41(8):1672–1677
[5] Matossian C. Effect of thermal pulsation system treatment on keratometry measurements prior to cataract surgery. Presented at the Annual Meeting of the American Society of Cataract and Refractive Surgery. May 6, 2019. San Diego, CA
[6] Trattler WB, Majmudar PA, Donnenfeld ED, McDonald MB, Stonecipher KG, Goldberg DF. The Prospective Health Assessment of Cataract Patients' Ocular Surface (PHACO) study: the effect of dry eye. Clin Ophthalmol. 2017; 11: 1423–1430
[7] Starr CE, Gupta PK, Farid M, et al. ASCRS Cornea Clinical Committee. An algorithm for the preoperative diagnosis and treatment of ocular surface disorders. J Cataract Refract Surg. 2019; 45(5):669–684
[8] Jones L, Downie LE, Korb D, et al. TFOS DEWS II Management and Therapy Report. Ocul Surf. 2017; 15(3):575–628
[9] Opitz D, Harthan J, Fromstein S, Hauswirth S. Diagnosis and management of meibomian gland dysfunction: optometrists' perspective. Clin Optom (Auckl). 2015; 7:59–69
[10] Qiao J, Yan X. Emerging treatment options for meibomian gland dysfunction. Clin Ophthalmol. 2013; 7:1797–1803
[11] Villani E, Garoli E, Canton V, Pichi F, Nucci P, Ratiglia R. Evaluation of a novel eyelid-warming device in meibomian gland dysfunction unresponsive to traditional warm compress treatment: an in vivo confocal study. Int Ophthalmol. 2015; 35(3):319–323

[12] Arita R, Morishige N, Shirakawa R, Sato Y, Amano S. Effects of eyelid warming devices on tear film parameters in normal subjects and patients with meibomian gland dysfunction. Ocul Surf. 2015; 13(4):321–330

[13] Wang MT, Jaitley Z, Lord SM, Craig JP. Comparison of self-applied heat therapy for meibomian gland dysfunction. Optom Vis Sci. 2015; 92(9):e321–e326

[14] Olson MC, Korb DR, Greiner JV. Increase in tear film lipid layer thickness following treatment with warm compresses in patients with meibomian gland dysfunction. Eye Contact Lens. 2003; 29(2):96–99

[15] Goto E, Monden Y, Takano Y, et al. Treatment of non-inflamed obstructive meibomian gland dysfunction by an infrared warm compression device. Br J Ophthalmol. 2002; 86(12):1403–1407

[16] Geerling G, Tauber J, Baudouin C, et al. The international workshop on meibomian gland dysfunction: report of the subcommittee on management and treatment of meibomian gland dysfunction. Invest Ophthalmol Vis Sci. 2011; 52(4):2050–2064

[17] Goto E, Endo K, Suzuki A, Fujikura Y, Tsubota K. Improvement of tear stability following warm compression in patients with meibomian gland dysfunction. Adv Exp Med Biol. 2002; 506 Pt B:1149–1152

[18] Stroman DW, Mintun K, Epstein AB, et al. Reduction in bacterial load using hypochlorous acid hygiene solution on ocular skin. Clin Ophthalmol. 2017; 11:707–714

[19] Liu R, Rong B, Tu P, et al. Analysis of cytokine levels in tears and clinical correlations after intense pulsed light treating meibomian gland dysfunction. Am J Ophthalmol. 2017; 183:81–90

[20] Yin Y, Liu N, Gong L, Song N. Changes in the meibomian gland after exposure to intense pulsed light in meibomian gland dysfunction (MGD) patients. Curr Eye Res. 2018; 43 (3):308–313

[21] Sambhi RS, Sambhi GDS, Mather R, Malvankar-Mehta MS. Intense pulsed light therapy with meibomian gland expression for dry eye disease. Can J Ophthalmol. 2020; 55(3):189–198

[22] Kassir R, Kolluru A, Kassir M. Intense pulsed light for the treatment of rosacea and telangiectasias. J Cosmet Laser Ther. 2011; 13(5):216–222

[23] Papageorgiou P, Clayton W, Norwood S, Chopra S, Rustin M. Treatment of rosacea with intense pulsed light: significant improvement and long-lasting results. Br J Dermatol. 2008; 159(3):628–632

[24] Asbell PA, Maguire MG, Pistilli M, et al. Dry Eye Assessment and Management Study Research Group. n-3 Fatty acid supplementation for the treatment of dry eye disease. N Engl J Med. 2018; 378(18):1681–1690

[25] Carson CF, Hammer KA, Riley TV. Melaleuca alternifolia (Tea Tree) oil: a review of antimicrobial and other medicinal properties. Clin Microbiol Rev. 2006; 19(1):50–62

[26] Gao YY, Di Pascuale MA, Li W, et al. In vitro and in vivo killing of ocular Demodex by tea tree oil. Br J Ophthalmol. 2005; 89(11):1468–1473

[27] Määttä M, Kari O, Tervahartiala T, et al. Tear fluid levels of MMP-8 are elevated in ocular rosacea: treatment effect of oral doxycycline. Graefes Arch Clin Exp Ophthalmol. 2006; 244(8):957–962

4 Topography and Tomography

Nandini Venkateswaran and Kendall E. Donaldson

Abstract

This chapter focuses on the importance of corneal topography and tomography in the preoperative planning and postoperative outcomes of refractive cataract surgery. Corneal imaging should be performed on all cataract surgery patients and the refractive cataract surgeon should thoroughly interpret these images to formulate surgical plans. Optimizing the ocular surface prior to obtaining corneal measurements and acquiring multiple sets of measurements utilizing various devices will assist the surgeon in determining a patient's candidacy for premium intraocular lens technology, optimizing postoperative visual outcomes, and increasing patient satisfaction.

Keywords: corneal topography, corneal tomography, refractive cataract surgery, ocular surface disease, corneal ectasia

4.1 Overview

Refractive cataract surgery is constantly evolving to demand greater levels of precision in refractive correction, creating high levels of spectacle independence for our patients. In the 1960s, successful cataract surgery simply involved the removal of the lens with little attempt to control residual refractive error. However, over the past 20 years, we have acquired more options for astigmatism correction with monofocal toric intraocular lenses (IOLs), and complex multifocal, trifocal, and accommodative toric lens designs. In addition, we have the ability to create precise corneal incisional plans which can be carried out through the use of the femtosecond laser or to create manual limbal relaxing incisions for cases involving smaller degrees of astigmatism correction not suitable for toric lens placement.

As cataract surgeons, we are fortunate to have a variety of instruments to measure the cornea preoperatively, allowing us to precisely define a patient's astigmatism in preparation for cataract surgery. This allows us to offer our patients very high levels of spectacle independence. While the precision achieved through improved technology has increased through the years, so have patient expectations. Thus, it is of utmost importance that we acquire the most accurate information through topography and tomography while also doing our best to communicate with our patients and set realistic expectations, discussing any limitations or challenges before surgery. Proper measurements are the essential foundation for all refractive cataract surgery.

In this chapter, we will focus on the importance and utility of corneal topography and tomography in the preoperative planning for refractive cataract surgery.

4.2 Topography

Corneal topography is a noninvasive imaging tool that is used to map the surface shape and curvature of the cornea.[1] There are two techniques used to obtain corneal topography: Placido disc and scanning slit beams.

4.2.1 Placido Disc

In the late 1800s, the Placido disc was developed to assess the shape of the anterior corneal surface. In this technique, dark and light concentric rings (referred to as mires) are reflected off the anterior corneal surface and the resultant pattern of rings is used to characterize the shape of the anterior surface of the cornea. This technique provides a two-dimensional analysis of the anterior surface of the cornea.[2] The normal Placido mires should be crisp and distinct and equally spaced over the entirety of the corneal surface (▶ Fig. 4.1). If the mires appear closer together on a certain portion of the cornea, they correspond to an area of steeper corneal curvature. In contrast, if the mires appear farther apart, they correspond to an area of flatter corneal curvature. Corneas with regular astigmatism often have Placido mires that are ovoid, with mires being more closely spaced in the meridian of the astigmatism (▶ Fig. 4.2). Placido mires suggestive of an area of corneal steepness can also help guide suture removal in patients with sutured wounds or corneal transplants (▶ Fig. 4.2). However, in corneas with irregular astigmatism or ocular surface pathology (i.e., dry eye disease or anterior basement membrane

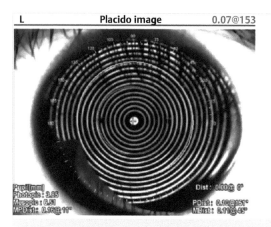
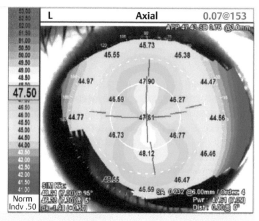

Fig. 4.1 OPD III (Nidek) Placido disc image showing clear crisp mires that are evenly spaced on the entire corneal surface. Axial curvature map generated from the corneal scan.

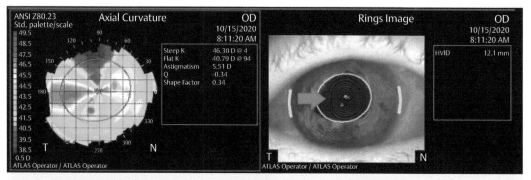

Fig. 4.2 Atlas 9000 (Zeiss) axial curvature image showing against-the-rule astigmatism secondary to sutures placed in the temporal cornea after corneal transplant surgery. The Placido mires are ovoid, with mires being more closely spaced in the meridian of the astigmatism (*blue arrow*).

dystrophy), the Placido mires can be diffusely blurred or distorted, providing a clue to proper triage and further decision and management.

Devices that employ Placido disc topography include the Atlas 9000 (Zeiss), Keratograph 5 M (Oculus), TMS-4N (Tomey), Galilei (Ziemer), and OPD III Scan (Nidek). These devices can produce axial and/or tangential curvature maps to measure corneal curvature (▶ Fig. 4.1, ▶ Fig. 4.3, and ▶ Fig. 4.4).

4.2.2 Scanning Slit Beam Technique

In the scanning slit beam method, reflections of rapidly scanned projected slit beams of light are captured by a camera and are used to indirectly construct a map of the anterior and posterior corneal surfaces. Unlike Placido disc images, scanning slit beams can image the posterior cornea.

The Orbscan (Bausch & Lomb) employs the scanning slit beam method to produce axial and tangential curvature maps as well as elevation maps of the anterior and posterior corneal surfaces.

4.2.3 Types of Topography Maps

Axial Maps

Axial maps, also referred to as power or sagittal maps, report reference distances across the corneal surface. They are created based on the assumption that all light rays striking the cornea are refracted, creating a reference axis through

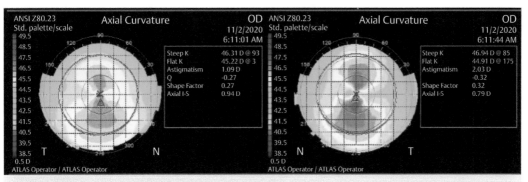

Fig. 4.3 Axial curvature maps generated on the Atlas 9000 (Zeiss) topographer showing regular with-the-rule astigmatism.

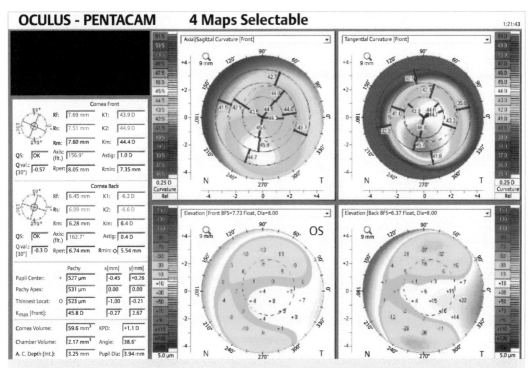

Fig. 4.4 4-map selectable display on the Pentacam (Oculus) that shows an axial curvature map (upper left), tangential curvature map (upper right), and elevation maps (bottom left and right). The tangential curvature map is able to highlight additional details in the central cornea as compared with the axial curvature map, notably the area of inferior steepening suggestive of keratoconus. The elevation maps show central elevation on the anterior and posterior surfaces of the cornea.

the optical axis. They do not represent values of dioptric power but rather run an average of scaled curvatures to produce outputs that create a global representation of corneal shape. These are the maps most often looked at by corneal surgeons; however, these maps tend to create "smoother" maps by averaging the data, rendering their outputs less accurate than tangential maps (see the next section). Details of the central cornea are more accurate as compared with details of the peripheral cornea with axial maps. Axial maps are often helpful to determine the base curve selection for contact lenses as the average central curvature is shown.[3]

Tangential Maps

Tangential maps, also referred to as instantaneous or local maps, also report reference distances across the corneal surface; however, they are based on the assumption that all refracted light does not fall on a central reference axis. As such, more extreme peripheral curvatures are included in the outputs and these maps are more sensitive to transitions in curvature of the corneal surface. Tangential maps show smaller patterns but are better at offering the true picture of the corneal shape. For example, tangential maps are very helpful in locating the apex of the cone in keratoconus.[3]

Elevation Maps

Elevation maps are maps that best convey the true shape of the cornea. Tomographers that use Scheimpflug imaging techniques directly measure elevation maps while placido disc-based topographers use algorithms to derive corneal elevation data. In elevation maps, elevation of the anterior and posterior cornea is compared to a reference best-fit sphere. The outputs then calculate areas of relative elevation and depression based on the deviations from the best-fit sphere. Elevation maps are often helpful to assess for posterior corneal elevation suggestive of keratoconus.

▶ Fig. 4.4 shows a printout of the axial, tangential, and elevation maps on the Pentacam (Oculus).

4.3 Tomography

Corneal tomography is also a noninvasive imaging tool that creates three-dimensional images of the entire cornea. This is primarily achieved through Scheimpflug imaging techniques.

4.3.1 Scheimpflug Imaging

In Scheimpflug imaging, a rotating camera is used to photograph cross-sections of the cornea illuminated by slit beams at differing angles. These cross-sectional images are used to create a three-dimensional image of the cornea and help characterize the anterior and posterior corneal surfaces along with corneal thickness distribution.

Devices that employ Scheimpflug imaging techniques include the Pentacam (Oculus), Galilei (Ziemer), and Sirius (CSO Ophthalmic). These devices can produce axial curvature maps, elevation maps of the anterior and posterior corneal surfaces, as well as corneal pachymetry maps. Tomographers such as the Pentacam can also provide information useful for IOL power calculations (i.e., white-to-white measurements, anterior chamber depth, and lens thickness). Enhanced ectasia displays can also be generated to further characterize and determine the likelihood of ectatic corneal disorders.

Tomographic images often provide simulated keratometry values, which are defined as the average keratometry calculated by using the standard keratometric index and the radius of anterior corneal curvature. Because the simulated keratometry values are derived from measurements and not true corneal power readings, we do not recommend using these values for IOL power calculations.[4]

▶ Table 4.1 outlines several of the currently available topography and tomography devices utilized by refractive cataract surgeons.

Table 4.1 Summary of currently available topography and tomography machines

Devices name	Manufacturer
Placido topography	
Atlas 9000	Zeiss
Keratograph 5 M	Oculus
OPD III	Nidek
Tomey	TMS-4N
Placido and scanning slit	
Orbscan	Bausch and Lomb
Scheimpflug tomography	
Pentacam	Oculus
Galilei	Ziemer
Sirius	CSO Ophthalmic
LED	
Cassini	i-Optics
Ray Tracing	
iTrace	Tracey Technologies

4.4 How to Make Proper Measurements/Avoiding Errors

One of the most important practices for the refractive cataract surgeon is to ensure that all preoperative measurements that are obtained are of the highest quality. It is essential that all preoperative testing be performed prior to manipulation of the ocular surface, which may occur during administration of eye drops, applanation tonometry, or measurement of manual corneal pachymetry. Patients are encouraged to remain out of soft contact lenses for approximately one week and out of rigid gas permeable contact lenses for several weeks (approximately one week per decade of contact lens wear) prior to any preoperative imaging to avoid any errors in keratometry measurements that may result from contact lens–induced corneal warpage. In patients receiving premium IOL technology, obtaining multiple sets of measurements is critical. Oftentimes, two serial sets of measurements spaced 2 to 4 weeks apart are obtained to verify reproducibility of measurements. Inconsistencies in measurements should prompt the surgeon to repeat measurements and to evaluate the patient for other underlying conditions such as ocular surface disease, or other forms of corneal dystrophies or degeneration. Patients need to be informed that just like building a new house, it takes time to get things ready. The same principle applies to getting prepared for the best possible quality eye surgery.

The most common causes of inaccurate or inconsistent preoperative measurements include dry eye disease, Salzmann nodular degeneration, anterior basement membrane dystrophy (▶ Fig. 4.5), and pterygia. Corneal topography is an excellent diagnostic tool for ocular surface disease in surgical patients. Oftentimes, ocular surface pathology can be subtle on clinical examination and may be easily overlooked, but a careful assessment of topographic images can help unveil these conditions. Looking for areas of dropout, irregular astigmatism, or inconsistent keratometry values can increase suspicion for ocular surface disease (▶ Fig. 4.6).

Studies have shown that dry eye disease is very common and often asymptomatic in patients presenting for cataract surgery evaluation.[5,6] Patients with hyperosmolar ocular surfaces have been shown to have a higher variability in the average corneal keratometry and anterior corneal astigmatism readings, with significant differences in IOL power calculations.[7] Similarly, in patients with anterior basement membrane dystrophy or Salzmann nodular degeneration, treatment with superficial keratectomy and/or phototherapeutic keratectomy led to normalization of the ocular surface with significant changes in keratometry as well as spherical and toric IOL power, axis, and meridian of astigmatism.[8] Timely diagnosis and management of ocular surface dysfunction in the preoperative period can help prevent refractive surprises and unhappy patients postoperatively.

4.5 How to Read Topography/Tomography Images

Having a systematic approach to reading topographic images is critical for a refractive cataract surgeon. Depending on which topography or tomography platform is utilized, the outputs may vary in appearance; however, having a step-by-step approach to analyze the important elements of the images can help the surgeon consistently identify outliers and abnormalities.

Steps:

1. Ensure that the scan is for the appropriate patient by verifying the patient's name and date of birth.
2. Verify that the scan is of good quality. Do not utilize scans that are incomplete due to poor patient fixation, blinking, or significant lid artifact.
   a) An easy way to check the quality of the scan is to look for eyelid artifact (where the top half of the scan is missing) or to look for irregular dropout of the Placido disc mires. Train office technicians to obtain multiple scans if these errors are noted. It is easy for beginning surgeons to utilize poor quality scans which can lead to inaccurate calculations.
3. Look at the color scale and identify the range and gradient of the values given. Different machines and scans can have different scales. A tighter color-coding scale may enhance patterns while a more widely spaced scale may hide important patterns.
4. Look at the flat and steep keratometry values as well as the maximum keratometry value (K_{max}), if reported. Determine if these values are average or abnormally steep or flat. Always concentrate primarily on the central 4 mm of

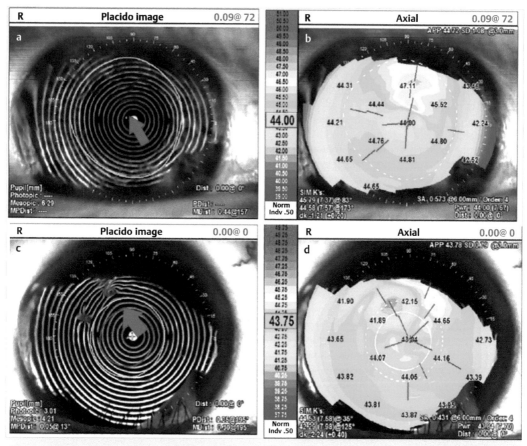

Fig. 4.5 (a) OPD III (Nidek) Placido disc image showing blurred mires in a patient with anterior basement membrane dystrophy (*red arrow*). (b) Axial curvature map shows irregular astigmatism with corneal steepening in the area of the corneal dystrophy. (c) OPD III (Nidek) Placido disc image showing distorted mires in a patient with Salzmann nodular degeneration (*red arrow*). (d) Axial curvature map shows marked corneal flattening in the area of the nodular degeneration. (Courtesy of Kathryn M. Hatch, MD.)

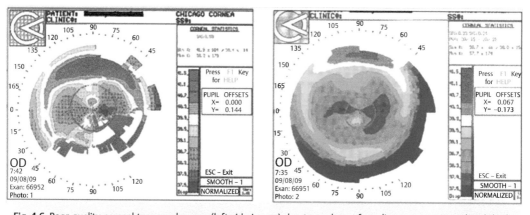

Fig. 4.6 Poor quality corneal topography scan (left side image) due to ocular surface disease as compared with high-quality scan (right side image). (Courtesy of Parag A. Majmudar, MD.)

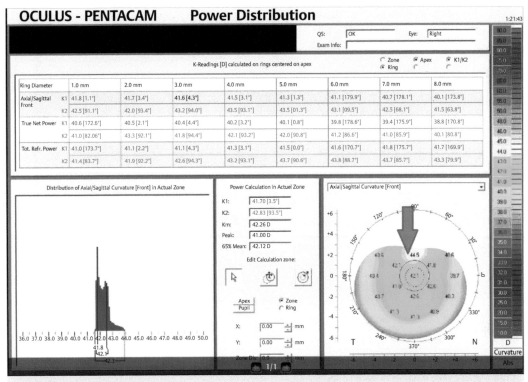

OCULUS - PENTACAM — Power Distribution

QS: OK   Eye: Right
Exam Info:

K-Readings [D] calculated on rings centered on apex

○ Zone ● Apex ● K1/K2
● Ring   ○   ○

Ring Diameter		1.0 mm	2.0 mm	3.0 mm	4.0 mm	5.0 mm	6.0 mm	7.0 mm	8.0 mm
Axial/Sagittal Front	K1	41.8 [1.1°]	41.7 [3.4°]	41.6 [4.3°]	41.5 [3.1°]	41.3 [1.3°]	41.1 [179.9°]	40.7 [178.1°]	40.1 [173.8°]
	K2	42.5 [91.1°]	42.0 [93.4°]	43.2 [94.0°]	43.5 [93.1°]	43.5 [01.3°]	43.1 [09.5°]	42.5 [68.1°]	41.5 [63.8°]
True Net Power	K1	40.6 [172.6°]	40.5 [2.1°]	40.4 [4.4°]	40.2 [3.2°]	40.1 [0.8°]	39.8 [178.6°]	39.4 [175.9°]	38.8 [170.8°]
	K2	41.0 [82.06°]	43.3 [92.1°]	41.8 [94.4°]	42.1 [93.2°]	42.0 [90.8°]	41.2 [86.6°]	41.0 [85.9°]	40.1 [80.8°]
Tot. Refr. Power	K1	41.0 [173.7°]	41.1 [2.2°]	41.1 [4.3°]	41.3 [3.1°]	41.5 [0.0°]	41.6 [170.7°]	41.8 [175.7°]	41.7 [169.9°]
	K2	41.4 [83.7°]	41.9 [92.2°]	42.6 [94.3°]	43.2 [93.1°]	43.7 [90.6°]	43.8 [88.7°]	43.7 [85.7°]	43.3 [79.9°]

Distribution of Axial/Sagittal Curvature [Front] in Actual Zone

36.0 37.0 38.0 39.0 40.0 41.0 42.0 43.0 44.0 45.0 46.0 47.0 48.0 49.0 50.0
41.8
42.1
42.3

Power Calculation in Actuel Zone

K1:   41.70 [3.5°]
K2:   42.83 [93.5°]
Km: 42.26 D
Peak: 41.00 D
65% Mean: 42.12 D

Edit Calculation zone:

Apex / Pupil   ● Zone ○ Ring

X: 0.00 mm
Y: 0.00 mm
Zone Dis: 0.0 mm

Axial/Sagittal Curvature [Front]

1/1

Fig. 4.7 Pentacam map highlighting the true net corneal power in the central 4 mm of the cornea (*blue arrow*).

the cornea (which is particularly important to remember in those postrefractive corneas, which may have more irregularities toward the periphery of the ablation zone) (▶ Fig. 4.7).

5. Look at the axial and tangential curvature maps as well as the anterior and posterior corneal elevation and thickness maps. Make note of the distribution of keratometry values, corneal pachymetry, and elevation differences on the anterior and posterior corneal surfaces. Look for patterns of corneal steepening or flattening.
   a) Central corneal flattening can be secondary to prior myopic LASIK/PRK (▶ Fig. 4.8) while central steepening can be secondary to previous hyperopic LASIK/PRK, corneal ectasia, or keratoconus.
6. Note the quantity of astigmatism and the steep axis.
   a) Look for irregular patterns of astigmatism, or patterns suggestive of ectasia such as an asymmetric bowtie appearance, prominent central or inferior corneal steepening, or an oblique meridian of astigmatism (▶ Fig. 4.9).
   b) Look for areas of prominent corneal flattening in the nasal or superior cornea, which could be secondary to a pterygium or a Salzmann nodule.
7. Assess the quality and symmetry of the Placido disc mires on topographic images. Areas of disruption or dropout can be suggestive of untreated ocular surface disease.
8. In tomographic images, make note of the corneal pachymetry (both in the central cornea and at the corneal apex) and evaluate for posterior corneal abnormalities. Look for a displacement of the thinnest point of the cornea and check to see if focal areas of corneal thinning correspond to posterior corneal abnormalities, consistent with ectasia (▶ Fig. 4.9).
9. Compare the tomography and topography measurements to measurements obtained from other devices such as a manual keratometer, automated keratometer, or biometer.

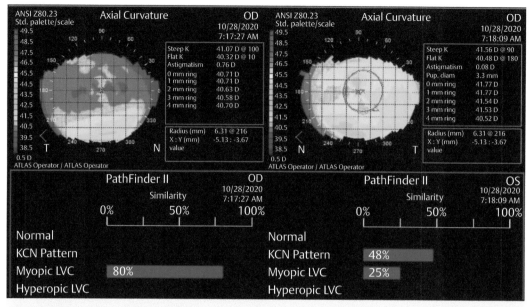

Fig. 4.8 Atlas 9000 (Zeiss) axial curvature images showing central corneal flattening consistent with prior myopic laser vision correction.

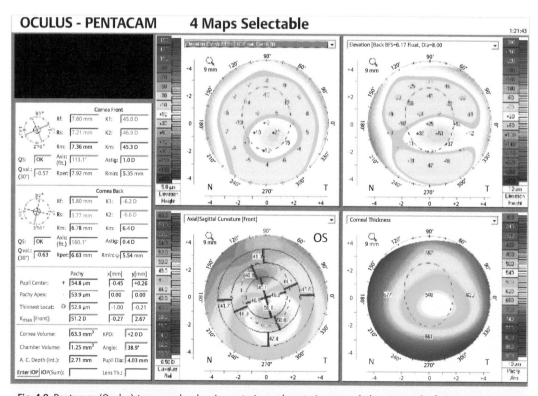

Fig. 4.9 Pentacam (Oculus) tomography showing anterior and posterior corneal elevation and inferior corneal steepening consistent with keratoconus.

10. It is important to look for symmetry in the topographic and tomographic images between both eyes. In most circumstances, symmetry is confirmatory for a lack of pathology.

4.6 Creating a Surgical Plan Using Topography and Tomography

The quality and accuracy of the information garnered from corneal topography and tomography is vital when generating surgical plans for refractive cataract surgery patients, particularly when determining the need for a toric or presbyopia correcting toric IOL.

Keratometry values play an essential role in IOL power calculation as well as in the estimation of the effective lens position of the implanted IOL. A 1 diopter error in corneal keratometry values can lead to a 0.9 diopter error in the predicted IOL power and 0.6 diopter error in the postoperative refractive error.[9] As such, it is important to obtain keratometry values using multiple methods (manual keratometry, automated keratometry, biometry, as well as topography and tomography), and compare these measurements to ensure there is consistency among all of these measurements. Inconsistencies may be a sign of underlying pathology and may indicate that a patient is not a good candidate for a toric or presbyopia correcting lens at the time of cataract surgery.

Particularly with astigmatism correction, accurate keratometry values are required to determine and confirm the quantity of astigmatism and the axis of astigmatism as well as to determine if the astigmatism is regular or irregular. Currently available corneal tomographers (Pentacam, Oculus) as well as biometers (IOL Master 700, Zeiss) can measure posterior corneal astigmatism, which has been shown to produce up to 0.3 diopters of against-the-rule astigmatism.[10]

Biometers, such as the IOL master 700, measure keratometry values in the central 2.5-mm zone of the cornea while corneal topographers/tomographers measure the whole cornea. The keratometry values obtained from the biometer are most accurate for use in IOL calculations while keratometry measurements obtained from topographers/tomographers are more critical for the overall evaluation of the regularity and symmetry of

corneal astigmatism, as well as to confirm the axis of astigmatism.

Refractive cataract surgeons will typically perform manual or femtosecond laser-assisted limbal relaxing incisions for less than 1.25 diopters of with-the-rule astigmatism and less than 0.75 diopters of against-the-rule astigmatism.[11] For higher values of with-the-rule and against-the-rule astigmatism, toric IOLs are generally considered. Alignment of toric IOLs on the correct axis is crucial to avoid a postoperative refractive surprise. For every 1 degree of axis rotation of a toric IOL, there is a 3.3% reduction in the effective cylinder correction of the toric IOL.[12] If the toric IOL is misaligned by 30 degrees, the toric IOL is essentially ineffectual (▶ Fig. 4.10). In addition to precise preoperative measurements, employing additional technologies such as intraoperative aberrometry (i.e., ORA Intraoperative aberrometry, Alcon) and intraoperative alignment tools (Callisto Eye, Zeiss) is helpful in confirming the correct orientation of toric IOLs in the operating room.

When performing toric IOL calculations, several methods can be used to seamlessly integrate posterior corneal measurement data to improve the validity and accuracy of the calculations. The IOL master 700 measures the total corneal keratometry (measurements of both the anterior and posterior cornea), referred to as the total cornea (TK) measurement. When obtaining printouts of IOL calculations, the Barrett TK toric formula can be applied for toric IOLs selection, producing a toric IOL calculation that takes into account the measured anterior and posterior corneal keratometry measurements. In general, patients who have against-the-rule astigmatism will have higher TK values as opposed to patients who have with-the-rule astigmatism (since the anterior cornea and posterior cornea have differing axes of astigmatism).

The Barrett toric IOL calculator can also be utilized to calculate toric IOL powers. On biometers such as the Lenstar (Haag Streit) and IOL master 700, the Barrett toric formula is automatically built in. The Barrett toric calculator by default uses a posterior cornea prediction based on theoretical models to predict the posterior corneal astigmatism for an individual eye. As an alternative, the online version of the calculator does allow the surgeon to enter directly measured posterior corneal values from Scheimpflug or swept source OCT devices. For surgeons who obtain

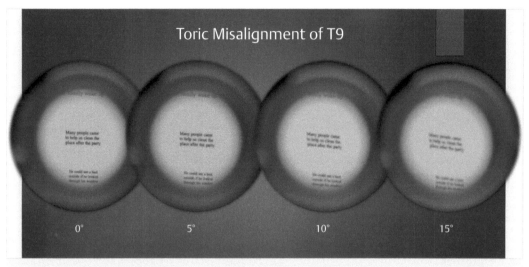

Fig. 4.10 Image depicting the visual blur associated with progressive misalignment of the axis of a toric IOL (Courtesy of John Berdahl, MD).

posterior corneal keratometry measurements with multiple devices, inputting this data can help improve the accuracy of their IOL selection, especially if they do not have access to intraoperative aberrometry.

Overlooking the posterior corneal astigmatism has been shown to adversely affect the outcome of astigmatic surgical interventions.[13] Notably, studies have shown that in patients with previous myopic excimer laser surgery, using the Barrett True-K formula in conjunction with measured posterior corneal power using Scheimpflug imaging resulted in the lowest standard deviation of prediction error.[14] Accounting for posterior corneal astigmatism helps surgeons more accurately determine the amount of total corneal astigmatism and select the most appropriate modality of astigmatism correction for a given patient. Incorporating direct measurements of the posterior corneal power will likely gain increasing popularity among refractive cataract surgeons to improve visual outcomes in patients.

Corneal topography and tomography can also be extremely helpful in identifying patients with corneal disorders such as keratoconus, pellucid marginal degeneration, or postrefractive corneal ectasia. Corneal ectatic disorders should be identified preoperatively to avoid postsurgical refractive surprises. Using toric IOLs in patients with irregular astigmatism can lead to suboptimal refractive outcomes. Aiming for a more myopic target at the time of cataract surgery in patients with keratoconus or pellucid marginal degeneration will help prevent a hyperopic refractive surprise and patient dissatisfaction.

Cornea tomographers, such as the Pentacam, also provide pachymetry measurements of the central and peripheral cornea. This enables the surgeon to determine if there are areas of corneal thinning and also helps plan the depth and location of a manual LRI if needed for astigmatic correction.

In devices such as the OPD-Scan III, which is a keratometer, corneal topographer, and integrated wavefront aberrometer, the surgeon can also make note of the degree of higher order aberrations as well as the angle alpha values, which if elevated, can render patients poor candidates for premium IOLs. Similarly, in devices such as the Pentacam, abnormal angle kappa values can also be noted, which can limit the tolerability and efficacy of premium IOLs in some patients.

Lastly, the iTrace (Tracey Technologies) combines autorefraction, corneal topography, autokeratometry, wavefront aberrometry, and pupillometry in one system to image the entire visual pathway (▶ Fig. 4.11a). In addition to providing keratometry values for corneal analysis, the platform can measure corneal as well as total higher order aberrations, and can enable surgeons to precisely plan toric IOL alignment as well as

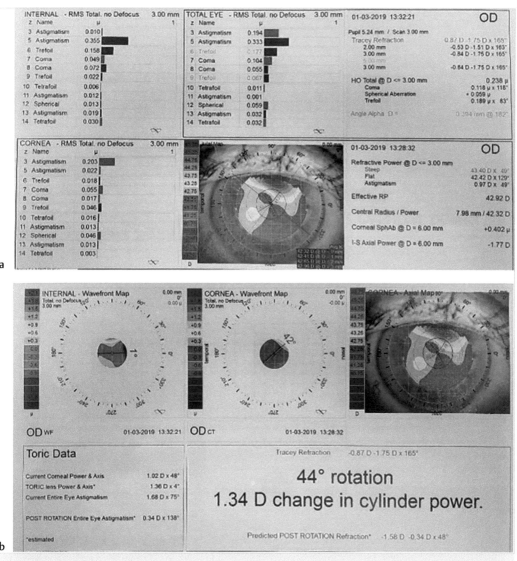

Fig. 4.11 (a) iTrace map showing total eye as well as internal and cornea higher order aberrations. (b) iTrace map indicating a 44-degree rotation of an implanted toric intraocular lens leading to a postoperative refractive surprise. (Courtesy of Florence Cabot, MD.)

determine the degree of postoperative toric IOL rotation (▶ Fig. 4.11b).

4.7 Postoperative Evaluation

Corneal topography and tomography can be utilized to monitor the effects of various surface treatments on keratometry values. Utilizing the same topographer and tomographer pre- and postoperatively is necessary for valid comparisons. Corneal imaging performed before and after dry eye disease treatment, superficial keratectomy for anterior basement membrane dystrophy, or Salzmann nodular degeneration (▶ Fig. 4.12), pterygium excision, or corneal crosslinking can highlight normalization of the corneal architecture and changes in corneal keratometry values. Difference maps can be used to monitor posttreatment

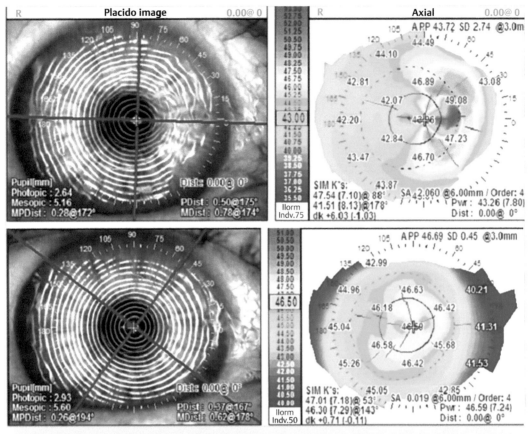

Fig. 4.12 OPD III (Nidek) Placido disc images and axial curvature maps before (top) and 1-month after (bottom) superficial keratectomy for Salzmann nodular degeneration. There is normalization of the corneal surface after the superficial keratectomy with a marked reduction in the irregular corneal astigmatism. (Courtesy of Elizabeth Yeu, MD.)

corneal flattening or steepening. Verifying stability of keratometry measurements with sequential scans is important as the cornea can continue to remodel for several weeks following procedures. Patients with irregular initial topographic and tomographic images often need multiple scans. Keratometry measurements should only be used for IOL calculations once they have shown definitive stability.

4.8 Summary

The art of refractive cataract surgery is one that requires high precision and attention to detail. Keratometry and biometry are the cornerstones of refractive cataract surgery, and high-quality measurements are essential to maximize visual outcomes. Preoperative corneal topography/tomography should be performed on all cataract surgery patients and the refractive cataract surgeon should know how to interpret these images and formulate thoughtful surgical plans. Optimizing corneal measurements, obtaining multiple sets of measurements, and utilizing multiple devices to obtain patient data will ultimately help the surgeon determine a patient's candidacy for toric or premium IOL technology and optimize postoperative visual outcomes and patient satisfaction. In addition to meticulous preoperative planning, postoperative assessment of outcomes helps refine one's nomogram for various subtypes of patients and helps improve outcomes over time.

References

[1] Moshirfar M, Duong A, Ronquillo Y. Corneal imaging. StatPearls. StatPearls Publishing LLC; 2020

[2] Fan R, Chan TC, Prakash G, Jhanji V. Applications of corneal topography and tomography: a review. Clin Exp Ophthalmol. 2018; 46(2):133–146

[3] Tummanapalli SS, Potluri H, Vaddavalli PK, Sangwan VS. Efficacy of axial and tangential corneal topography maps in detecting subclinical keratoconus. J Cataract Refract Surg. 2015; 41(10):2205–2214

[4] Kamiya K, Kono Y, Takahashi M, Shoji N. Comparison of simulated keratometry and total refractive power for keratoconus according to the stage of amsler-krumeich classification. Sci Rep. 2018; 8(1):12436

[5] Trattler WB, Majmudar PA, Donnenfeld ED, McDonald MB, Stonecipher KG, Goldberg DF. The Prospective Health Assessment of Cataract Patients' Ocular Surface (PHACO) study: the effect of dry eye. Clin Ophthalmol. 2017; 11:1423–1430

[6] Gupta PK, Drinkwater OJ, VanDusen KW, Brissette AR, Starr CE. Prevalence of ocular surface dysfunction in patients presenting for cataract surgery evaluation. J Cataract Refract Surg. 2018; 44(9):1090–1096

[7] Epitropoulos AT, Matossian C, Berdy GJ, Malhotra RP, Potvin R. Effect of tear osmolarity on repeatability of keratometry for cataract surgery planning. J Cataract Refract Surg. 2015; 41(8):1672–1677

[8] Goerlitz-Jessen MF, Gupta PK, Kim T. Impact of epithelial basement membrane dystrophy and Salzmann nodular degeneration on biometry measurements. J Cataract Refract Surg. 2019; 45(8):1119–1123

[9] Lee AC, Qazi MA, Pepose JS. Biometry and intraocular lens power calculation. Curr Opin Ophthalmol. 2008; 19(1):13–17

[10] Koch DD, Jenkins RB, Weikert MP, Yeu E, Wang L. Correcting astigmatism with toric intraocular lenses: effect of posterior corneal astigmatism. J Cataract Refract Surg. 2013; 39(12):1803–1809

[11] Vickers LA, Gupta PK. Femtosecond laser-assisted keratotomy. Curr Opin Ophthalmol. 2016; 27(4):277–284

[12] Potvin R, Kramer BA, Hardten DR, Berdahl JP. Toric intraocular lens orientation and residual refractive astigmatism: an analysis. Clin Ophthalmol. 2016; 10:1829–1836

[13] Koch DD, Ali SF, Weikert MP, Shirayama M, Jenkins R, Wang L. Contribution of posterior corneal astigmatism to total corneal astigmatism. J Cataract Refract Surg. 2012; 38(12):2080–2087

[14] Savini G, Hoffer KJ, Barrett GD. Results of the Barrett True-K formula for IOL power calculation based on Scheimpflug camera measurements in eyes with previous myopic excimer laser surgery. J Cataract Refract Surg. 2020; 46(7):1016–1019

5 Marking the Limbal Reference and Steep Axes

Fuxiang Zhang, Alan Sugar, and Lisa Brothers Arbisser

Abstract

The accuracy and precision of astigmatism correction can be affected by many steps. Preoperative marking is part of surgical astigmatism correction which is the core of refractive cataract surgery. This chapter will discuss the important steps of marking the limbal reference and steep axes, including the basic orientation of corneal meridians. More advanced quantitative digital imaging systems have recently become available which allows toric IOL alignment without preoperative corneal marking; beginners, however, are more likely to start with the manual method, so this chapter will focus on the manual technique. Cost-effective manners will be described, including steps to prevent head tilt, chin up/down, and marks becoming smudged and washed out.

Keywords: marking, limbal reference, steep axis, manual marking, digital marking, Verion, Callisto

5.1 Introduction

Managing astigmatism is one of the key components of refractive cataract surgery. Even when presbyopia remains, refractive cataract surgery patients can function with over-the-counter reading glasses and see perfectly well without prescription glasses at a chosen distance. One would never prescribe glasses without including a needed astigmatism correction! In considering risk versus benefit there is virtually no risk other than an inaccurate outcome necessitating that the patient choose between still needing glasses and further intervention to correct the result. Therefore, this refractive surgery can even be offered to monocular patients and those with comorbidities. Although safety glasses may be preferred, should they break or be lost, the monocular patient can function while waiting for a new pair. Due to emmetropization, a rare patient may have "latent astigmatism"; meaning the corneal curvature is compensated for by the crystalline lens. These patients may have a spherical refraction. Without topography or careful analysis of their biometry, this can be tragically missed. Upon nonrefractive cataract surgery, such rare patients will have

manifest astigmatism for the first time in their lives and be miserable or even irate.

For that reason, sometimes some surgeons may even provide a toric lens for free to such individuals, if they are unable to pay. Some may just offer free limbal relaxing incision (LRI) to avoid the toric lens cost. We hope that in the future Medicare will be able to cover the cost of intraoperative astigmatism correction during cataract surgery.

Astigmatism is a common condition. A study of 4540 eyes in 2415 patients with a mean age 60.6 years noted that more than one-third of these cases had more than 1 diopter (D) of astigmatism.[1] A large cataract database showed that more than 60% of patients had 0.75 D of corneal astigmatism or greater prior to cataract surgery.[2] Per the ASCRS Cataract Clinical committee, "Astigmatism management is vital to the performance of multifocal IOLs. A rule of thumb is that these IOLs perform best with less than three-quarters of a diopter (D) of cylinder. Beyond this, the image may degrade below satisfactory levels to achieve proper visual function."[3]

The accuracy and precision of astigmatism correction can be affected by many steps. This chapter will discuss the important steps for marking the limbal reference and steep axis.

5.2 Is the Corneal 360-Degree Map Symmetrical between OD and OS?

The answer is yes and no. Let us review the orientation. Imaging in ▸ Fig. 5.1 represents a patient facing you. 90 degrees is always at the top and 270 is at the bottom. From this perspective, it is symmetrical. The 0 degree for the right eye (OD) is at the eye's nasal side and for the left eye (OS) is at the eye's temporal side, so we can say OD and OS are not symmetrical. If you remember this pattern, you know the 360-degree orientation.

Some beginners hesitate to initiate refractive cataract surgery simply because of being confused about the orientation of corneal meridians. This basic but essential topic is not often discussed. The impact of lack of understanding of this orientation can be significant. Some are even reluctant

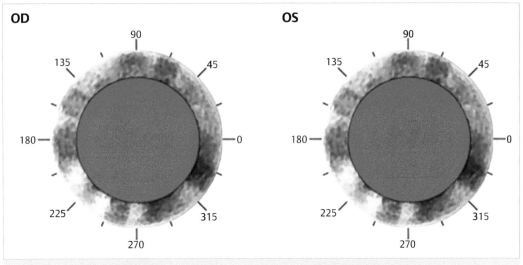

Fig. 5.1 Eye background 360-degree orientation. Used with permission from ASCRS.

to ask this question because "it is basic knowledge" (▶ Fig. 5.1).

5.3 Digital versus Manual Marking Systems

Because of the variable degree of ocular cyclotorsion (either incyclotorsion or excyclotorsion) upon patients becoming recumbent compared to sitting upright, one cannot count on accurately identifying the 90- or 180-degree axes (let alone the steep axis which is referenced to this measurement in the upright position) once the patient is on the table under the drape. This is why an independent system is required or reference marks must be made prior to the patient laying down, usually in the preoperative area with or without a slit lamp.

In addition, transcription errors or mistaken identification of studies can lead to tragic mistakes. This possibility is mitigated by developing the habit of always having the patient's topography hung on the microscope or digitally referenced in the OR at the time of surgery. The time-out prior to beginning surgery should include the recognition of these data.

Marking can be divided into two types: basic manual and advanced digital. Beginners are more likely to start with the manual method, so this section will focus on the manual technique.

5.3.1 Manual Marking

- Approximately 75% of responders use manual marking systems according to a 2017 ESCRS survey.[4]
- Basic manual marking consists of two parts: first, the reference orientation marking in the preop area with a marking pen with or without a slit lamp, and second, marking the steep axis with a handheld instrument under the microscope in the operating room.
- How to prevent marks becoming smudged and being washed out quickly?
  - Dry technique:
    Using a dry technique is easy and adds no cost. It works well.
    Have an assistant hold the lids while the surgeon does the marking. Have the patient use the fellow eye to look at a distance target straight ahead at eye level. After applying a topical anesthetic, with a regular cotton-tipped applicator, dry the peripheral cornea near the limbus at the reference locations (12:00/6:00, or 3:00/9:00, see ▶ Fig. 5.2), then use a marking pen (see ▶ Fig. 5.3) to make a nice clear mark. Continue to hold the lids for about 10 seconds to let the marks dry. With this simple dry technique, the marks will stay

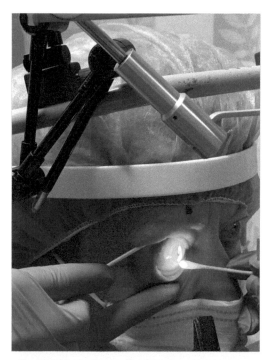

Fig. 5.2 Using a Q-tip to dry first.

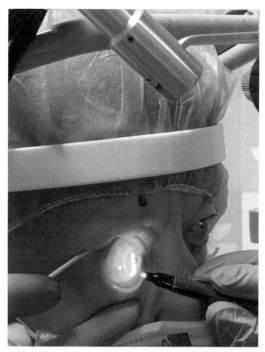

Fig. 5.3 Once the peripheral corneal spots are dried, a marking pen (green color in the picture; Devon Skin Marker, Covidien/CardinalHealth, Dublin, Ohio; Dual ends; Made in Japan; KS77642410) is used to make the marks.

clear longer, rather than smudge and washout quickly. A smudged mark can easily spread 5 to 10 degrees. From this perspective, we know a few extra minutes with this dry technique has merit.
○ Needle picking:
  Another option for a more discrete and long-lasting mark which won't spread, fade, or disappear entirely after the prep: a 25-gauge needle can be coated with ink from a pad or pen. Only at the slit lamp, of course, with the patient well pressed against the headband, a tangential approach with the needle is used to create a tiny epithelial defect or scratch at the limbus. Care must be taken to avoid any corneal or deep injury. Appropriate antisepsis requires a new needle and pen for each patient.
○ Thermal-burn[5]:
  Dr. Robert Osher presented this technique at the 20/Happy, Refractive Cataract Surgery online course, 2020 ASCRS. The extra benefit of this technique is the ability to check PO1 toric IOL alignment. Of course, this needs topical anesthesia.

• Does use of a slit lamp improve accuracy of marking?
  ○ The downside of using a slit lamp is the use of an extra few minutes, but it is more accurate. With a slit lamp, patient head position (no tilt) as well as chin-down or chin-up can be squared off in both planes. At least two studies have shown that with the slit lamp, the accuracy increases compared to without a slit lamp.[6,7] We recommend it as a routine (see ▸ Fig. 5.2 and ▸ Fig. 5.3). By the way, the same principle should be applied to corneal photography, LenStar and IOLMaster biometry. The patient's head should be straight without tilt. Technician staff education is important to avoid this kind of human error.
• How to mitigate tilt during marking?
  ○ Without any conscious attention or any extra help, small head tilt can easily induce 5 to 10 degrees of misalignment.

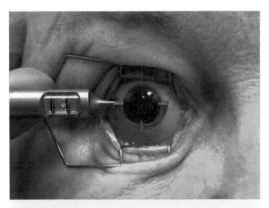

Fig. 5.4 Nuijts-Lane Pre-Op Toric Marker With Bubble REF#: AE-2791TBL. Used with permission from ASICO.

○ Dr. Graham Barrett's cell phone method is a very good one.
○ Slit lamp is easy to use and proven to be valuable.
○ Nuijts-Lane Pre-Op Toric Marker (▶ Fig. 5.4) with a leveling bubble as part of the marker to help assure proper positioning when not using a slit lamp, but this kind of device will still have accuracy issues if the head is tilted. We do use this marker with a slit lamp to secure the head position. It is also difficult to view the bubble while a slit lamp is used if the view is through the microscope. Caution is needed to avoid corneal scratch from the device.
• Do we have to mark two points (12/6 or 3/9) for limbal reference marking?
Dr. Rubenstein[5] marks only one point at 6 o'clock. If the accuracy is secured, this should be fine too. It can save time and efforts. Under the table, 12 o'clock should be easily identified if the 6 o'clock is accurately marked.
• How to mark the good eye if the patient has amblyopia?
If a patient has one amblyopic eye and we are going to use a toric lens for the nonamblyopic eye, there is a trick for marking the limbal reference mark at slit lamp. The mark may not be accurate if we ask the patient to use the amblyopic eye looking straight ahead while we are marking the nonamblyopic eye because the good eye may not be in the normal fixation position. A better way is to have the good eye looking straightforward as a fixation position while marking that eye.
• Study at Baylor College in Houston found that a manual method was as good as a digital one.[8]
• Making a limbal reference is still often needed even for digital marking.
• So, beginners should not feel inferior when manual marking is used. More important factor is to pay attention to details.

5.3.2 Digital Marking

Robert Osher, MD, should be credited for his pioneering work on the digital imaging system and iris fingerprinting concept a decade ago, which captures a photo of reference vessels or iris landmarks. (Please refer to Chapter 1, "A Career of Refractive Cataract Surgery" for detail). Needless to say, this great idea has led to the development of more advanced quantitative digital imaging systems.

More advanced quantitative digital imaging systems have recently become available which allow toric IOL alignment without preoperative corneal marking.[9,10] Verion V-Lynk (Alcon) and Callisto (Zeiss) are the two commonly used in the past few years.

The Verion Image-Guided System (Alcon) consists of a measurement module and digital marker. Preoperatively, a color reference image of the patient's eye is obtained using the measurement module in the office. These images are transferred to the digital marker with an USB device. Using multiple reference points on the conjunctiva and limbus, a digital overlay of the imported preoperative image and live-surgery image is created. With the eye-tracking navigation of the system, cyclotorsion and eye movement effects are theoretically eliminated, allowing the desired implantation axis of the toric IOL to be accurately projected in the right ocular of the surgeon's microscope.

There have been many studies in the literature favoring the digital marking methods.[9,10,11,12,13] A prospective study by Solomon et al noted that a manual blue mark was not inferior to the Verion.[14] Another prospective comparative study,[15] ($n = 54$ patients) between IOLMaster (Zeiss) and Verion suggested that the two devices seemed to present differences in IOL calculation and surgical planning that could lead to unexpected residual refractive error. When discrepancy is detected in IOL calculation, IOLMaster should be used as the primary biometry. Our own clinical practice (FZ) with Verion V-Lynk (Alcon) did not give us a remarkable impression of accuracy or reliability and we are now back to traditional manual marking while still exploring other electronic marking options.

5.4 Which Device to Use to Mark the Steep Axis?

Once under the microscope in the operating room, based on the reference marks from the slit lamp, with a second device such as Mendez gauge (▶ Fig. 5.5) or Barrett Dual Axis Marker (▶ Fig. 5.6; Duckworth & Kent) mark the limbus at the desired angle location for toric IOL placement or LRI (▶ Fig. 5.5).

A retrospective case series by Lipsky et al found that the Barrett Dual Axis Toric Marker was more accurate than the commonly used Mendez gauge, with a significantly higher percentage of eyes achieving a manifest refraction astigmatism within ±0.50 D: 80.6% versus 53.8% achieved a manifest refractive astigmatism of 0.50 D or less.[16] In that study, the Barrett Dual Axis Marker (36 eyes of 35 patients) had the mean absolute error (intended vs. achieved axis of alignment) toric alignment of 4.0 degrees ±2.9 (SD) versus the Mendez gauge group (36 eyes of 25 patients) which had 8.4 ± 6.5 (SD). The Barrett Dual Axis Marker is smaller than the Mendez and other rings and the gradations are finer. The main advantage however is that the outer ring can be set independently for the reference axis

from the inner mark which is for the desired Toric axis. The marker is then inked and pressed onto the cornea. This is particularly useful if the Tori-CAM app is used to accurately determine the reference axis after the cornea has been marked[16] (▶ Fig. 5.6).

5.5 What Is a Keratoscope?

There have been basic cost-effective systems to qualitatively confirm the steep axis at the surgical microscope; these are vital adjuncts to one's marks. Chief among these is a sterile safety pin which is available to all. The circular part at the end of the pin can be used to show a mire determined by the corneal reflex under the microscope when held between the cornea and the microscope lens. When the cornea is spherical, the mire is circular. When there is astigmatism of 1 D or greater, the mire will appear oval with the short diameter indicating the steep axis. With a little experience one can see even 0.75 D and the greater the astigmatism the more obvious the ability to pinpoint the steep axis. A more sophisticated qualitative instrument is a keratoscopy ring of lights (▶ Fig. 5.7) such as the Mastel Illuminating Surgical Keratoscope. This device attaches to the surgical microscope and presents three concentric rings of LEDs (36 LEDs per ring, every 10 degrees) with adjustable illumination intensity. This not only provides a corneal mire but also shows a separate mire reflected from the IOL once in place. One can then not only confirm the steep axis but also the toric IOL's astigmatic correction which must be positioned 90 degrees away for effective cancelling of corneal astigmatism (▶ Fig. 5.7).

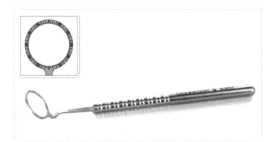

Fig. 5.5 Mendez Gauge. Used with permission from Duckworth & Kent.

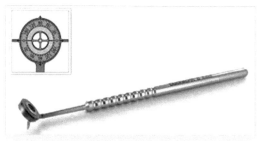

Fig. 5.6 Barrett Dual Axis Marker. Used with permission from Duckworth & Kent.

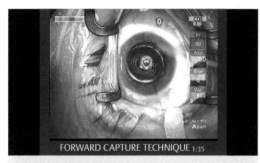

FORWARD CAPTURE TECHNIQUE 1:35

Fig. 5.7 Keratoscopy ring of lights. Used with permission from Mastel.

References

[1] Ferrer-Blasco T, Montés-Micó R, Peixoto-de-Matos SC, González-Méijome JM, Cerviño A. Prevalence of corneal astigmatism before cataract surgery. J Cataract Refract Surg. 2009; 35(1):70–75

[2] Abulafia A, Hill WE. The toric intraocular lens, successful strategy. In: Hovanesian JA, ed. Refractive cataract surgery. 2nd ed. Thorofare, NJ: Slack; 2017:157–166

[3] Braga-Mele R, Chang D, Dewey S, et al. ASCRS Cataract Clinical Committee. Multifocal intraocular lenses: relative indications and contraindications for implantation. J Cataract Refract Surg. 2014; 40(2):313–322

[4] Nuijts R. ESCRS Clinical Survey Data: Maximizing Outcomes with Presbyopia and Toric IOLS. ESCRS Supplement: Focusing on Premium, IOL Advances and Best Practices. December 2018/January 2019: 1

[5] Weikert M, Hill W, Barret G, et al. Hitting the refractive target: achieving 20/20 in 2020. 20/Happy in 2020 webinar. August 15, 2020. https://ascrs.org/20 happy/agenda/hitting-the-refractive-target

[6] Abulafia A. Toric IOLs: How to choose them and where to put them. Presented at ASCRS. Washington DC, April 13–17, 2018

[7] Popp N, Hirnschall N, Maedel S, Findl O. Evaluation of 4 corneal astigmatic marking methods. J Cataract Refract Surg. 2012; 38(12):2094–2099

[8] Montes de Oca I, Kim EJ, Wang L, et al. Accuracy of toric intraocular lens axis alignment using a 3-dimensional computer-guided visualization system. J Cataract Refract Surg. 2016; 42(4):550–555

[9] Varsits RM, Hirnschall N, Döller B, Findl O. Evaluation of an intraoperative toric intraocular lens alignment system using an image-guided system. J Cataract Refract Surg. 2019; 45(9):1234–1238

[10] Webers VSC, Bauer NJC, Visser N, Berendschot TTJM, van den Biggelaar FJHM, Nuijts RMMA. Image-guided system versus manual marking for toric intraocular lens alignment in cataract surgery. J Cataract Refract Surg. 2017; 43(6): 781–788

[11] Elhofi AH, Helaly HA. Comparison between digital and manual marking for toric intraocular lenses: a randomized trial. Medicine (Baltimore). 2015; 94(38):e1618

[12] Mayer WJ, Kreutzer T, Dirisamer M, et al. Comparison of visual outcomes, alignment accuracy, and surgical time between 2 methods of corneal marking for toric intraocular lens implantation. J Cataract Refract Surg. 2017; 43(10): 1281–1286

[13] Zhou F, Jiang W, Lin Z, et al. Comparative meta-analysis of toric intraocular lens alignment accuracy in cataract patients: Image-guided system versus manual marking. J Cataract Refract Surg. 2019; 45(9):1340–1345

[14] Solomon KD, Sandoval HP, Potvin R. Correcting astigmatism at the time of cataract surgery: toric IOLs and corneal relaxing incisions planned with an image-guidance system and intraoperative aberrometer versus manual planning and surgery. J Cataract Refract Surg. 2019; 45(5):569–575

[15] Labiris G, Panagiotopoulou EK, Ntonti P, et al. Level of agreement of intraocular lens power measurements between an image-guided system and partial coherence interferometry. J Cataract Refract Surg. 2020; 46(4): 573–580

[16] Lipsky L, Barrett G. Comparison of toric intraocular lens alignment error with different toric markers. J Cataract Refract Surg. 2019; 45(11):1597–1601

6 Limbal Relaxing Incisions

Fuxiang Zhang, Alan Sugar, and Lisa Brothers Arbisser

Abstract

Limbal relaxing incision (LRI) is a misnomer. Peripheral corneal relaxing incision (PCRI) is a better term, but in most of the literature, as of what we know, LRI has been used. Also, in all other chapters in this book, LRI is used. So, we are going to leave it unchanged. LRI is one of the commonly used clinical modalities to manage astigmatism during or after cataract surgery. It is one of the prerequisites for any refractive cataract surgeon before considering the engagement of premium intraocular lenses (IOLs). This chapter will focus on basic knowledge and skills of this seemingly simple manual procedure. It will cover basic definitions, blade choices, candidate selection, nomogram introduction, guideline for LRI versus toric IOL, and introduction of femtosecond laser-created arcuate keratotomy (AK).

Keywords: limbal relaxing incision, LRI, peripheral corneal relaxing incision, astigmatism correction, laser-created arcuate keratotomy, AK

6.1 How Do We Define Regular versus Irregular Astigmatism?

If the two main meridians, the lowest and the highest refractive power, are located perpendicular to each other, the astigmatism is regular. If an optical system has more than two main meridians, or if the two main meridians are not perpendicular (90 degrees away), the astigmatism is categorized as irregular. Neither spectacles nor toric implants can correct irregular astigmatism to form a clear image. Similarly, we cannot expect to ameliorate irregular astigmatism with manual peripheral keratotomy incisions, although phototherapeutic laser keratotomy can potentially improve the quality of vision in such patients. A rigid contact lens or pinhole gives the patient with significant irregular astigmatism the sharpest vision.

6.2 How Do We Logically Define WTR/ATR?

The steepest meridian positions define the types of astigmatism. The following three layout distributions have been commonly used in our profession and they are useful for communication, validation, and comparison. Why is it important to know these different layout distributions? It might be important and helpful to have a uniform classification. Another thing is for clinical purposes. For example, generally speaking, we should overcorrect against-the-rule (ATR) and undercorrect with-the-rule (WTR), and neutral for oblique. If the steep K is at 20 degrees, it belongs to oblique astigmatism based on ▶ Fig. 6.1, but it belongs to ATR based on ▶ Fig. 6.3.

One assigns WTR and ATR each 1/6 (30 degrees) of the 180-degree arc as in ▶ Fig. 6.1.[1] If the steepest meridian is positioned between 75 and 105 degrees, it is WTR, and if the steepest meridian is positioned between 165 and 195 degrees, it is ATR. If the steepest meridian is positioned between 15 and 75 or 105 and 165 degrees, it is oblique astigmatism. This definition gives 1/6 for WTR, 1/6 for ATR, and 4/6 for oblique in terms of angle coverage (▶ Fig. 6.1).

Another definition is as in ▶ Fig. 6.2: WTR steep axis at 45–135 and ATR 0–30/150–180 as in the NAPA (Nichamin-Age and Pachymetry Adjusted) nomogram in ▶ Fig. 6.8. This definition gives 3/6 to WTR, 2/6 to ATR, and 1/6 to oblique in terms of angle coverage. In ▶ Fig. 6.12, another system is used for FLACS: 0–44/136–180 ATR, 45–135 WTR.

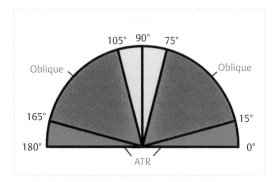

Fig. 6.1 With-the-rule (WTR) and against-the-rule (ATR) each only has 1/6 (16.7%).

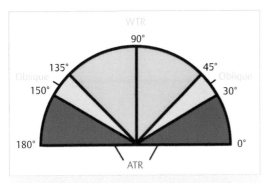

Fig. 6.2 This definition gives 3/6 to with-the-rule (WTR), 2/6 to against-the-rule (ATR), and 1/6 to oblique in terms of angle coverage.

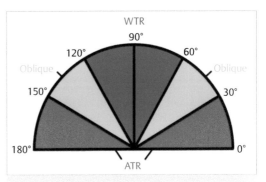

Fig. 6.3 In this system all three categories are evenly distributed.[2,3]

The following definition may be more logical and reasonable, to evenly divide 1/3 for each: 0–30 ATR, 31–59 oblique, and 60–90 WTR[2,3] (▶ Fig. 6.3).

6.3 On-Axis Incision and Its Limitation

When the cornea of a cataract surgery patient has significant regular astigmatism, the most common intraoperative modalities used are toric intraocular lenses (IOLs) and limbal relaxing incisions (LRIs). On-axis incision or dual symmetric full-thickness penetrating limbal/clear corneal incisions have also been used to flatten the steep meridian if the astigmatism magnitude is suitable for incision alone. This method has other concerns and may cause other issues, such as a need for rotating the surgical table, an uncomfortable surgical position, and difficulty in deep set eyes. With modern small incision techniques, the impact from the main cataract surgery incision is limited. Also, the predicted surgery-induced astigmatism (SIA) is often very small. So, an on-axis incision is not the mainstay for astigmatism correction for most of our patients.

6.4 When to Use Toric IOL or LRI?

With the consideration of posterior corneal astigmatism (PCA), ATR astigmatism of 0.50 D or more, and WTR astigmatism of 1.50 D or more, toric IOLs will usually correct astigmatism better than LRIs. We usually use measurements from multiple instruments, if most of them agree well. When calculations recommend a T2 toric IOL (Alcon toric IOLs range from T2 to T9 with 1–6 D of cylinder at the IOL plane), we use LRI to correct it since we do not have the T2 toric version in the United States. If calculations suggest a T3 IOL (1.5-D cylinder at IOL plane, and 1.03 D at corneal plane) or greater, we use a toric lens. For premium IOLs or for the distance eye in IOL monovision, anything close to 0.50-D cylinder or higher is significant when corneal posterior astigmatism is also considered.

Due to a rise in toric IOL use, the incidence of LRI has decreased from 2013 to 2019 based on American Academy of Ophthalmology IRIS registration data.[4]

Well-done LRIs are safe,[5,6] although it is almost universally agreed that toric IOLs correction of cylinder is more predictable and durable than with LRIs.[7,8,9,10,11] More higher order aberrations are observed in LRI-treated patients due to the corneal surface change,[8] although a different conclusion has also been drawn.[12] The most concerning issues for LRIs are predictability, durability, and interpatient variations. The healing process and the corneal stiffness may play significant roles in predictability and durability. We recommend that toric IOLs be used whenever significant astigmatism correction is indicated. Use of toric IOLs requires longer OR times when compared with using LRIs, but the long-term outcome is typically better.

The main function of LRI is widely considered to be treatment of low-level astigmatism and residual astigmatism. It is rare to use LRI to manage significant corneal astigmatism anymore, but residual astigmatism can often be managed with manual LRI in the operating room or office. We also sometimes have situations when we are not able to use a toric IOL, such as intraoperative complications in complex cases, or zonulopathy as in pseudoexfoliation where postoperative IOL position change may occur.

6.5 What Happens If Corneal Perforation Occurs from LRI?

Some beginners want to do a full range of refractive cataract surgery with multifocal IOLs (MFIOLs), extended depth of focus (EDOF) IOLs, and trifocal IOLs but are reluctant to initiate manual LRIs. They are afraid of corneal perforation and infection. Perforations are rare due to choosing a safe depth and most dedicated blade designs (see ► Fig. 6.4 and ► Fig. 6.5). Even if microperforation happens, it may not always require suturing if the leak is minimal. Bandage contact lenses and topical antibiotics with careful observation typically can resolve questionable leaks. The preferred way is always to suture it. Careful hand positioning will generally keep the surgeon out of trouble. Leaking from arcuate incisions heals faster than from radial incisions because of cor-

neal shape. Topical antibiotics should be used until there is no fluorescein staining (► Fig. 6.4 and ► Fig. 6.5).

6.6 Where Should be the LRI Located?

The LRI should be centered on the steep axis, just anterior or central to the limbal vascular arcade. LRI is actually a misnomer since the real location should be in clear corneal tissue. More centrally located corneal arcuate incisions are more powerful, but they are less forgiving and may have a greater chance of causing irregular astigmatism and secondary aberration. Too peripheral incisions are not recommended either. If there are limbal conjunctival vascular arcades involved with the LRI, they may result in undercorrection due to a stronger healing process associated with the rich blood supply. Occasionally, a large peripheral vessel's ingrowth will force you to cut into limbal vessels. Undercorrection of corneal astigmatism is easier to handle than overcorrection. LRIs can be extended in length or another more central LRI done to manage undercorrection, but overcorrection more likely will need laser vision correction.

6.7 When to Do the LRI?

An LRI can be done at the beginning or at the end of the surgery. This is an individual surgeon's choice. We prefer to do it prior to the phaco surgery when the eye is firm and orientation marks are clear. The only exception is when there is need for a long ATR LRI when a temporal clear corneal

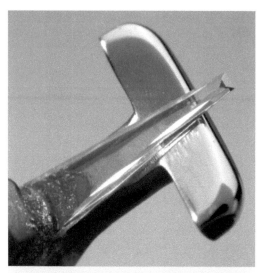

Fig. 6.4 Nichamin preset depth limbal relaxing incision (LRI) diamond blade from Mastel. Used with Permission from Mastel.

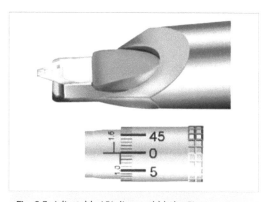

Fig. 6.5 Adjustable LRI diamond blade. Picture provided courtesy of Katena Products Inc., © 2020.

incision is used. In this situation, a tunneled three-plane phaco incision is used to complete the phaco surgery. Once the cataract surgery is done, the phaco incision line (not the tunnel part) will be extended with the LRI blade at the desired depth. If this long temporal LRI is performed at the beginning of the surgery, it may cause significant corneal edema or intraoperative leaking.

6.8 What Is the Typical Depth and the Length of LRI?

The depth of the LRI blade is typically 85 to 90% of the thinnest pachymetry reading. Increasing LRI length increases the effect of astigmatism correction, but it is commonly believed that the maximum length for LRI is about 3 clock-hours. When the incision is longer, the coupling ratio for spherical equivalence will tend to be more than 1.0, meaning it may cause hyperopic change for the final spherical equivalent. This is similar when we compare curved arcuate LRI with straight tangential incisions.[13] There is a limit to the length of incisions before they start to cancel out their own effect. When astigmatism correction is mild to moderate, the coupling ratio is typically 1.0 and you do not need to adjust for the spherical equivalent.[14,15] Degrees of arc is used to express the length of the incision, rather than millimeters, due to the variation in corneal diameter. The Nichamin Age and Pachymetry Adjusted (NAPA) intralimbal Arcuate Astigmatic Nomogram is one of the most commonly used guides (▶ Fig. 6.8).

6.9 What Are the Commonly Used LRI Blades?

Diamond knives are recommended rather than metal ones. Mastel, Katena, and other manufacturers have excellent diamond knives. Preset 500-or 600-µm or adjustable blades are common options (see ▶ Fig. 6.4 and ▶ Fig. 6.5). Choose a single-footplate LRI blade which does not obscure your view of the blade as you create the incision. Some older styles of blades have dual footplates, the advantage of which is that it controls the angle of approaching to the tissue. The downside of dual footplates is blocking of the direct view of the blade by the footplate. The blade must be visible with the handle tilted so the handle and the blade are perpendicular to the cornea. Most peripheral corneas measure thicker than 600 µm

and preset 600 µm blades can be used for most cases. While an adjustable blade may not be needed, it can be a source of operator error. Another pitfall can be the inaccuracy of corneal pachymetry measurement. Central corneal thickness is used for glaucoma management and Fuchs corneal dystrophy and peripheral thickness for LRIs. The central cornea is typically thinner than the peripheral cornea. Surgeons should educate their technicians about this difference. Ideally, numbers from a machine that measures peripheral pachymetry at the intended incision location is used but the thickness may vary on the table based on the time the speculum has held the eye open as desiccation or overhydration can grossly affect the thickness at the moment of incision. Intraoperative pachymetry can be time consuming and difficult and has not been definitively shown to yield superior results.

6.10 Should We Consider Posterior Corneal Astigmatism When We Do LRIs?

Should we count on the impact of posterior corneal astigmatism (PCA) as we do for toric IOLs? We should, simply because we will overcorrect WTR and undercorrect ATR astigmatism for most of our patients if we do not count on the impact of PCA, which is not measurable with corneal topography, LenStar, or manual keratometry based on Dr. Douglas Koch and his colleagues' research. This PCA does not drift with age.[16] We are not aware of peer-reviewed studies which have updated LRI nomograms to integrate PCA. We expect this will be addressed in the near future. If your IOLMaster or LenStar device can automatically print Barrett toric calculations, you can use the recommended toric axis and magnitude as a reference because it has already accounted for both PCA and SIA. If you do not use the Barrett Toric system, and if you do not directly measure the posterior cornea, simply add 0.3 D to ATR cases and subtract about 0.5 D for WTR cases when you plan to use LRI. No need to make adjustments if astigmatism is oblique.[17]

6.11 Should We Consider Age and Gender When We Plan for LRI?

Age is known to play a significant role in the effect of LRI due to related elasticity changes in corneal tissue. An 80-year-old may have almost twice the response of a 30-year-old patient. The Nichamin Age and Pachymetry Adjusted (NAPA) intralimbal Arcuate Astigmatic Nomogram (▶ Fig. 6.8) is one of the best and most commonly used nomograms. We are not aware of a difference in response between genders.

6.12 Should We Aim to Treat Corneal Astigmatism or Refractive Astigmatism?

When we use a nomogram, we always need to be guided by corneal astigmatism instead of refractive astigmatism. The cataract can significantly alter the amount of astigmatism measured on manifest refraction. Two to three diopter astigmatism caused by cataract is not rare clinically.

6.13 Are Single LRIs as Good as Paired Ones?

LRIs are usually paired to optimize the symmetrical corneal flattening effect and limit the length of the required incision. Single incisions also work well and have been popular. A single LRI paired with the phaco incision also works well. Some surgeons also use paired full-thickness penetrating incisions on the steep axis and that also seems to work well. One study in Brazil,[18] however, noted that the single LRI group did not achieve as significant a reduction of astigmatism as the paired group. That study could not conclude that the suboptimal outcome in the one LRI incision group was due to the single versus paired pattern. It could have been due to the nomogram or other factors. The sample size of that study was rather small, only five patients in the single LRI incision group. One author (LBA) always used paired incisions except for ATR astigmatism where the clear corneal incision was centered on the steep axis.

6.14 Should We Always Use Our Dominant Hand to Do LRI?

Probably not. If the dominant hand is the only one doing LRI, it will require a lot of position change and it will significantly decrease OR efficiency. You need to spend some time practicing with your nondominant hand so that the LRI arc cut will be as nice, smooth, and perpendicular to the tissue as the one made by your dominant hand. There is no shortcut except practice and practice. How to practice? If your right hand is dominant and you hold the LRI blade as the same way as you hold a pen, then you can use your nondominant hand to hold a pen and draw an arc line mimicking a cut. The curved line from the nondominant hand is typically not as good as one from the dominant hand, especially if its length reaches 2 o'clock hours or more. Practice makes perfect.

6.15 Should the Blade be Perpendicular to the Corneal Surface or Iris Plane?

The blade and the handle of the blade should be perpendicular to the corneal surface where the LRI is planned, not the iris plane. It will cause a beveled incision if it is not perpendicular to the corneal surface. That means, when you view through the microscope, the handle should be tilted and you should be able to see the blade. Care should be taken to make the entire incision at the same depth as much as possible. Without conscious attention to this detail, there is a tendency for it to be deepest (and most effective) at the center of the incision. AK incisions (including LRIs) often span approximately 30 degrees to 75 degrees of arc (3 mm to 6 mm in length). if the diamond knife has an angled end face (as is typical), the ends of the incision are necessarily shallower where the blade end itself is angled, even if the blade tip has penetrated to full depth. There are designs to avoid this added variable.

6.16 Who Are Good Candidates for the First Few Cases of LRI?

Please refer to ▶ Table 6.1 (▶ Fig. 6.6 and ▶ Fig. 6.7).

6.17 Manual LRI versus Laser-Created Arcuate Keratotomy (AK)

Every refractive cataract surgeon should know how to do a manual LRI, because a small amount

Table 6.1 Candidate selection pearls for beginners' first few cases of manual LRI

	Good candidates	Try to avoid
Cornea	Healthy, clean, and regular Placido image rings	Dry eyes, moderate MGD, any noticeable EBMD, any noticeable Salzmann nodules
Limbus	Clear and no new blood vessels	Irregular changes or with new blood vessels invading limbus
Regularity	Regular astigmatism on topography	These should be contraindications for any LRI: significant irregular astigmatism on topography, such as keratoconus, pellucid marginal degeneration, s/p RK
Length of LRI	1–2 o'clock hours	More than 2 o'clock hours
LRI location	Fit your dominant hand	Nondominant hand may be more difficulty for your first few cases
Axial length	Normal range	Extreme axial length, especially very short eyes, ELP will be more critical and harder to hit refractive target and make the overall outcome less predictable
IOL options	Monofocal IOL	MFIOL, trifocal, or EDOF will add extra challenges for beginners
Simple LRI vs. combined with Toric	Simple LRI alone	LRI combined with toric IOL
Overlapping with main incision	No overlapping of phaco incision, see ▶ Fig. 6.6	Overlapping of phaco incision, see ▶ Fig. 6.7
History of autoimmune disorders	No	History of active or advanced rheumatoid arthritis or lupus
Personality	Easy going	Demanding

Abbreviations: EBMD, epithelial basement membrane dystrophy; EDOF, extended depth of focus; ELP, effective lens position; IOL, intraocular lens; LRI, limbal relaxing incision; MFIOL, multifocal intraocular lens; MGD, Meibomian gland dysfunction; RK, radial keratotomy.

of astigmatism may be better managed with LRI rather than with a toric IOL, especially while T2 toric IOLs are not available in the United States. Not all surgeons use femtosecond lasers for a variety of reasons. The need to correct residual astigmatism increases as our patient expectations increase. Some special situations may not be suitable for laser AK, such as in patients with filtering blebs. Sometimes, we may have to abandon FLACS, such as in a patient with an unacceptably small pupil or a narrow palpebral aperture where we are not able to dock the laser interface. Learning manual LRI is often the first step for beginners in refractive cataract surgery. Years ago, our OR nurse forgot to order the backup T5 toric but the ORA measurement recommended T5, so an LRI

was added with T4 Toric and the patient was doing very well postoperatively with excellent uncorrected distance vision.

We believe that manual LRI may have some downsides when compared with a laser-created AK in terms of consistency of depth, location, configuration, symmetry, and repeatability/predictability. Another unique advantage is the integration of digital registration to transfer preoperative corneal topography to the laser system accurately with less chance of human error.

Optical coherence tomography-controlled corneal pachymetry is performed directly in the area of the intended incisions, which increases the safety (less chance of perforation). True intrastromal LRI incisions are only possible with

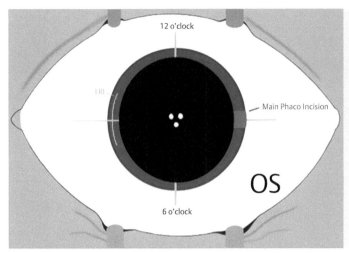

Fig. 6.6 Limbal relaxing incision (LRI) paired with main incision.

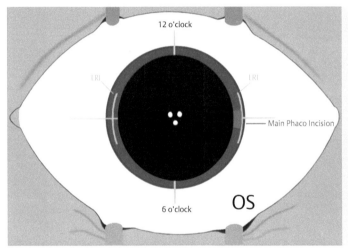

Fig. 6.7 Limbal relaxing incision (LRI) overlap the main phaco incision.

femtolaser and may cause less postoperative foreign body sensation and irritation. Theoretically, they should also have less chance of infection, although the manual LRI infection rate is also very low.[19,20]

A randomized comparison study from the United Kingdom with 51 eyes of 51 patients with manual LRI and 53 eyes of 53 patients with femtosecond AK noted better outcomes in the laser group: 42% of patients attained a postoperative cylinder less than 0.50 D while only 20% in the manual LRI group did so ($p = .01$).[21] Another large retrospective study of 189 eyes in 143 patients demonstrated that femtosecond laser-assisted cataract surgery (FLACS) was a safe and effective method for astigmatism correction at the time of cataract surgery, with proven stability of correction for at least one year postoperatively.[22] There was a study indicating that long-term stability and predictability from laser-created stromal AK could be still a concern.[23]

6.18 Pearls on Laser-Arcuate Keratotomy for Beginners

- Laser arcuate keratotomy (AK) incisions have opened and nonopened options. The laser can create a purely stromal incision without breaking through the superficial epithelium. Such incisions do not achieve full refractive

The "NAPA" Nomogram

Nichamin Age & Pachymetry-Adjusted Intralimbal Arcuate Astigmatic Nomogram Louis D. "Skip" Nichamin, MD ~ The Laurel Eye Clinic

With-the-Rule (Steep Axis 45 degrees to 135 degrees)

Preoperative Cylinder (diopters)	Paired Incisions in Degrees of Arc					
	20 to 30 years old	31 to 40 years old	41 to 50 years old	51 to 60 years old	61 to 70 years old	71 to 80 years old
0.75	40	35	35	30	30	
1.00	45	40	40	35	35	30
1.25	55	50	45	40	35	35
1.50	60	55	50	45	40	40
1.75	65	60	55	50	45	45
2.00	70	65	60	55	50	45
2.25	75	70	65	60	55	50
2.50	80	75	70	65	60	55
2.75	85	80	75	70	65	60
3.00	90	90	85	80	70	65

Against-the-Rule (Steep Axis 0 to 30 degrees/150 to 180 degrees)

Preoperative Cylinder (diopters)	Paired Incisions in Degrees of Arc					
	20 to 30 years old	31 to 40 years old	41 to 50 years old	51 to 60 years old	61 to 70 years old	71 to 80 years old
0.75	45	40	40	35	35	30
1.00	50	45	45	40	40	35
1.25	55	55	50	45	40	35
1.50	60	60	55	50	45	40
1.75	65	65	60	55	50	45
2.00	70	70	65	60	55	50
2.25	75	75	70	65	60	55
2.50	80	80	75	70	65	60
2.75	85	85	80	75	70	65
3.00	90	90	85	80	75	70

Blade depth setting is at 90% of the thinnest pachymetry

Fig. 6.8 The Nichamin Age & Pachymetry Adjusted (NAPA) intralimbal Arcuate Astigmatic Nomogram. (latest version). Used with permission from Louis D. "Skip" Nichamin.

effect until they are opened. We can open them intraoperatively if the ORA determines that the correction is not enough or leave it unopened until a few weeks postoperatively when manifest refraction and corneal topography are used to find out if the correction is adequate. They can be opened many months postoperatively. If the correction is not enough, the cut can be opened with a sterile Sinskey hook or a sterile lacrimal punctum dilator. It is easier to use the equipment pushing down rather than pulling out to avoid epithelial peeling (▶ Video 6.1).

Unopened incisions have the merit of less foreign body sensation postoperatively and retaining the option of fine adjustment of undercorrections. We assess all stromal AK patients in 3 to 4 weeks with corneal topography and an accurate refraction. If the measured steep meridian is at approximately the unopened AK location, open the incision(s) to get 100% effectiveness if undercorrection is present.

- It is very common to use an optical zone between 8 and 9 mm when AK is performed with the femtosecond laser. Mainly due to the decreased optical zone diameter, the length of the AK will need to be shortened compared with manual LRI. Roughly about 30% reduction, compared to conventional manual LRI, can be employed.[24,25] The more central, the greater effect, but be careful not to be too close to the central cornea to create more cut-induced aberration. An optical zone bigger than 9 mm will have more chance to involve the limbal conjunctival vascular arcade, especially in short and small eyes. The commonly used nomograms are good starting points, but each surgeon should pay attention to his/her own outcomes and make modifications accordingly. A study comparing laser-created anterior penetrating AK with laser-created intrastromal AK noted that intrastromal AK tends to have more undercorrection.[26] Our personal experience is that there is a greater chance of undercorrection than of overcorrection if we make a 30% reduction due to the smaller optic zone diameter. This may be due to the use of unopened laser AK cuts. Postoperative topography is highly recommended for every single case although it is not billable.

- The computer software automatically determines the desired depth of the incision at the set location of the incisions. Typical depth is 85 to 90%.

- The impact of PCA should be considered, although most, if not all, of the current nomograms may not actually integrate this important factor. So, a logical adjustment is advisable. Recommendations from Baylor can be considered. What we use is based on the toric IOL level from the Barrett toric calculator from the biometer (such as LenStar or IOLMaster) printout. If our two technicians' printouts both recommend a T2 toric lens and are consistent with the other two corneal topography measurements, we will do an AK. The Barrett toric calculator takes into account the PCA and SIA impact.

- The Nichamin Femto-LRI Nomogram in ▶ Fig. 6.12[27] presumes epithelial penetration along the entire arc length of the incision (personal communication), so if the incisions are created intrastromally without manually breaking through the epithelium, the arc length may need to be increased. We have noted that when we keep the FLACS-AK unopened, there is more undercorrection and very rarely overcorrection with current femto-LRI nomograms, both Nichamin's and Donnenfeld's. That is another reason to integrate our personal follow-up data to make necessary adjustments.

- We need to spend more time discussing prevention of a potentially very significant mistake. Human error choosing the wrong axis may occur, but we cannot undo the AK. It is worse than the insertion of a wrong power IOL, for which we can do IOL exchange or the wrong axis for a toric IOL which can be realigned. We recommend that the AK location be double checked preoperatively and recorded in a red color to warn the surgeon in the OR. In the laser room, as after a careful "time-out," laser treatment will be performed after a quick laser parameter check. A little bit of extra homework can almost completely avoid this problem of an inaccurate FLACS's AK location. Here is a sample:

Draw the location of the AK in relation to the main phaco incision and the sidedness of the eye to be operated on as in ▶ Fig. 6.9 and attach this form to

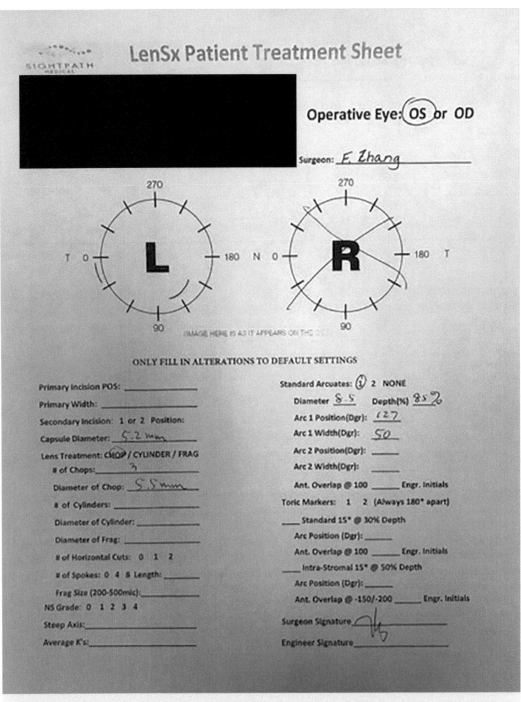

Fig. 6.9 Preoperative drawing to display the relationship of the main phacoemulsification incision and the arcuate keratotomy (AK). The main incision is at 10 degrees and the single AK incision is at 127 degrees. Of note, the reason why 90 degree is at the bottom (sounds conflicted with Chapter 5, "Marking the Limbal Reference and Steep Axes," ▶ Fig. 5.1) is due to the fact that the patient is lying under the laser machine, with the head toward the surgeon and the feet away from the surgeon. See ▶ Fig. 6.11 for the positional relationship of the surgeon and the patient.

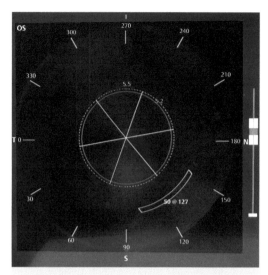

Fig. 6.10 Real-time LenSx image display for one line arcuate keratotomy (AK) incision length and location.

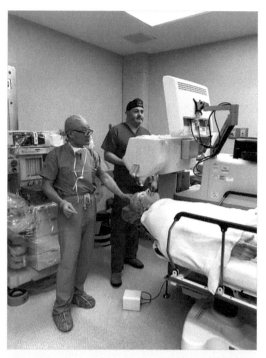

Fig. 6.11 The surgeon is standing in front of the patient in the LenSx laser room. Used with permission from Dave Coon.

the laser machine. The laser computer screen display as in ▶ Fig. 6.10 should match exactly the office-drawn picture from ▶ Fig. 6.9. This quick check takes only a few seconds but it gives the surgeon peace of mind. ▶ Fig. 6.9 is the orientation drawing from the office. The main phacoemulsification incision is at 10 degrees in this case and there is a planned single AK incision at 127 degrees. Hanging this form on the front of the laser machine allows comparison of this preoperative drawing with the screening of the laser machine as in ▶ Fig. 6.10. *If the two pictures have the same orientations*, we know the AK we are going to make with the laser will have the *correct* axis, unless there is a mistake in the preoperative drawing. If there is a wrong axis 90 degrees away, the preoperative drawing (▶ Fig. 6.9) and the laser computer screen display (▶ Fig. 6.10) will not match.

Beginners may be confused here and ask why the 90-degree location is not at the top as

discussed earlier with ▶ Fig. 5.1 in Chapter 5. The reason for this is that the patient is lying down and the surgeon is standing at the patient's head. So the surgeon is viewing the 270-degree mark at the top. See ▶ Fig. 6.11 where the surgeon is standing in front of the patient and the patient is lying under the laser machine with head toward the surgeon. The one-line AK cut is in the supero-nasal quadrant of the patient's left eye. The main phaco incision is at 10 degrees, which is *not* shown here on this real-time image in ▶ Fig. 6.10 because the author (FZ) still preferred a manually created main incision to a laser-created one at the time this book was written.

Nichamin Femto – LRI Nomogram
Louis D. "Skip" Nichamin, M.D.

WITH-THE-RULE
(Steep Axis 45°–135°)

PREOP CYLINDER (Diopters)	Paired Incisions in Degrees of Arc					
	20–30 yo	31–40 yo	41–50 yo	51–60 yo	61–70 yo	71–80 yo
0.75	39	34	30	27	25	23
1.00	44	39	35	33	31	28
1.25	50	45	41	38	35	33
1.50	55	51	47	43	40	37
1.75	60	56	52	48	44	41
2.00	65	60	56	52	48	45
2.25	70	64	60	56	52	48
2.50	75	69	64	60	56	52
2.75	80	70	68	64	60	56
3.00	85	78	73	69	65	60

AGAINST–THE-RULE
(Steep Axis 0–44°/136–180°)

PREOP CYLINDER (Diopters)	Paired Incisions in Degrees of Arc					
	20–30 yo	31–40 yo	41–50 yo	51–60 yo	61–70 yo	71–80 yo
0.75	40	35	31	28	26	25
1.00	46	41	38	36	33	31
1.25	52	48	45	41	37	35
1.50	58	54	50	46	42	39
1.75	63	59	55	51	47	43
2.00	67	63	59	55	51	47
2.25	71	67	63	59	55	51
2.50	75	71	67	63	59	55
2.75	80	75	71	67	63	59
3.00	85	79	75	71	67	63

Approximate 9.0 mm OZ   85% Depth

Fig. 6.12 Nichamin Femto-LRI Nomogram.[27] Used with permission from Louis D. "Skip" Nichamin.

References

[1] Kohnen T, Derhartunian V, Kook D, Klaproth OK. Toric intraocular lenses for correction of astigmatism in primary cataract surgery. In Kohnen T, Kock DD, eds. Cataract and refractive surgery. Essentials in ophthalmology. Berlin, Heidelberg: Springer; 2009:67–80

[2] Koch DD, Jenkins RB, Weikert MP, Yeu E, Wang L. Correcting astigmatism with toric intraocular lenses: effect of posterior corneal astigmatism. J Cataract Refract Surg. 2013; 39 (12):1803–1809

[3] Abulafia A, Barrett GD, Kleinmann G, et al. Prediction of refractive outcomes with toric intraocular lens implantation. J Cataract Refract Surg. 2015; 41(5):936–944

[4] Registration Snapshot IRIS. Use of relaxing incisions. EyeNet. 2020: 42

[5] Budak K, Friedman NJ, Koch DD. Limbal relaxing incisions with cataract surgery. J Cataract Refract Surg. 1998; 24(4):503–508

[6] Lim R, Borasio E, Ilari L. Long-term stability of keratometric astigmatism after limbal relaxing incisions. J Cataract Refract Surg. 2014; 40(10):1676–1681

[7] Lam DK, Chow VW, Ye C, Ng PK, Wang Z, Jhanji V. Comparative evaluation of aspheric toric intraocular lens implantation and limbal relaxing incisions in eyes with cataracts and ≤ 3 dioptres of astigmatism. Br J Ophthalmol. 2016; 100 (2):258–262

[8] Ouchi M. High-cylinder toric intraocular lens implantation versus combined surgery of low-cylinder intraocular lens implantation and limbal relaxing incision for high-astigmatism eyes. Clin Ophthalmol. 2014; 8:661–667

[9] Freitas GO, Boteon JE, Carvalho MJ, Pinto RM. Treatment of astigmatism during phacoemulsification. Arq Bras Oftalmol. 2014; 77(1):40–46

[10] Leon P, Pastore MR, Zanei A, et al. Correction of low corneal astigmatism in cataract surgery. Int J Ophthalmol. 2015; 8 (4):719–724

[11] Gauthier L, Lafuma A, Robert J. Long term effectiveness of limbal relaxing incision (LRI) during cataract surgery to correct astigmatism. Value Health. 2011; 14 (7):A261

[12] Monaco G, Scialdone A. Long-term outcomes of limbal relaxing incisions during cataract surgery: aberrometric analysis. Clin Ophthalmol. 2015; 9:1581–1587

[13] Incisional Corneal Surgery. In: Hamill MB, ed. Refractive surgery, basic and clinical science course 2017–2018. Vol. 13. San Francisco, CA: American Academy of Ophthalmology; 2017:54

[14] Intraocular Refractive Surgery. In: Hamill MB, ed. Refractive surgery, basic and clinical science course, 2017–2018. Vol. 13. San Francisco, CA: American Academy of Ophthalmology; 2017:147

[15] Nichamin LD. Management of astigmatism in conjunction with clear corneal phaco surgery. In: Gills JP, ed. A complete surgical guide for correcting astigmatism: an ophthalmic manifesto. Thorofare, NJ: Slack; 2003:41–47

[16] Stodola E. Handling posterior corneal astigmatism. EyeWorld. https://www.eyeworld.org/article-handling-posterior-corneal-astigmatism. Published August 2015. Accessed April 27, 2020

[17] Sheen Ophir S, LaHood B, Goggin M. Refractive outcome of toric intraocular lens calculation in cases of oblique anterior corneal astigmatism. J Cataract Refract Surg. 2020; 46 (5):688–693

[18] Arraes JC, Cunha F, Arraes TA, Cavalvanti R, Ventura M. Incisões relaxantes limbares durante a cirurgia de catarata: resultados após seguimento de um ano. [Limbal relaxing incisions during cataract surgery: one-year follow-up]. Arq Bras Oftalmol. 2006; 69(3):361–364

[19] Haripriya A, Smita A. A case of keratitis associated with limbal relaxing incision. Indian J Ophthalmol. 2016; 64(12): 936–937

[20] Haripriya A, Syeda TS. A case of endophthalmitis associated with limbal relaxing incision. Indian J Ophthalmol. 2012; 60(3):223–225

[21] Roberts HW, Wagh VK, Sullivan DL, Archer TJ, O'Brart DPS. Refractive outcomes after limbal relaxing incisions or femtosecond laser arcuate keratotomy to manage corneal astigmatism at the time of cataract surgery. J Cataract Refract Surg. 2018; 44(8):955–963

[22] Visco DM, Bedi R, Packer M. Femtosecond laser-assisted arcuate keratotomy at the time of cataract surgery for the management of preexisting astigmatism. J Cataract Refract Surg. 2019; 45(12):1762–1769

[23] Chang JSM. Femtosecond laser-assisted astigmatic keratotomy: a review. Eye Vis (Lond). 2018; 5:6

[24] Donnenfeld ED. Correcting corneal astigmatism with laser incisions. Cataract & Refractive Surgery Today. 2014:30–31. https://crstoday.com/articles/2014-may/correcting-corneal-astigmatism-with-laser-incisions/#. Published May 2014

[25] Donaldson KE. Femtosecond laser-assisted cataract surgery. In: Hovanesian JA, ed. Refractive cataract surgery. 2nd ed. Slack; 2017. Chapter 9 The toric intraocular lens. Page 95–113

[26] Ganesh S, Brar S, Reddy Arra R. Comparison of astigmatism correction between anterior penetrating and intrastromal arcuate incisions in eyes undergoing femtosecond laser-assisted cataract surgery. J Cataract Refract Surg. 2020; 46(3):394–402

[27] Nichamin LD. Limbal relaxing incisions transition to femtosecond laser-based technique. Ocular surgical news U.S. edition. August 10, 2014

7 Toric Intraocular Lenses

Fuxiang Zhang, Alan Sugar, and Lisa Brothers Arbisser

Abstract

Astigmatism management is one of the two main objectives for refractive cataract surgery and toric intraocular lens (IOL) implants are the main intraoperative cornerstone modality for the treatment of astigmatism. This chapter focuses on many key topics, such as how to determine if a toric IOL is suitable and indicated (the magnitude and the axis of astigmatism), how to determine surgically induced astigmatism, how to help those surgeons who still do not integrate posterior corneal astigmatism when they use toric IOLs, the advantages and disadvantages of direct measurement of posterior corneal astigmatism, the roles of femtosecond laser and intraoperative aberrometry related to toric IOL implantation, the reasons for toric IOL rotation and detailed discussions about how to prevent and manage misalignments, and toric IOL selection criteria for the beginners.

Keywords: toric IOL, astigmatism correction, refractive cataract surgery, toric IOL rotation, capsular tension ring, reverse optic capture, posterior corneal astigmatism

7.1 Introduction

The first commercial toric intraocular lens (IOL) in the United States was the STAAR Toric IOL which received FDA approval in 1998.[1] In 2017, the European Society of Cataract and Refractive Surgery (ESCRS) survey noted that 7% of IOLs implanted were toric and 6% were presbyopia-correcting IOLs.[2] By the 2018 ESCRS survey,[3] 11% of cataract patients with clinically significant astigmatism were implanted with a toric IOL, while 44% (rather than 11%) would receive a toric IOL if cost were not an issue. 2019 ESCRS clinical survey noted a sharp increase in toric IOL usage during cataract surgery to correct astigmatism to 14% while the percentage of using multifocal IOLs was 9% in 2019, which did not increase much compared to the percentage of previous years.[4] Respondents from the 2018 American Society of Cataract and Refractive Surgery (ASCRS) survey reported that on average only 20% of these patients received toric IOLs. The most common reasons cited for not implanting a toric IOL were cost to the patient, not enough surgical training, and toric IOLs not being available. Per Dr. David Chang's comments regarding the 2018 ASCRS Survey, "more than 30% of respondents do not feel sufficiently trained to integrate toric IOLs into their practices." Among American respondents, this number surprisingly jumps to 39%, which may reflect a major knowledge gap in residency training.[5]

7.2 How to Decide the Astigmatism Magnitude and the Axis of the Steep Meridian?

How much of the astigmatism should be corrected and where should the axis be placed? The principles discussed here also apply to manual limbal relaxing incision (LRI)/laser arcuate keratotomy (AK). No matter how advanced our tools are, K-values can differ since different machines measure by different algorithms and at different locations on the cornea. Even with the same equipment, for the same eye at different times, intradevice agreement may vary. Assuming an overall healthy cornea and acceptable ocular surface however, though measurements vary somewhat, the axis and magnitude should be similar. Most surgeons use multiple tools to measure astigmatism. A study by Browne and Osher[6] found that, by eliminating outliers, the use of multiple measurement devices increased the precision and accuracy of the cylinder meridian and magnitude.

For many years, manual keratometry was considered the preferred method, if not the gold standard, for measuring corneal astigmatism. This method is technician dependent and time consuming. Newer technologies have made it virtually obsolete. According to the 2018 ESCRS survey, 64% used optical biometry while only 25% mainly depended on manual keratometry.[7] In 2019 ASCRS survey, the percentage of those who mainly depended on manual keratometry was 15% (▶ Fig. 7.1).[8]

How much astigmatism to correct and where the axis should be placed are generally determined by optical biometers such as the LenStar and IOLMaster, but these are not sufficient; topog-

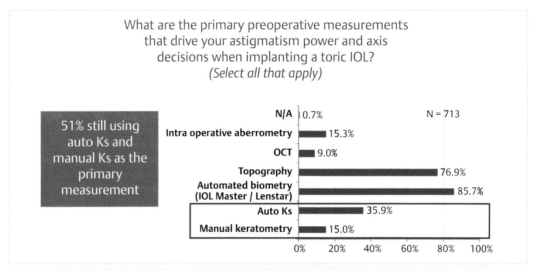

Fig. 7.1 2019 ASCRS survey. When asked about the primary preoperative measurements that drive the surgeon's astigmatism power and axis decisions when implanting a toric IOL, 85.7% said they use automated biometry. Additionally, 76.9% use topography. The survey found that 51% of respondents were still using auto Ks and manual Ks as the primary measurement. Used with permission from ASCRS.

raphy is an essential study to achieve the outcomes we require. Tomography will likely dominate in the future due to the fact that it also measures the posterior cornea. Intraoperative aberrometer such as optiwave refractive analysis (ORA) is helpful to measure the posterior cornea, but it is better to know it prior to the surgery and integrate it in the surgical plan.

Keratometry numbers will be based on our biometry, but a standard topographic axial curvature map deserves attention to the topographic power distribution. Ideally, the astigmatism should be both regular and symmetrical, meaning a central line can be drawn through each of the two astigmatism lobes while passing through the center of the corneal vertex. It is like the "credit card meridian," meaning that you put a straight line (like the edge of a credit card or a ruler) along the steep axis and see where that fits best to bisect the topographic hourglass of the steep measurement. (See more discussion in *Chapter 4, Topography and Tomography for Refractive Cataract Surgery.*)

The method we use is to lay out all the tests on a large table (despite electronic health records [EHR]), including the patient's current spectacle refraction if the cylinder correction in the glasses is significant. The average level of the cylinder is usually considered. The magnitude differences should not vary significantly. For the axes, if two

or more of them, especially corneal topography and LenStar/IOLMaster, agree with each other within 10 degrees, then the axis should be within that small zone. The key is consistency. Generally speaking, we use a biometer for power/meridian and topography for meridian/power. When the cylinder information on the patient's longstanding spectacle (if the astigmatism is significant) matches your biometry and topography or tomography, you should feel very comfortable that you are all set and ready to go, although sometimes lenticular astigmatism can impact the whole picture. If the measured axes from these different instruments are located far apart, and if the measurements are accurate and the ocular surface condition is acceptable, that typically tells us that either the astigmatism is very low or irregular and no toric IOL or LRI should be considered.

If we do not get great refractive outcomes from toric IOLs, we should always carefully explore the reasons. Of course the toric axis alignment and the lens position should be observed. The result could be due to residual astigmatism, or early posterior capsular opacification (PCO), ocular surface disorders, maculopathy, or aberration/coma issues. Sometimes, we find the error was at the very first step of identifying astigmatism: the astigmatism was not perfectly regular; or the steep meridian was not symmetrically displayed on corneal topography. The manual keratometer, IOLMaster, and LenStar are great for looking at the central cornea, but the topography will give us the whole picture. Just think about this, how difficult is it to rule out keratoconus and peripheral marginal degeneration with a manual keratometer, IOLMaster, or LenStar? Biometers only measure a small region of the central cornea while topographers measure the whole cornea. Corneal topography determines corneal regularity, symmetry, and is our most accurate tool to show the orientation of the steep axis. "In 90% of cases the IOLMaster or LenStar will be accurate enough so that topography can be ignored."[9]

Because of these differences in algorithms, multiple equipment measurements have merit and are part of the due diligence required for successful refractive cataract surgery (RCS). Generally speaking, lots of things in nature follow probability theory. A normal distribution (Bell curve) is a type of continuous probability distribution for the true value of a random variable. When most of the measurements agree for certain parameters and we delete the outliers, we have a better chance of hitting the target.

7.3 Should We Keep the Conventional Concept of Surgically Induced Astigmatism (SIA) or Use the Centroid Value?

Cataract surgeons using toric IOL calculators may have better outcomes when using a centroid value for their surgically induced astigmatism (SIA), rather than the traditional method of measurement: the difference of preoperative and postoperative means of the magnitude from a series of cases. The traditional method focuses on the magnitude of astigmatism but ignores the fact that the direction of the vector is quite variable and may be unpredictable. Especially with incisions under 3 mm, the practice of calculating a surgeon's particular mean change for left and right eyes is marginally productive. The centroid value in contrast is the geometric mean of a group of vectors. As such it also takes into account the axis of each vector which is quite unpredictable when calculating SIA. The impact of SIA in these small corneal incisions with centroid analysis seems to be much less than the traditional average magnitude analysis. Recent studies and presentations seemed to

favor using the centroid value for SIA rather than the traditional method.[10,11,12,13]

Typically, the centroid value for SIA is ~0.1 D and this value is more appropriate when performing calculations for a toric IOL. Based on over 35,000 cases, the calculated centroid value ranges from 0.08 to 0.14 D.[10] The centroid concept is now applied for SIA among commonly used toric IOL calculators, such as the Barrett Toric Calculator and ASCRS online toric calculator. Currently there is no accurate method to measure the total corneal astigmatism. Hence there is no accurate method to measure the actual SIA on the cornea.[14] The magnitude of SIA is usually small and it is not necessary to directly measure and calculate it.

A study in Japan observing incision-related corneal change with video-keratography also demonstrated that the flattening in the total and anterior cornea and the steepening in the posterior cornea around the clear cornea incision were obvious on postoperative day 2, but rapidly decreased within a few months.[15]

The point of discussing this topic is that the status quo can be very strong and resistant to change. Consider that nearly 30% of cataract surgeons queried in the 2018 ASCRS survey still did not integrate the impact of posterior corneal astigmatism (PCA) into their plan when they corrected astigmatism despite the critical study by Douglas Koch and colleagues showing its profound significance published about a decade ago. In a 2019 ESCRS survey, 31% of responders still do not consider PCA when they use toric IOLs and less than 70% do.[16] Prior to the centroid concept era, my routine was adding −0.35 D against-the-rule (ATR) astigmatism due to my temporal clear cornea incision. For example, if the LenStar and Tomey/Atlas topographers showed the eye to have 0.50 D at 180, then I would not do anything in those days since I believed that the incision would flatten the 180 axis (SIA would add −0.35 D and therefore compensate for most of the 0.50×180). Most likely, that eye would be left with significant uncorrected ATR astigmatism.

7.4 Why Is It Important to Consider Posterior Corneal Astigmatism (PCA)?

We all know that if we want to have an eye see well uncorrected for distance with a monofocal

IOL, or if we want to use multifocal IOL (MFIOL)/extended depth of focus (EDOF)/trifocal IOLs to best advantage, we must provide effective astigmatism correction. Leaving residual astigmatism at 0.75 D is less likely to provide a satisfactory outcome. Based on studies[17,18] by Koch et al, if we do not consider posterior corneal astigmatism, we will overcorrect with-the-rule (WTR) astigmatism by 0.5 D and undercorrect ATR by 0.3 D. Among the 715 eyes of 435 patients, they found that 86.6% of the eyes, steep corneal meridian was aligned vertically. Since the posterior cornea is a negative lens, the vertical steep meridian results in ATR astigmatism. This prediction was actually realized when evaluating our patients for their annual follow-up. Many patients had overcorrected WTR and undercorrected ATR astigmatism before this revelation. The discovery of astigmatism from the posterior corneal contribution by Koch and his colleagues has perceptibly improved the clinical outcome of the toric IOL.[19,20] How about oblique astigmatism? A recent study in Australia has confirmed the understanding that toric IOL calculation with oblique anterior corneal astigmatism does not need adjustment for the impact of posterior corneal astigmatism.[21]

According to the 2018 ASCRS survey, 29% of respondents do not know how to calculate PCA or do not understand its significance.[5] Outside of the United States, the percentage is even higher. In the 2018 ESCRS survey[3] there were still 35% of respondents who did not consider PCA in toric IOL power calculation. This must change, and largely has changed, especially for those reading this book!

Other factors can also cause the overcorrection of WTR and the undercorrection of ATR. There is an inherent tilt of roughly 5 degrees for the crystalline lens and for in-the-bag IOLs with the nasal aspect rotated anteriorly along the vertical meridian, which can cause what is called lenticular astigmatism.[22] Toric IOLs for WTR astigmatism are aligned vertically and have their higher power aligned horizontally. A horizontal tilt in this case increases ATR astigmatism and can cause overcorrection of WTR. On the other hand, toric IOLs that are aligned horizontally for correcting ATR astigmatism have their higher power aligned vertically; the horizontal tilt position can cause undercorrection of ATW.[22]

7.5 Is It Necessary to Directly Measure Posterior Corneal Astigmatism (PCA)?

With currently available corneal topography and most biometry, the posterior curvature contribution is not directly measured. Rather, we now depend on formulas to make this correction. Newer IOL calculation formulas that take into account the effect of the PCA in toric IOL calculations with a theoretical model, such as the Barrett Toric calculator and the Abulafia-Koch/Hill-RBF toric calculator, have significantly improved clinical outcomes, resulting in significantly lower levels of residual refractive cylinder than might be expected with standard calculators.[23,24,25,26,27]

The ideal scenario would be to obtain accurate direct measurements of the posterior cornea because the distribution or variation can be from 0 to 0.8 D of astigmatism[28] although most of the population fall into what we know as the average. Current methods include Scheimpflug technology, such as the Galilei (Ziemer, Port, Switzerland), Pentacam (Oculus Pentacam, South San Francisco, CA), and swept-source optical coherence tomography (OCT) such as the IOLMaster 700 (Zeiss Meditec, Jena, Germany), etc. Accuracy and reproducibility, however, may still be a concern for these instruments as of this writing.

A retrospective study by Serels et al[29] was recently presented at the 2020 ASCRS meeting, looking into whether the Barrett True-K formula with anterior keratometry is as good as total corneal power (TK) measurement. There were 109 postmyopic LASIK eyes, out of which 46 that had TK power available were analyzed. Using TK, the Wang-Koch formula had the highest percentages of eyes with expected spherical equivalent refractive errors within 0.50 and 1.00 D of plano (57 and 87%, respectively). The anterior Ks and Barrett True-K formula had the highest percentages within 0.50 and 1.00 D of plano (64 and 92%, respectively), but was not significantly better than the Wang-Koch with TK within 0.50 and 1.00 D ($p > 0.2$). The authors concluded that using measured total corneal (TK) power in existing post-LASIK formulas did not appear beneficial. The best expected results were obtained with the Barrett True-K formula and anterior keratometry.

There are many other studies and presentations showing that more accurate results were obtained with the Barrett Toric Calculator than with a direct measurement,[12,19,24,25,27,30,31,32] suggesting that we still cannot reliably and consistently measure the posterior cornea for individual patients.[13,33,34,35,36]

The future trend, however, will be direct measurement of the PCA. With technology advances, we expect direct measurement will become more accurate than predicted value in the future. Currently, direct measurement may provide extra value in certain subsets of patients, such as post-corneal refractive surgery, keratoconus, etc.

A recent study in the December 2020 issue of JCRS revealed that the IOLMaster 700 is also highly repeatable with regard to measuring posterior corneal keratometry and even exceeds the repeatability of its own anterior keratometry readings, but posterior keratometry measurements obtained with the IOLMaster 700 are consistently flatter than those obtained using the Galilei G4 (a dual Scheimpflug–Placido (S-P) disk-based tomographer/topographer) and cannot be considered interchangeable.[37]

A recent study[38] ($n = 50$ eyes of 50 patients) published in the July 2020 Issue of JCRS compared four modules: with history and measured posterior corneal power, with history and predicted posterior corneal power, no history with measured posterior corneal power, and no history with predicted posterior corneal power. The Barrett True-K formula with history and measured posterior corneal power by Scheimpflug camera (Pentacam) resulted in the lowest standard deviation of the prediction error (PE), lowest median and mean absolute errors, and highest percentage of eyes within ±0.25D (54%) ±0.50D (70%) and ±0.75D (84%). The Barrett True-K no-history formula with predicted posterior corneal power yielded the worst refractive outcomes. When the four options were compared, statistically significant differences were detected among the median absolute errors ($p = .0017$) and the percentage of eyes with a PE within ±0.25 D ($p < .0001$).

Another retrospective consecutive comparison cohort study ($n = 50$ patients 75 eyes) also suggested that accuracy of IOL power calculations in post-laser eyes can be improved by the addition of posterior corneal values as measured by the IOLMaster 700. The use of total keratometry plus the Barrett True-K formula may supplement outcomes when no prior refraction history is known.[39]

7.6 The Concept of Single-Angle and Double-Angle Plots

The traditional way to present astigmatism data is to use the single-angle plot. Correct astigmatism analysis requires doubling the angle to transform the astigmatism date into 360-degree Cartesian coordinates.[14] It is easier to show the data and read the literature with a double-angle plot. In a single-angle plot, the ATR astigmatism eyes are laid out separately (▶ Fig. 7.2). With a single-angle plot, ATR data is split on either side of the graph. With the double-angle plot, both WTR and ATR data are grouped accordingly, allowing easy visualization of trends, data centroids, confidence intervals, and standard deviations.

7.7 Can Severe Ocular Surface Disease (OSD) Patients be Good Candidates for Refractive Cataract Surgery (RCS)?

OSDs are very common in the cataract patient population. Can they still be good candidates for RCS? It depends on several factors. If simple and maintainable/sustainable management can keep the ocular surface healthy enough, the patient can still be a reasonable candidate for RCS. Some patients can do well with a punctal plug, periodic antibiotic ointment at bed time or hypochlorous acid such as Avenova sprayed twice a day on the lids which doesn't select for resistant organisms, is hypoallergenic, and kills demodex, and with the use of oral omega 3 supplements. That is our standard for a maintainable and sustainable protocol.

OSD may be much improved only after intensive management, such as daily warm compresses, lubricant drops/gel/ointment, punctal plugs, lid cleaners, topical steroid/cyclosporine, and oral omega fatty acids supplements. These daily intensive treatments are often done by patient family members. In this case, repeated corneal topography can show significant improvement, but we need to ask, "is this kind of management sustainable and realistic for the rest of the life of this patient and his/her family?" Very often, patients are

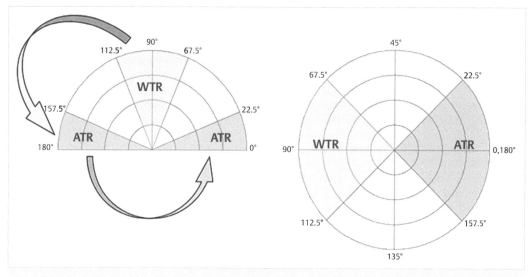

Fig. 7.2 Single-angle plot on the left versus double-angle plot on the right.[26] In a double-angle plot, the with-the-rule (WTR) eyes are grouped together on the left side of the figure and the against-the-rule (ATR) eyes are grouped together on the right. Used from Abulafia A, Koch DD, Holladay JT, Wang L, Hill W. Pursuing perfection in intraocular lens calculations IV. Rethinking astigmatism analysis for intraocular lens-based surgery: Suggested terminology, analysis, and standards for outcome reports. J Cataract Refract Surg 2018;44(10):1172, with permission from Elsevier.

not going to continue treatment once the perioperative period is over and severe OSD returns.

Our approach is that after reasonable management of OSD, if corneal topography is improved with good repeatability and if such management is not overwhelming to the patient (it should not depend on family member because this is not realistic in most situations), then we would consider the patient as an RCS candidate. If the OSD and repeated topography are acceptable, but the treatment is not sustainable for the patient and the family, we would not recommend expensive procedures/premium IOLs, simply because it is less likely to realistically result in long-term ideal outcomes.

7.8 Can Femtosecond Laser Surgery Help with Toric IOLs?

The IntelliAxis feature of the LENSAR platform outperforms other femtosecond laser machines in this regard because it can make permanent visible alignment marks at the continuous curvilinear capsulorhexis (CCC) rim. The marks on the cornea are not as easy to accurately align as those at the CCC rim due to the eye/head position as well as

due to the distance between the cornea and the toric IOL (parallax). The IntelliAxis feature seems to give the most accurate marks for toric IOLs among all ophthalmic equipment at this point without compromising capsulotomy strength and integrity. With accurate preoperative measurements and the most accurate IOL formula, the IntelliAxis can let you have great outcomes even without the need for an intraoperative aberrometer and save many extra surgical steps (▶ Fig. 7.3).[40]

Other laser machines such as LenSx (Alcon) find it helpful to make a 15-degree 30 to 50% corneal thickness cut at the steep axis. It actually can save one step intraoperatively because we do not have to mark again with other equipment such as a Cionni ring or Mendez gauge, although the mark is 15 degrees width, not a point mark. For purely intrastromal cuts, the bubbles created by the laser can dissipate so they may not be visible when you need to see them. Going with the superficial toric marks seems to be more helpful because if necessary, we can use fluorescein stain to make them visible. There are other advantages that femtosecond laser-assisted cataract surgery (FLACS) can offer to help with toric IOLs: a near-perfect

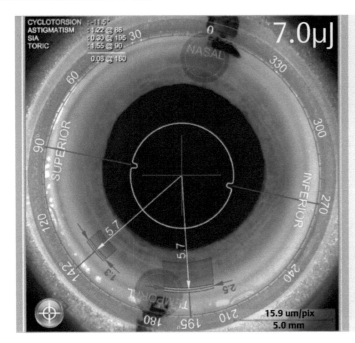

Fig. 7.3 The LENSAR Laser System's proprietary Streamline software with IntelliAxis Refractive Capsulorhexis. Used with permission from LENSAR.

capsulorhexis, data automatically inputted eliminating transcription errors and management of cyclotorsion when the patient is lying down. (See more discussion in Chapter 17 Femtosecond Laser Assisted Cataract Surgery [FLACS].)

7.9 Is It Necessary to Get No Rotation Recommended (NRR) Every Single Case?

The ORA will present NRR if the toricity magnitude is less than 0.5 D, *or* if the axis is within 5 degrees. (Please pay attention to "or," not "and," meaning imperfection for this intraoperative aberration system.) (Personal communication with ORA team, Alcon.) Some surgeons often skip the pseudophakic measurement phase, just using the aphakic version measurement of the toric IOL without pseudophakic version to achieve NRR. IOL centration, lens tilt, and other factors can affect achieving NRR. A prospective randomized study in New York[41] consisted of 40 bilateral cataract surgeries with toric IOLs, one eye with aphakic measurement only, and the fellow eye with both aphakic and pseudophakic measurements. No difference was noted between the two methods in terms of residual astigmatism. The average pseudophakic measurement was 3 minutes and 46 seconds.

7.10 How Much Postoperative Rotation Is Acceptable?

Residual astigmatism can occur for a variety of reasons. A European review summarized 20 studies from 2000 to 2011 and noted that > 10% of eyes still had more than 1.0 D and 30% more than 0.5 D of residual astigmatism after toric IOLs.[42]

Rotation of the implanted toric IOL has a significant impact on the cylindrical power of the toric IOL. The literature has suggested that 10 degrees off axis will decrease one-third of the correction; 15 degree off axis will decrease the correction to 50%, and 30 degrees off will decrease the correction by 100%. Ninety degrees off axis will double the original preoperative astigmatism.[43] How much is 30 degrees? We all know: one clock hour measures 30 degrees.

Németh challenged the validation of this statement in his paper in the JCRS 2020 March issue.[44] Based on Alpins' vector analysis and other literature reviews, the author believes that 45-degree misalignment will cause a 100% loss of toric correction, rather than the longstanding belief of

30 degrees. Thirty-degree rotation may lead to 50% loss of toric correction and less than 10 degrees of misalignment affects image quality only minimally. The paper concludes that dogma with false numbers was embedded into common knowledge as a consequence of the improper use of the literature. In response to Németh's statement, Holladay and Koch replied with further discussion and clarification suggesting that the original statement was correct.[45]

The question should be asked in a different way. Lower cylinder power toric lenses are different from higher level corrections. A T3 toric (cylinder power of 1.03 D at corneal plane) may tolerate a 10-degree rotation well but a T6 (cylinder power of 2.57 D at corneal plane) may present significant vision issues. The residual astigmatism is six times greater for the same angular misalignment for 6 D of IOL toricity compared with 1 D of toricity.[45] We believe <5 degrees is desirable, especially for high-level toric IOLs. If the patient is satisfied with visual function, even with a greater rotation, we do not have to realign the toric lens since it may be hard to predict what the outcome of the second procedure will be. Patient age, the fellow eye situation, and other factors should also be considered when weighing the decision to realign the rotated toric IOL. Forty-seven percent (47%) of ESCRS delegates believed that 10 degrees off is acceptable according to the 2017 survey.[2] The 2018 ASCRS survey for the same question revealed that more than 65% of respondents think 5 degrees or less is acceptable while 16% respondents think 10 degrees or more is acceptable.[5]

7.11 What Is the Most Vulnerable Time for a Toric IOL to Rotate?

A study was done in Japan to detail when and how much rotation happens within one year of surgery.[46] They included 72 Tecnis toric eyes (slit lamp ink mark), with digital photos immediately after surgery, and then POH1, POD1, POM1, POM3, and PHY1. The mean rotation was 6.67 degrees by POY1. Intraoperative surgical misalignment 1.87 degrees (28%); POH1, first hour 4.09 degrees (61%), POY1, 0.71 degrees (11%). So 89% of the total rotation occurred within and during the first one hour after the surgery (▶ Fig. 7.4).

7.12 What Is the Better Way to Realign a Rotated Toric IOL?

If realignment of a toric IOL is necessary, the Berdahl and Hardten calculator (http://astigmatismfix.com) can be helpful and it is straightforward. This back-calculator is also available at the ASCRS website in the online tool section. The tutorial is very educational and informative. The Barrett Rx formula can also be used to determine the ideal axis of alignment to which repositioning of the IOL will reduce the residual astigmatism. If

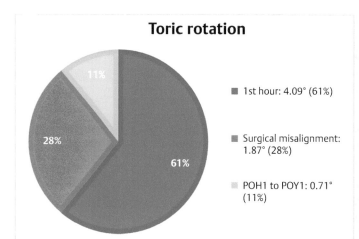

Toric rotation

- 1st hour: 4.09° (61%)
- Surgical misalignment: 1.87° (28%)
- POH1 to POY1: 0.71° (11%)

Fig. 7.4 Most toric rotation (89%) happens within the first hour postoperatively.[46] POH1: postop hour 1. POY1: postop year 1. Used with permission from Tetsuro Oshika, MD.

you use astigmatismfix.com, the following information will be needed:
• Manifest refraction.
• IOL model and power.
• Originally calculated IOL axis (degrees).
• Current IOL axis (degrees).

The key factor is the manifest refraction, which should be as accurate as possible. The calculator will tell you the amount of residual astigmatism and give the suggested new axis location.

Sometimes you may need to exchange the toric IOL due to too much residual astigmatism or due to incorrect spherical power. If the patient's SE is less than ±0.50 D, an IOL rotation to the ideal axis of astigmatism can be performed to reduce or eliminate the residual astigmatism. If the predicted residual SE is greater than ±0.50 D, an IOL exchange and/or rotation of the secondary IOL to the ideal meridian may be warranted to refine the refractive target. We can change the toric IOL power in the astigmatismfix.com program to find out if such a change will yield a better outcome, closer to the refractive target and closer to zero residual refractive astigmatism. The other options can be manual LRI or laser vision correction.

The astigmatismfix.com also has imperfections. There is room to optimize this very helpful and popular tool. One is "the originally calculated IOL axis." If the IOL calculation formula for the originally calculated IOL axis did not account for posterior corneal astigmatism, the accuracy of the recommendation from astigmatismfix.com will be compromised. So, the web software can give the user two options: toric formula with PCA considered and toric formula without PCA considered. The software can then automatically integrate the average PCA data for those who did not use the newer formula. Another step to optimize the accuracy is to integrate the PCA component into its own calculation system. (Personal communication with John Berdahl, MD.)

It is also important to understand that toric IOL rotation may not be the only contributing factor for the residual astigmatism. There may be a combination of a number of factors: incision position and healing, posterior corneal astigmatism, lens decentration, lens tilt, etc., as what was proposed as the total SIA.[47] Even the physiologic tilt of the eye (angle alpha = 5.2 degrees) and mean temporal decentration (0.2 mm) can result in approximately 0.20 D of refractive ATR astigmatism.[47]

7.13 At the Final Stage of Positioning Toric IOL, If You Have to Make a Small Amount of Turnaround Count Clockwise Direction, How Do You Do It?

There are at least three ways to do it.
• You can turn clockwise 360 degrees.
• You can pull the leading haptic toward you with a Sinskey hook so you can turn the IOL counter clockwise a little bit.
• You can put the I/A handpiece in through the main incision, which will inflate the AC and the capsular bag, which will make the IOL rotation easier. This seems to work best in our hands.

7.14 What Can We Do to Prevent Toric IOLs from Rotating?

• Completely remove the ophthalmic viscosurgical devices (OVDs) from behind the lens.
• Gently press the lens to let it touch and "sit" on the posterior capsule.
• Avoid overinflating the eye at the end of surgery, which will leave more space for the IOL to rotate. Underinflating the eye is not desirable either. For glaucoma patients, we usually leave the eye less firm. This is not good for the toric IOL. The less firm eye is prone to IOL rotation if the patient squeezes or rubs the eye.
• Have the patient lie supine for 20 to 30 minutes immediately once the surgery is done.
• Have the patient sleep on their back on the first postoperative night.
• Have them avoid strenuous physical activities during the first week.
• Consider a capsular tension ring (CTR), either a regular CTR or Henderson CTR. A Henderson CTR may be better than a regular CTR due to its undulatory shape. We have been very happy with the new type 15 "regular" CTR with the feature of a gentle elbow of the leading end which provides a broad area of contact that glides more easily against the equator, reducing risk of snagging or puncturing capsular bags.[48]
• The unique future of the EyeJet CTRs, type 15 preloaded CTR, is a prominent, gentle, leading elbow. It is often visible during the insertion so

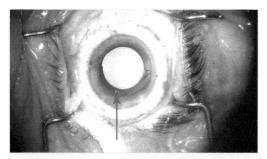

Fig. 7.5 EyeJet new type 15 with a prominent, gentle, leading elbow.

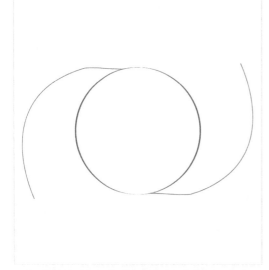

Fig. 7.6 A new concept of combining capsule tension rings to form a 360-degree PCIOL.

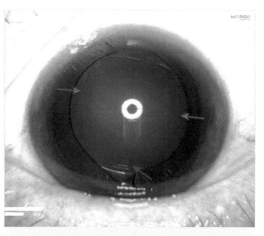

Fig. 7.7 Reverse optic capture to prevent potential postop toric intraocular lens (IOL) rotation. *Red arrows* indicate the continuous curvilinear capsulorhexis (CCC) rim behind the optic. *Blue arrows* show toric marks and CCC is in front of the IOL.

For large eye *or* large capsule patients, CTRs have been reported to be helpful.[49,50,51] The rationale for implanting a CTR to improve toric IOL stability is that it theoretically enforces symmetry on the bag, stretching the bag's equator and thus flattening the bag in the anterior–posterior axis. The CTR may also increase friction on the IOL haptics and thus increase stability.[49] The CTR rounds out the oval shape of the capsular bag, reducing the tendency for the IOL to rotate toward the narrowest position.[51] It is easier to understand this rationale if we imagine two oval shapes in a parallel relationship, which will make it easier to rotate. But if the outside oval shape becomes a round shape, then rotation will be more difficult.

- Reverse optic capture (ROC; see ► Fig. 7.7): Another option is to use ROC as shown in ► Fig. 7.7. This patient had an axial length of 28.32-mm OD and 26.92-mm OS. Preoperative Manifest: OD was −12.75 + 3.00 × 065 and OS was −9.75 + 2.75 × 075. OD was also s/p retinal detachment surgery with a scleral buckle. WTW was 13.55-mm OD and OS. The CCC size was 5.2 mm created with the LenSx laser. I hydrated the main incision and made a reasonable IOP and then with a Sinskey hook, pushed the CCC rim at the two red arrow locations as in ► Fig. 7.7 to move the CCC rim below the optic.

the surgeon has no concern about the risk of snagging or puncturing the capsular bag. Please see the visible leading elbow during insertion in ► Fig. 7.5, *red arrow* and **Video 7.1**.

- A new design (► Fig. 7.6): In the presence of zonulopathy or for toric IOL implantation, a CTR is often placed in the capsular bag and then followed by a posterior chamber intraocular lens (PCIOL). We can combine these two procedures into one, even for toric IOLs. Toric IOLs are typically one-piece lenses, but this proposed 360-degree haptic three-piece IOL may be a reasonable solution. IOL companies are welcome to explore this design by contacting fzhang1@hfhs.org.

This can be easier said than done. With cohesive OVD filled in AC, it will be easier to create an ROC.

- CCC pioneer Howard Gimbel, MD, introduced a new technique he calls *haptic tuck for reverse optic capture* to fix the toric IOL in cases of a posterior capsular rent.[52] This is a new technique for capsule fixation of one-piece acrylic toric IOLs in the presence of a large posterior capsule tear resulting in an open capsule. "The toric lens was delivered into sulcus first. Each of the two haptics was separately tucked through the anterior CCC opening, leaving the optic edges above the capsule. The beauty of this innovative technique is to skip delivering the IOL in the bag when there is a posterior capsule opening risking dislocation."[52] The final result is the same as standard ROC.

7.15 Can Reverse Optic Capture (ROC) Cause Pigment Dispersion Syndrome (PDS) and Do We Need to Change the Implant Power?

There is concern whether ROC will cause pigment dispersion due to interaction of the iris and the squared edge one-piece acrylic lens, but in our anecdotal experience this seems to be quite safe. We have used this technique for over a decade and have not seen a single case of PDS. It could be due to the fact that the haptics are within the bag and those eyes are typically larger than average with a deep space between the iris and the capsule. We are not saying PDS cannot happen, but it is probably rare.

Iris chafing with pigment dispersion, uveitis-glaucoma-hyphema (UGH) syndrome, and recurrent vitreous hemorrhage can be the consequence of placement of the whole one-piece acrylic IOL in the sulcus. The problem is believed to be due to the presence of bulky and thick haptics in the sulcus and their tacky hydrophobic acrylic surface. The ASCRS committee published a paper about complications due to single-piece acrylic IOLs in the sulcus in 2009.[53] The bulky single-piece haptics are large and thick enough to contact the posterior iris when placed in the sulcus. Contact between the sharp edges and the posterior iris

vasculature may also cause chronic uveal inflammation and recurrent microhyphema that can impair vision and abruptly raise IOP—the UGH syndrome.

Jones et al evaluated the clinical results of ROC with single-piece posterior chamber acrylic IOLs in cases of phacoemulsification cataract and IOL surgery with posterior capsular rupture.[54] Sixteen eyes that underwent ROC were reviewed and analyzed. The fellow eyes of 12 patients undergoing uneventful phacoemulsification without optic capture served as the control group. Over a mean of 19 months' follow-up, 94% of eyes in the ROC group and 92% in the control group achieved a best-corrected visual acuity of 20/25 or better. Ninety-four percent of eyes in the ROC group and 100% in the control group had postoperative spherical equivalent within ±1.00 D of the intended refraction. Refraction was stable between 1 month and final follow-up in both groups. In all eyes with ROC, the IOL remained well centered with a securely captured optic. There were no vision-threatening complications throughout the follow-up.[54]

Do we need to decrease the spherical power of the IOL due to the anterior shift? Theoretically yes, especially for high-power IOLs, but most of the long eyes will need lower power IOLs. It is quite safe not to change the power for those long eyes. When both haptics are placed in the bag behind the CCC with ROC, the anterior shift of the optic position and the consequence of myopic shift is minimal.[52,54] We do not adjust IOL power in this scenario.

7.16 Is It Better to Aim for Zero Astigmatism or Undercorrection versus Overcorrection?

Patients unhappy with their uncorrected distance vision typically have > 0.50 D astigmatism left at the spectacle plane.

- For most premium IOLs and for the distance eye of IOL monovision patients, we aim for zero astigmatism. Multifocal, EDOF, and trifocal IOLs can cause some loss of contrast sensitivity that can be worsened by any residual astigmatism.
- Leaving small amounts of with-the-rule (WTR) astigmatism if you are not able to get to zero astigmatism correction is a good option. We still try to get zero astigmatism correction for most elderly patients, because we prefer to have great

vision right away in the immediate postoperative period. For patients in their 60 s or younger, we should consider leaving a bit closer to 0.3-D WTR to compensate for future astigmatism drift. A small amount of ATR astigmatism, average around 3/8 D, occurs during a 10-year period.[55,56] This is important for young patients with toric IOLs. Flipping the axis in this scenario is logical and reasonable.

• Leave as little ATR astigmatism as possible for any age group.

For the near eye of conventional IOL monovision, zero astigmatism correction is not necessary. A small amount of astigmatism affects distance vision more than near vision. Particularly WTR may actually confer better depth of focus and help reading accordingly. Residual astigmatism has also been shown to enhance depth of focus and actually to be good for near vision.[57] Let us think about $-2.0 + 1.00 \times 90$ (same as $-1.0 - 1.0 \times 180$) as the near eye in a pseudophakic monovision case. This patient should be expected to do well if the dominant eye is emmetropic with good distance vision and this near eye will do well without correcting the 1-D cylinder. The near eye has -1.0 D at the 90-degree meridian and has -2.0 at 180 degrees, resulting in increased depth of focus. This can be a win-win scenario; it saves money not to buy a toric lens or to pay for an LRI with an increased depth of focus. If we use a nonspherical aberration correction lens (without built-in minus SA) such as SN60AT/SA60AT (Alcon) and Sensar 1-piece AABOO (Johnson & Johnson) for the near eye, the near vision eye can be expected to have better depth of focus.

7.17 Do You Use Toric IOLs or LRIs for Keratoconus Patients?

Theoretically, keratoconus patients are not good candidates for either toric or LRI astigmatism correction due to their irregular nature. We do not use toric lenses or LRIs for these patients if the cornea has a noticeable scar or if they wear contact lenses and can't be corrected by glasses. We never did laser LRIs in any of our keratoconus patients because we are afraid the manipulation may actually further weaken the keratoconus cornea leading to unstable and unpredictable results. Manual LRIs may have an increased risk of perforation due to the uneven thickness of the cornea. We did have good success using toric IOL in a few keratoconus eyes when the cylinder magnitude and axis were pretty consistent and stable for a few years. The outcome will not be as perfect as we would expect from classic bowtie astigmatism cases, but the astigmatism can be significantly mitigated and patients can still be very happy as long as a good preoperative consultation is carried out. They must understand they will never again be able to wear a rigid contact lens over the toric IOL and therefore cannot use this method to reduce irregularity and improve visual sharpness.

7.18 Who Can Be the First Few Cases of Toric IOL Patients?

Refer to ▶ Table 7.1 for candidate selection of the first few toric IOL cases for beginners.

Table 7.1 Candidate selection for the first few toric IOL cases for beginners

	Good candidates	Try to avoid
Refractive status	Hyperopic patients are easy to please	Severe hyperopia may have amblyopia or have very short eyes
Ocular history	No history of laser vision correction	S/P LASIK/PRK/RK
Ocular surface	Healthy with good tear film	Significant dry eye and/or MGD, or with noticeable EBMD, Pterygium, Salzmann nodules
Placido rings	Clear	Significant irregularity
AC depth and axial length	Within normal range	Extreme length eyes; ELP can be critical for very short eyes; toric IOLs rotate easily in very large eyes

(Continued)

Table 7.1 (*Continued*) Candidate selection for the first few toric IOL cases for beginners

	Good candidates	Try to avoid
Pupil	Dilate well	Flomax and other Alpha-1 blocker can shrink pupil and make it hard to view toric marks intraoperatively
Toric implant	Monofocal	Toric version of MFIOL/EDOF/trifocal; still requiring LRI for supplement
Toricity of the IOL	Lower to medium, such as T3 to T4	High, such as T6 or higher; high toricity can be very sensitive to rotations
Personality	Easy going	Perfectionist

Abbreviations: EBMD, epithelial basement membrane dystrophy; EDOF, extended depth of focus; ELP, effective lens position; IOL, intraocular lens; LRI, limbal relaxing incision; MFIOL, multifocal intraocular lens; MGD, meibomian gland dysfunction.

References

[1] Bylsma S. Staar toric IOL. Cataract & refractive surgery today. Published August 2009. Accessed April 19, 2021. https://crstoday.com/articles/2009-aug/crst0809_15-php/

[2] ESCRS 2017 Clinical trends survey. EuroTimes. Accessed April 19, 2021. https://www.eurotimes.org/escrs-2017-clinical-trends-survey-results/

[3] 2018 ESCRS Clinical trends survey. EuroTimes. Accessed April 19, 2021. https://www.eurotimes.org/escrs-2018-clinical-trends-survey-results/

[4] Presbyopia & astigmatism correcting IOLs: Key clinical opinions & practice patterns. EuroTimes. Published July 2020. Accessed April 19, 2021. https://www.eurotimes.org/presbyopia-astigmatism-correcting-iols-key-clinical-opin-ions-practice-patterns/

[5] ASCRS Clinical survey 2018. EyeWorld. Published November 20, 2018. Accessed April 19, 2021. https://supplements.eyeworld.org/eyeworld-supplements/december-2018-clin-ical-survey

[6] Browne AW, Osher RH. Optimizing precision in toric lens selection by combining keratometry techniques. J Refract Surg. 2014; 30(1):67–72

[7] Morselli S. Precise preoperative planning optimizes premium IOL outcomes. Strategies for success with toric & presbyopia correcting IOLs. EuroTimes. 2019 April Suppl:1–2

[8] ASCRS. 2019 Clinical survey. ASCRS Database

[9] Arshinoff S. Turning to topography. EuroTimes. 2020; 25 (10):13

[10] Hill WE. Centroid value, posterior cornea info adds game for toric calculators. Ophthalmology Times. Published May 18, 2017. Accessed April 19, 2021. https://www.ophthal-mologytimes.com/view/centroid-value-posterior-cornea-info-adds-game-toric-calculators

[11] Koch DD. Presented at EyeWorld/ASCRS reporting live from the BRASCRS meeting. Sao Paulo, Brazil. May 18, 2018

[12] Chayet A, et al. Treating astigmatism: how low can you go? Rev Ophthalmol. 2018; XXV(7):48–50

[13] Koch DD. Astigmatism correction. EyeWorld. 2018;23 (7):68–73. Reporting from the 2018 BRASCRS annual meeting

[14] Abulafia A, Koch DD, Holladay JT, Wang L, Hill W. Pursuing perfection in intraocular lens calculations: IV. Rethinking astigmatism analysis for intraocular lens-based surgery: Suggested terminology, analysis, and standards for outcome reports. J Cataract Refract Surg. 2018; 44(10):1169–1174

[15] Hayashi K, Yoshida M, Hirata A, Yoshimura K. Changes in shape and astigmatism of total, anterior, and posterior cornea after long versus short clear corneal incision cataract surgery. J Cataract Refract Surg. 2018; 44(1):39–49

[16] ESCRS Clinical Trends Survey 2019. EuroTimes. Accessed April 19, 2021. https://www.eurotimes.org/escrs-2019-clinical-trends-survey-results/

[17] Koch DD, Jenkins RB, Weikert MP, Yeu E, Wang L. Correcting astigmatism with toric intraocular lenses: effect of posterior corneal astigmatism. J Cataract Refract Surg. 2013; 39 (12):1803–1809

[18] Koch DD, Ali SF, Weikert MP, Shirayama M, Jenkins R, Wang L. Contribution of posterior corneal astigmatism to total corneal astigmatism. J Cataract Refract Surg. 2012; 38(12): 2080–2087

[19] Koch DD. The enigmatic cornea and intraocular lens calculations: the LXXIII Edward Jackson Memorial Lecture. Am J Ophthalmol. 2016; 171:xv–xxx

[20] Reitblat O, Levy A, Kleinmann G, Abulafia A, Assia EI. Effect of posterior corneal astigmatism on power calculation and alignment of toric intraocular lenses: comparison of methodologies. J Cataract Refract Surg. 2016; 42(2):217–225

[21] Sheen Ophir S, LaHood B, Goggin M. Refractive outcome of toric intraocular lens calculation in cases of oblique anterior corneal astigmatism. J Cataract Refract Surg. 2020; 46 (5):688–693

[22] Jacob S. Everything you ever wanted to know: toric IOL implantation. EuroTimes. 2020; 25(9):12–13

[23] Gundersen KG, Potvin R. Clinical outcomes with toric intraocular lenses planned using an optical low coherence reflectometry ocular biometer with a new toric calculator. Clin Ophthalmol. 2016; 10:2141–2147

[24] Abulafia A, Koch DD, Wang L, et al. New regression formula for toric intraocular lens calculations. J Cataract Refract Surg. 2016; 42(5):663–671

[25] Abulafia A, Hill WE, Franchina M, Barrett GD. Comparison of methods to predict residual astigmatism after intraocular lens implantation. J Refract Surg. 2015; 31(10):699–707

[26] Abulafia A, Barrett GD, Kleinmann G, et al. Prediction of refractive outcomes with toric intraocular lens implantation. J Cataract Refract Surg. 2015; 41(5):936–944

[27] Abulafia A, Koch DD, Wang L, et al. A novel regression formula for toric IOL calculations. Paper presented at: European Society of Cataract and Refractive Surgeons Congress; September 5–9, 2015; Barcelona, Spain

[28] Weikert M, Hill W, Findl O, et al. Hitting the refractive target. ASCRS 20/Happy in 2020 webinar. August 15, 2020. https://ascrs.org/20happy/agenda/hitting-the-refractive-target

[29] Serels CM, Sandoval HP, Potvin R, Solomon KD. Evaluation of IOL power calculation formulas using different keratometries in post-refractive surgery cases. Paper presented at: ASCRS Virtual Annual Meeting. May 16–17, 2020. https://ascrs.org/clinical-education/cataract/2020-pod-sps-110-65874-evaluation-of-iol-power-calculation-formulas-using-different-kerato

[30] Ho YJ, Sun CC, Lee JS, Lin KK, Hou CH. Comparison of using Galilei Dual Scheimpflug Analyzer G4 and Barrett formula in predicting low cylinder preoperatively for cataract surgeries. Eur J Ophthalmol. 2020; 30(6):1320–1327

[31] Hill WE. Toric IOL planning and alignment. 2020 spotlight on cataract: complicated phaco cases: Part II. Presented at American Academy of Ophthalmology 2020 Virtual Conference. November 15, 2020. https://www.aao.org/annual-meeting-video/2020-spotlight-on-cataract-complicated-phaco-cases-2

[32] Abulafia A. Managing astigmatism. Euro Times. 2018; 23(2):6

[33] Savini G, Negishi K, Hoffer KJ, Schiano Lomoriello D. Refractive outcomes of intraocular lens power calculation using different corneal power measurements with a new optical biometer. J Cataract Refract Surg. 2018; 44(6):701–708

[34] Savini G, Hoffer KJ, Lomoriello DS, Ducoli P. Simulated keratometry versus total corneal power by ray tracing: a comparison in prediction accuracy of intraocular lens power. Cornea. 2017; 36(11):1368–1372

[35] Dell S. Diagnostics in refractive cataract surgery: corneal topography. EyeWorld. 2018; 23(7):57–58

[36] Wang L, Cao D, Vilar C, Koch DD. Posterior and total corneal astigmatism measured with optical coherence tomography-based biometer and dual Scheimpflug analyzer. J Cataract Refract Surg. 2020; 46(12):1652–1658

[37] Lu AQ, Poulsen A, Cui D, et al. Repeatability and comparability of keratometry measurements obtained with swept-source optical coherence and combined dual Scheimpflug-Placido disk-based tomography. J Cataract Refract Surg. 2020; 46(12):1637–1643

[38] Savini G, Hoffer KJ, Barrett GD. Results of the Barrett True-K formula for IOL power calculation based on Scheimpflug camera measurements in eyes with previous myopic excimer laser surgery. J Cataract Refract Surg. 2020; 46(7):1016–1019

[39] Lawless M, Jiang JY, Hodge C, Sutton G, Roberts TV, Barrett G. Total keratometry in intraocular lens power calculations in eyes with previous laser refractive surgery. Clin Exp Ophthalmol. 2020; 48(6):749–756

[40] Visco DM, Hill WE, Mckee Y. Prospective evaluation of iris registration-guided femtosecond laser-assisted capsular marks for toric IOL alignment during cataract surgery. Paper presented at ASCRS Virtual Annual Meeting. May 16–17, 2020

[41] Modi SS. Clinical outcomes after aphakic versus aphakic/pseudophakic intraoperative aberrometry in cataract surgery with toric IOL implantation. Int Ophthalmol. 2020; 40(12):3251–3257

[42] Visser N, Bauer NJ, Nuijts RM. Toric intraocular lenses: historical overview, patient selection, IOL calculation, surgical techniques, clinical outcomes, and complications. J Cataract Refract Surg. 2013; 39(4):624–637

[43] Kohnen T, Derhartunian V, Kook D, Klaproth OK. Toric intraocular lenses for correction of astigmatism in primary cataract surgery. In: Kohnen T, Kock DD, eds. Cataract and refractive surgery. Springer; 2009:67–80

[44] Németh G. One degree of misalignment does not lead to a 3.3% effect decrease after implantation of a toric intraocular lens. J Cataract Refract Surg. 2020; 46(3):482

[45] Holladay JT, Koch DD. Residual astigmatism with toric intraocular lens misalignment. J Cataract Refract Surg. 2020; 46(8):1208–1209

[46] Inoue Y, Takehara H, Oshika T. Axis misalignment of toric intraocular lens: placement error and postoperative rotation. Ophthalmology. 2017; 124(9):1424–1425

[47] Holladay JT, Pettit G. Improving toric intraocular lens calculations using total surgically induced astigmatism for a 2.5 mm temporal incision. J Cataract Refract Surg. 2019; 45(3):272–283

[48] Zhang F. New type 15 EyeJet ® capsular tension ring. Industrial Case Show. Presented at American Academy of Ophthalmology 2020. November 13–15, 2020

[49] Sagiv O, Sachs D. Rotation stability of a toric intraocular lens with a second capsular tension ring. J Cataract Refract Surg. 2015; 41(5):1098–1099

[50] Zhao Y, Li J, Yang K, Li X, Zhu S. Combined special capsular tension ring and toric IOL implantation for management of astigmatism and high axial myopia with cataracts. Semin Ophthalmol. 2018; 33(3):389–394

[51] Rastogi A, Khanam S, Goel Y, Kamlesh, Thacker P, Kumar P. Comparative evaluation of rotational stability and visual outcome of toric intraocular lenses with and without a consular tension ring. Indian J Ophthalmol. 2018; 66(3):411–415

[52] Gimbel HV, Marzouk HA. Haptic tuck for reverse optic capture of a single-piece acrylic toric or other single-piece acrylic intraocular lenses. J Cataract Refract Surg. 2019; 45(2):125–129

[53] Chang DF, Masket S, Miller KM, et al. ASCRS Cataract Clinical Committee. Complications of sulcus placement of single-piece acrylic intraocular lenses: recommendations for backup IOL implantation following posterior capsule rupture. J Cataract Refract Surg. 2009; 35(8):1445–1458

[54] Jones JJ, Oetting TA, Rogers GM, Jin GJC. Reverse optic capture of the single-piece acrylic intraocular lens in eyes with posterior capsule rupture. Ophthalmic Surg Lasers Imaging. 2012; 43(6):480–488

[55] Hayashi K, Hirata A, Manabe S, Hayashi H. Long-term change in corneal astigmatism after sutureless cataract surgery. Am J Ophthalmol. 2011; 151(5):858–865

[56] Ho JD, Liou SW, Tsai RJ, Tsai CY. Effects of aging on anterior and posterior corneal astigmatism. Cornea. 2010; 29(6):632–637

[57] Kieval JZ, Al-Hashimi S, Davidson RS, et al. ASCRS Refractive Cataract Surgery Subcommittee. Prevention and management of refractive prediction errors following cataract surgery. J Cataract Refract Surg. 2020; 46(8):1189–1197

8 Engage Successfully in Pseudophakic Monovision

Fuxiang Zhang, Alan Sugar, and Lisa Brothers Arbisser

Abstract

Monovision, though in common usage, is a misnomer; blended vision may be a better term. Pseudophakic monovision is one of the most commonly used modalities for the management of presbyopia in cataract patients. Because of its high quality of image contrast, high yield of spectacle independence, low cost, and low intraocular lens (IOL) exchange rate, it can and should be the starting point for most novice refractive cataract surgeons. This chapter will focus on some commonly asked questions with the goal of helping beginners engage and do well with a solid foundation in refractive cataract surgery. More details can be found in our previous publication, *Pseudophakic Monovision: A Clinical Guide.*[1] IOL monovision is not going to disappear in the United States and worldwide even when we have more, and, better, IOLs in the future. With the knowledge and skills of IOL monovision, the road to refractive cataract surgery will be much wider. It will also make other premium IOL practices easier with more flexibility.

Keywords: refractive cataract surgery, pseudophakic monovision, IOL monovision

8.1 Pseudophakic Monovision Is Widely Used by Cataract Surgeons in Refractive Cataract Surgery (RCS)

As science and technology advance, more and more presbyopia-correcting intraocular lens (IOLs) come to market, but pseudophakic monovision is still one of the most common surgical modalities for the management of presbyopia in cataract patients. The European Society of Cataract and Refractive Surgery (ESCRS) 2016 survey noted that 6% used presbyopia-correcting IOLs while 43% used IOL monovision.[2] As indicated by the 2019 ASCRS clinical survey, minimonovision (15% < 1.0 D myopic defocus; ▶ Fig. 8.1) and "true" monovision (12% 1.0 D or higher; ▶ Fig. 8.2) together represent 27% of cataract surgeries while only about 10% (▶ Fig. 8.3) use presbyopia-correcting IOLs in the United States.[3] The cost, vision quality, patient satisfaction, etc., are the reasons behind these numbers (▶ Fig. 8.1, ▶ Fig. 8.2, and ▶ Fig. 8.3).

Monovision, especially minimonovision (−0.50 to −0.75 D) and moderate monovision (−1.0 to

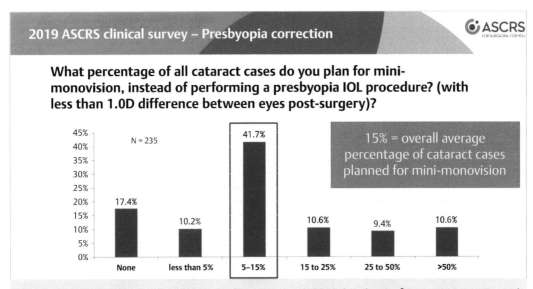

Fig. 8.1 2019 American Society of Cataract and Refractive Surgery (ASCRS) clinical survey.[3] Minimonovision 15%. Used with permission from ASCRS.

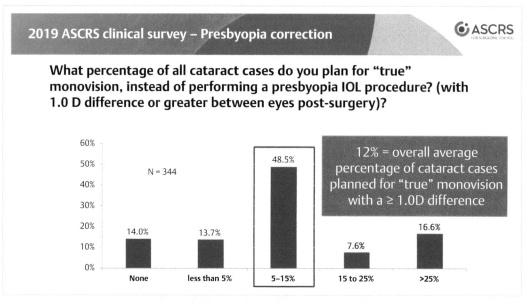

Fig. 8.2 2019 ASCRS clinical survey.[3] "True" monovision 12%. Used with permission from ASCRS.

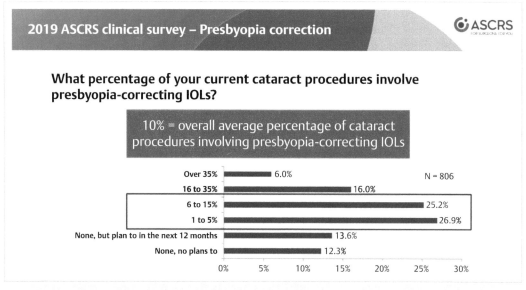

Fig. 8.3 2019 ASCRS clinical survey.[3] Presbyopia-correcting IOLs 10%. Used with permission from ASCRS.

−1.50 D), provides high-quality vision, low cost, and is responsible for a very low rate of IOL exchange. Patient satisfaction and spectacle independence rates are very high. Depending on which study, it is reasonable to expect a satisfaction rate at or above 80% and almost complete independence from glasses or need for backup glasses only at 70 to 90%.[1,4,5,6,7] There is hardly any major downside. Most IOL monovision patients still have good stereovision,[4,5,6,8] and its mild decrease does not affect patients' daily activities. Patients can always have a pair of backup glasses to regain full bilateral stereovision, should that become necessary (so long as we avoid anisometropia by staying within the recommended limits)—the unique beauty of IOL monovision compared to multifocal IOLs where IOL exchange may become the only option for management or else the patient may have to live with the complaints.

Patient selection is also much wider for IOL monovision than other premium IOLs. A demanding personality is not as big an issue for monovision as long as a thorough preoperative consultation is performed. IOL monovision is better tolerated in the presence of preexisting ocular pathology than are multifocal IOLs. The same is a favorable factor in postoperative years. As our patients get older, age-related ocular comorbidities, such as age-related macular degeneration (ARMD), epiretinal membrane (ERM), diabetic retinopathy, and dry eye syndrome, may become progressively worse. Patients may also develop more against the rule astigmatism. As we have long known, these ongoing changes have a much bigger negative impact in eyes with current multifocal IOLs than with monofocal IOLs.

Considering the above merits of monofocal pseudophakic monovision, it is not surprising to learn that most surveyed practicing ophthalmologists would choose monofocal pseudophakic monovision for their own eyes, should they need cataract surgery.[9,10]

8.2 Why Do We Recommend that Beginners Start with Monofocal IOLs?

Compared with monofocal IOLs, multifocality has many more hurdles to overcome for residents and beginners. These include:
• Reduced image contrast sensitivity.
• Dysphotopsia, especially under low light condition.
• Image gap between distance and near vision in traditional multifocal IOLs.
• Impact of pupil size.
• Challenges due to IOL centration and tilt.
• Demand for healthier ocular surface and macula.
• Neuroadaptation does not always work.
• Angle alpha and kappa concerns.

• Backup glasses typically do not work for unhappy patients.

8.3 When I Start with Monofocal IOLs, What Else Can I Do Besides Pseudophakic Monovision?

One of the common practices is to have our patients fill out a survey before we see them. Patients are asked to tell us what their needs are, including for the following:
• Their jobs.
• Their hobbies.
• Life styles, including nighttime driving.
• Preference of no spectacles for far, for near, intermediate distance, or all of them.
• Willingness to wear readers.
• Willingness to use backup spectacles if needed.
• Personality, easy going or perfectionist.

Based on the survey, we discuss more details with patients and their family members, if they prefer spectacle independence, partial or complete.

If the patient prefers standard surgery and IOLs, we do not deed to discuss too much further, but we do ask the patient to sign and acknowledge the fact that we did offer the presbyopia-correction option.

If the patient prefers to have good vision for distance but does not mind wearing readers, we can plan to aim both eyes for distance or micro monovision (one eye aimed for plano and fellow eye aimed for −0.25 to −0.50 regardless of dominance to allow an unaided view of an automobile dashboard and GPS).

If the patient prefers to have good vision for near but does not mind wearing glasses for driving, then we can aim the first eye for −1.50. Where to aim for the second eye will depend on how well the first eye can see clearly without glasses at postoperative week 2. If the patient is happy at near with the operated eye monocularly, then we can aim the second eye at −1.25 or −1.75 D depending on his/her preference. Sometimes, the patient can change their mind and want to have the second eye see far without glasses. Of note, it is also very important to ask the patient's input about the reading distance. For example, high myopia patients typically tend to prefer the near eye to be at −2.0 to −2.50 D rather than −1.5 D.

These strategies all qualify as RCS because we are trying to decrease spectacle dependence. We consider this pattern partial RCS, and that can certainly be the starting point for residents and beginners. In this scenario, we only need to correct astigmatism with monofocal toric IOLs or limbal relaxing incision (LRI) and we do not need to use any multifocal intraocular lens (MFIOL), trifocal, or extended depth of focus (EDOF) lenses.

If a patient does require full spectacle independence but does lots of nighttime driving and hates glare and halo with demanding personality, what is the best option? Pseudophakic monovision is likely the option of choice with one eye at plano, although newer IOLs, such as Vivity (Alcon) and Eyhance DIBOO (Johnson & Johnson) also work well.

8.4 What Three Main Downsides of Monovision Must You Tell Your Patients during Preoperative Counseling?

Every RCS conversation should include the fact that we are working with live human tissue and do not have full control, despite the most modern equipment and science, over how the eye and the brain may behave. Therefore no one on the planet can promise or be promised a certain result. Even if something is 95% sure, someone must be in the 5% with suboptimal outcomes. We can promise that we will do everything known to control the variables and be with the patient until they have the best result possible. Some variation on this conversation should be had in our opinion.

- The single most important thing you have to tell prospective IOL monovision patients is that the distance vision of the near vision eye will not be as sharp as the distance vision eye, if they compare the two for distance vision without glasses. This seems to be the number one "negative" comment, if you fail to make your patients understand and remember that fact before the surgery. It is also the clinician's job to reduce worry about that phenomenon since we live our lives with both eyes open and also the near vision eye has the potential to have good distance vision if a pair of glasses is given. Because of this drawback, there are some patients who do not like the idea of traditional IOL monovision. One of the ways to compensate the distance vision of the near vision eye is to use an EDOF lens as what we called modified or hybrid IOL monovision, where an EDOF lens is used for the second eye to cover both distance

and intermediate vision. See discussion later in this chapter, "What Is the Concept of Modified IOL Monovision?"

A Case Report (1): A 70-year-old woman came for cataract evaluation. She had an ERM in her OD but an unremarkable OS. (See ▸ Fig. 8.4 and ▸ Fig. 8.5.) Preoperative refraction OD was −1.00 + 0.50 × 10 giving 20/40 distance vision; OS was + 1.25 + 0.75 × 180 giving 20/30 distance vision. OD was her dominant eye with the "hole-in-card" test. "My right eye has always been my dominant eye." She did not want to deal with any dysphotopsia. OD surgery was done in November 2017 aiming for plano. OS was done one month later aiming for −1.50D. She was very happy with her right eye but pretty upset at two weeks after her OS surgery. "My left eye cannot see as good as my right eye." UDVA was 20/25 OD and 20/50 OS; UNVA 20/200 OD and 20/30 OS. Refraction of −0.50 + 0.25 × 127 gave 20/20 distance vision OD and −1.50 sphere gave 20/25 distance vision OS. Good UNVA in OS did not make her happy. The teaching point of this case is that even when clearly explained prior to the surgery, patients may still have complaints: the near eye does not see as well for distance as the distance vision eye. Another teaching point is that an eye with coexisting ocular pathology can still be chosen for distance vision if the patient has a history of clear dominance in one eye. Her only complaint was "My left eye cannot see as good as my right eye." She never came back for follow-up (▸ Fig. 8.4 and ▸ Fig. 8.5).

- Patients still need to know the fact that spectacle freedom is not 100% guaranteed. They may still need glasses, although usually the glasses are for backup only, such as for nighttime driving and/or prolonged small print reading. Based on our own 10-year IOL monovision deidentified survey data,[1] approximately 42% are completely spectacle free, 39% need backup only, 18% need glasses sometimes but less often than prior to surgery and 1.5% need glasses all the time. In the same survey, about one-third of our IOL monovision patients needed glasses for nighttime driving while two-third did not need any glasses for nighttime driving.

- There is a compromise in fine stereovision. The patient may need glasses to thread a needle, but for gross depth perception, such as steps, stairs,

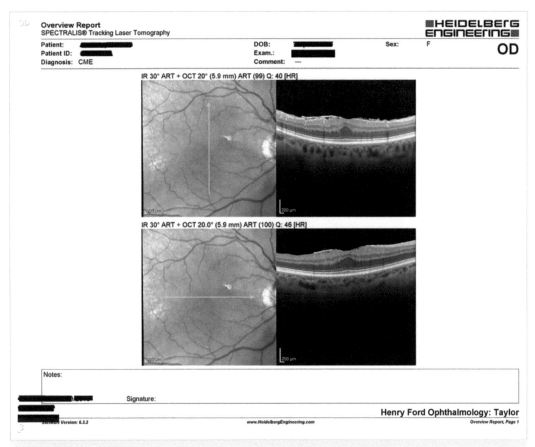

Fig. 8.4 Optical coherence tomography (OCT) showed epiretinal membrane (ERM) OD.

and curbs, they should be fine. Based on our own 10-year deidentified survey data, only 0.5% of IOL monovision patients had to wear glasses all the time for better stereopsis.[1] This subject becomes very important in certain situations, such as pilots, professional golfers, baseball and billiards players. Full preoperative discussion is absolutely necessary. Our guideline for these situations is not to have more than −0.50 myopic defocus. It is also important to explain clearly the rationale of this defocus is to cover dashboard and GPS. We have noted that some of these patients prefer not to have any negative impact from monovision, and then they choose aiming both eyes at plano, while most of these patients at our practice choose −0.25 to −0.50 D. Mistakes may actually happen if we miss patients' occupation/hobby at the beginning,

rather than aiming for plano both eyes versus a micro defocus aim. For that reason, every single patient coming for cataract evaluation will need to fill out a preoperative survey in which they will tell us their jobs and three main hobbies.

8.5 Which Three Preoperative Tests Are Highly Recommended?

8.5.1 Cover and Uncover Test

This test is essential to achieve a high IOL monovision success rate. Mild phoria works fine but tropia is a disassociated vision category and should not be considered for presbyopia-correction IOL monovision. If we skip this test, monovision can make the extraocular muscle (EOM) alignment worse, an iatrogenic complication if the patient

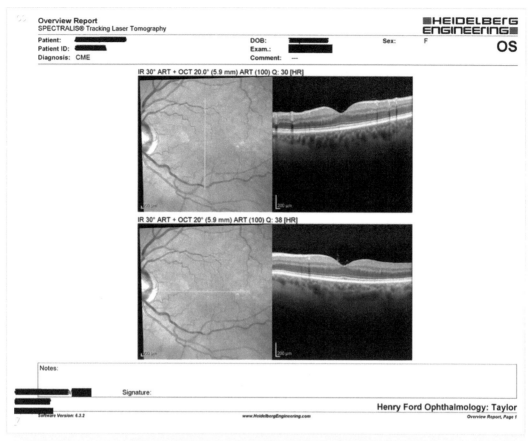

Fig. 8.5 Optical coherence tomography (OCT) showed an almost normal macula OS.

has significant phoria, although some patients may not be aware of this side effect being the consequence of the monovision.

We should be able to perform this test in most cataract patients in the United States and developed countries although it does not work in patients with very dense cataracts when the vision is not good enough to fix a distant target. If one eye has been very poor due to advanced cataract or trauma for a long time and we expect to rehabilitate it there needs to be a discussion of possible diplopia that can be transient after surgery or permanent, requiring strabismus surgery. This scenario may be one in which we might consider avoiding monovision so that we give the brain a chance to overcome the sensory exotropia or exophoria which may have developed.

8.5.2 Dominant Eye Test with Hole-in-Card Method

This test will let you know if you are going to do conventional IOL monovision versus crossed IOL monovision. Crossed monovision has more contraindications than conventional monovision. If you fail to avoid contraindications, the patient will not only not get spectacle independence, but they may need more surgery to reverse IOL monovision. See more discussion later in this chapter, "What Are the Concerns if We Choose Crossed Pseudophakic Monovision?"

8.5.3 Plus-Lens Mimic Test

There are several ways to do this preoperative monovision simulating test.[1] The mainstay is to give the patient a chance to experience the mimicked monovision status: place a +1.50 D lens in front of the near vision eye. The patient will be experiencing the mimicked monovision status of seeing better for near while not so clear for far for his/her near vision eye. The feedback from the patient is important for decision making. If the patient does not like this when either sitting/reading or walking, IOL monovision probably should not be offered. This test also has the merit of informing the patient that IOL monovision is not perfect but it does have some tradeoffs.

8.6 I Have Known a Cataract Surgeon Who Also Does a Lot of Monovision for His Cataract Patients, but He Did Not Seem to Do Any Tests that You Recommended in Your Presentation. How Important Are Those Tests? Do You Do All These Tests Yourself or Your Staff Do It?

With these three tests, you will surely have a much higher success rate and happier patients than if you do not do any of them. Routinely doing the worse eye first aiming for plano and the fellow eye aiming for near without any preoperative tests regardless of dominance is not recommended because this will have more chance of causing what literature termed "fixation switch diplopia" if we missed potential contraindications, such as monofixation syndrome, significant phoria, and amblyopia, which may be asymptomatic. In our team, my technician staff do the first two of the three routine tests but I personally do the cover and uncover test when the pupils are not dilated. These tests do take time and typically are not billed, but the outcomes will be better. We have also included stereopsis test as our routine, but that is probably not necessary for most of the routine cases.

8.7 Is It Necessary to Offer a Contact Lens Trial Test for Most Pseudophakic Monovision Patients?

A contact lens trial test is not necessary for most routine IOL monovision decisions. Although it is a very common practice pattern for laser-vision refractive surgery such as LASIK/PRK to offer a contact lens trial test, IOL monovision is different from laser vision-induced monovision. Our anecdotal experience tells us that elderly patients find it much easier to adapt to IOL monovision than younger patients. A study in Japan also suggested that elderly patients have a higher success rate with pseudophakic monovision.[11] Contact lens trials can be difficult or not realistic in the following conditions:

- There is severe astigmatism.
- The patient is unable to use a contact lens due to a systemic or ocular condition.
- Advanced age.
- The patient does not want to go through the process.
- The cataract is dense with very poor vision. The process of a contact lens trial itself can be difficult and it can be discouraging for most elderly patients if they have never used contact lenses before.

For many years, when we received questions from surgeons who had just started to do pseudophakic monovision, a frequent question was "is it necessary to have a contact lens trial prior to the surgery?" Our answer was, typically, "theoretically it is reasonable, but practically it is not necessary for the majority of our patients." It is probably reasonable or even advisable to conduct a contact lens trial for those patients with very demanding personalities. Among several thousand IOL monovision cases over two decades, I (FZ) have had only two patients who had a contact lens trial prior to decision-making.[1] A well-known pseudophakic monovision pioneer, Jay McDonald MD, never used a contact lens trial for his monovision patients.[12]

8.8 Which Eye for Distance and Which Eye for Near?

For this topic, the following factors should be considered:
1. Sighting dominance test.
2. Distance vision and the cataract density of each eye.
3. Refractive status of each eye.
4. History of monovision.
5. Longstanding weaker eye.
6. Ocular comorbidity.

8.8.1 Sighting Dominance Test

Correcting the dominant eye for distance and the nondominant eye for near is the conventional monovision approach, although this convention is largely based on information and tradition from the optometric literature not the ophthalmic literature. To our knowledge, there is no prospective randomized peer-reviewed evidence that validates this convention. Correcting the dominant eye for near and the nondominant eye for far is called crossed monovision. There is evidence that the conventional approach yields a high level of satisfying results for vision and spectacle independence, with the assumption that it is easier for the dominant eye to suppress the blur induced in the nondominant eye during distance viewing.[13,14] There are also studies to suggest that crossed monovision works well,[7,15] but crossed monovision may have a higher chance of causing fixation switch diplopia if you fail to consider potential contraindications, such as monofixation syndrome, borderline phoria, and amblyopia, which may be asymptomatic.[16,17,18,19] Except for specific conditions discussed later, choosing the dominant eye with the hole-in-card test for distance is recommended.

8.8.2 Distance Vision and the Density of the Cataract of Each Eye

There is no fixed pattern of vision and sighting dominance,[20,21] but we usually see that better distance vision is with the sighting dominant eye. The denser cataract eye typically causes worse preoperative vision. It is not hard to decide if the vision and lens density match the sighting dominance hole-in-card test; but if they do not match, we would still make the decision to follow the hole-in-card test.

8.8.3 Refractive Status

The less myopic eye is often preferred for distance and the more myopic eye for near in the preoperative stage. This is similar in hyperopia, but it seems to be more variable. The eye with no astigmatism or less astigmatism is usually the better seeing eye in the preoperative stage. It is reasonable to keep the same pattern for postoperative goals.

8.8.4 History of Monovision

If a patient has a history of monovision with good results and no complaints, or is currently using monovision, especially for a long duration, no matter whether due to natural monovision, contact lenses, or laser vision correction, stick to the same pattern, regardless of the dominant eye test. It does not seem to matter if the monovision is conventional or crossed from the dominance point of view. When there is a conflict between the history of long duration of monovision and the eye dominance test, our anecdotal experience tells us to follow the history.

A Case Report (2): A woman in her 70s had a history of contact lens monovision OS for near for about 10 years. "Never had any problem with monovision." She wore no contact lens for the past few years due to "dry eye." She wanted cataract surgery and to resume monovision. She had no contraindications for IOL monovision by history and by cover and uncover test. Her vision in OD was worse than OS at presentation due to a denser cataract and likely some myopic shift. OS was her dominant eye with the hole-in-card test at presentation. The decision was to choose the dominant eye OS for far and the nondominant eye OD for near based on the hole-in-card test. Surgery was uneventful in both eyes and there was no need to correct astigmatism in either eye. Postoperative vision was good OD for near and OS for far without correction.

After she recovered from a long hospitalization for chronic obstructive pulmonary disease (COPD), she came back complaining that "something is not right. I do not feel comfortable when I am reading." Ocular examination was unremarkable without tropia or phoria.

A pair of customized reading glasses was prescribed to yield good reading vision for OS. The patient did not have any ocular complaint at the follow-up visit except that she did not like the reading glasses: "They hurt my ears because of my O2 line on my ears." She refused to use contact lenses again. She took the option of a piggyback IOL to reverse OS for reading and OD for distance. She was basically wheelchair bound from her COPD and reading was her main hobby, so a piggyback IOL was first done in her OS for reading. She remained complaint free after OS reversal for reading, so the plan to reverse OD for far was cancelled.

The lesson was learned. She had enjoyed 10 years of contact lens–induced monovision with OS for near prior to her cataract formation. Her OD most likely was her real motor sighting dominant eye. Her OS became the dominant eye when OD became more myopic with denser cataract formation and worse vision. It has been shown that ocular dominance can change when vision changes.[22] The teaching point from this case is that it is probably advisable to keep the prior monovision pattern if the patient was doing well in the past with contact lens–induced or laser vision correction–induced monovision. This is our clinical experience only and we are not aware of peer review studies in the literature in this regard. A sighting dominance test such as the hole-in-card can be plastic as the vision changes and/or as the refractive status changes.

8.8.5 Longstanding Weaker Eye

It is advisable for IOL monovision practice to consider this question for any prospective patient: Can you recall if you have one eye which was always weaker than the other eye? If yes, pay close attention to the cover and uncover test; do a stereopsis test with the best manifest correction and then include the reading add; do a Worth 4 Dot test and 4ΔBO test to make sure that that patient does not have amblyopia, or a monofixation syndrome. If no contraindication is found, then avoid choosing that weaker eye for the distance eye. The "weaker" eye could be due to greater astigmatism, or a more myopic or hyperopic refractive error. We should avoid that weaker eye for the choice of the distance eye.

8.8.6 Ocular Comorbidity

Patients with severe ocular comorbidities are not good candidates for IOL monovision. Some patients are very motivated, such as those with a history of laser vision correction, to get as much spectacle independence as possible; in these situations, it is quite reasonable to consider IOL monovision if potential UCDVA of 20/30 to 20/40 can be expected. But the patient must also understand the limitations and the likelihood of needing glasses in the future. The eye with greater ocular comorbidity, as in macular pathology, is usually chosen for the near vision eye, if there is no other

priority. This can be re-evaluated after we see the result in the first eye.

8.9 What Level of Anisometropia Is Preferred?

A customized approach is the best option. There is no consensus in terms of classification. The following classification for IOL monovision in terms of focal length separation between the two eyes has been recommended in the literature.[1]
1. Minimonovision (sometimes referred to as Micro or Nano): −0.50 to −0.75 D
2. Modest monovision (sometimes referred to as Medium): −1.00 to −1.5 D
3. Full monovision (sometimes referred to as Traditional or Classical): −1.75 to −2.5 D

8.9.1 Mini-IOL Monovision −0.50 to −0.75 D

The majority of minimonovision patients (anisometropia less than 1.00 D) do well for far and intermediate focal distances, but usually need some help for reading, especially for prolonged small print reading.

Generally speaking, patients with minimonovision are universally happy as long as we hit the target for the distance eye at or close to plano, astigmatism is corrected and they are informed at the preoperative consultation that they will need reading glasses for small print. There should be no stereopsis or contrast issues for these patients. The concern for conventional versus crossed monovision in this group is negligible if contraindications are excluded. Preoperative screening becomes less important in this group compared to the modest and full monovision groups. Minimonovision works very well for those patients who are taxi drivers and truck drivers and those who do not have reading as their hobby. We predict that this option will increase in popularity in the future because of increased use of modern digital devices such as computers, tablets, cell phones, and GPS.

We usually do not target both eyes for exact emmetropia, even when the patient desires to have good vision for far in both eyes. In this situation we prefer to have the distance eye aimed at plano and the fellow eye at around −0.25 to −0.50. We do explain the rationale to the patient preoperatively. We have had a few patients with complaints in the past who had perfect distance vision for far, with each eye at plano, but they were not perfectly happy with their view of the dashboard when driving. This issue becomes worse if the refractive outcome unintentionally ends in the low hyperopic range. One has the option of picking up a pair of reading glasses for digital reading at home, which can be a challenge during driving.

8.9.2 Modest IOL Monovision −1.0 to −1.50 D

Most pseudophakic monofocal monovision falls in this subgroup. Our clinical experience has been consistent with studies in the literature. The sweet spot for the anisometropic level for a successful IOL monovision patient who wants to have spectacle freedom without significant downsides seems to be located somewhere between −1.25 and −1.50 D.[7,23,24,25] Anisometropia of 1.00 to 1.50 should work well for the majority of patients with good binocular stereopsis and contrast sensitivity, although they may still have to use backup glasses for prolonged reading of small print. It is a good idea to advise these patients to get a pair of prescription glasses with bifocals with the explanation: You may need them for driving at night in

the rain for your best vision although you would pass a driver's test without, or for reading fine print for long periods without tiring though OTC readers will work well enough. Medicare actually pays for the first pair of prescription glasses after cataract surgery.

What are the merits? At this level of anisometropia, even in patients with strong ocular dominance, which is not always easy to pick up in preoperative testing, asthenopia is unlikely to be a concern. This degree of anisometropia can be considered almost physiological, allowing fusion and binocular summation rather than the suppression that may be necessary with higher levels of anisometropia (▶ Fig. 8.6).

This group of patients had the highest complete spectacle freedom when compared with minimonovision and full monovision.[1] Even with modest monovision, high spectacle independence and patient satisfaction were achievable for most patients in both conventional and crossed pseudophakic groups.[7] It is a common assumption that low anisometropia has a high chance of needing glasses, but our study[7] suggests that a modest anisometropia level (average about 1.15 D) can still achieve a high patient satisfaction rate (more than 95% were "happy" or "very happy" among 60 participants in that study) with both conventional and crossed IOL monovision patterns.

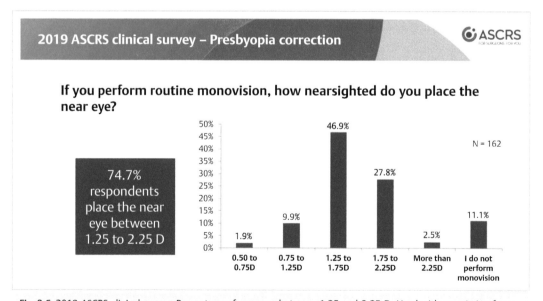

Fig. 8.6 2019 ASCRS clinical survey. Percentage of near eye between 1.25 and 2.25 D. Used with permission from ASCRS.

8.9.3 Traditional Monovision −1.75 to −2.50 D

With the near eye at −1.75 to −2.50 D, patients typically can have a high rate of reading glasses independence but may have a more noticeable impact on fine stereopsis and nighttime driving. Typical happy patients are older with main hobbies such as reading/crocheting/word puzzles, who do not drive much at night but still prefer no spectacles for most of their routines at home, such as watching TV.

These patients have the highest rate of needing glasses for nighttime driving when compared with minimonovision and modest monovision subgroups.[1] For high myopia patients, it is important to ask what postoperative reading distance they prefer. They may not be happy if the reading eye is set at −1.25 D because they are used to a short reading distance prior to their cataract surgery. If they prefer a short reading distance, we can aim the reading eye at −2.0 D or a bit more, but we will also need to warn these patients that they will have more chance of needing glasses for driving, especially at night. The body height and arm length of the patient should also be considered. For example, the reading eye for a 6-foot-tall gentleman can be set at −1.25 D, but for a short-stature 5-foot-tall older patient it may need to be set at −1.75 D. This often can be one of the factors affecting patient happiness. The pros and cons of full monovision should be fully explained prior to any decision-making.

Duke-Elder taught that each 0.25 D difference between the refraction of the two eyes causes 0.5% difference in size between the two retinal images and a difference of 5% is the limit which can usually be tolerated with ease.[26] He also mentioned that patients might experience discomfort due to an artificial heterophoria when they have more than 2.00 D of anisometropia.

A Case Report (3)[1]: A 65-year-old well-educated woman payroll accountant presented in 2014 for cataract evaluation. She complained of decreased vision in both eyes, especially when driving. Her uncorrected distance vision was OD 20/200 and OS 20/100; uncorrected near vision was OD J1 and OS J1 +. Her corrected distance vision was OD 20/40 and OS 20/30. Preoperative refraction was OD −2.75 D and OS −2.25 D. Hole-in-card and camera tests showed that the right eye was dominant. Past ocular history and the cover and uncover test revealed no contraindication for IOL

monovision. She had been wearing a contact lens for OD only for 15 years and her OS was her near eye without a contact lens.

She wanted to keep her monovision. Her three main hobbies were cooking, biking, and shopping. The decision for her refractive goal was made based on these main hobbies: OD plano and OS −1.25 D. The right eye was done in June 2014 and left eye in July 2014.

She came back 2 years later, with OD 20/20 plano and OS 20/20 −1.00 D sphere. Near vision without correction OD was J16 and OS J7. She wore +1.50 D readers. She was not happy with the reading ability of her left eye. She wanted to know if she could get rid of the readers. "Make my left eye stronger so I do not have to wear readers." To make sure that full permanent monovision was what she really liked, a trial contact lens was offered. She preferred +1.75 D contact lens rather than +1.50 D for her OS. Popular piggyback IOLs with 0.50-D increments, such as the Staar AQ5010 were no longer available at that time, so we had to choose either a +2.00-D or a +3.00-D Alcon MA60MA three-piece sulcus lens. A +2.00-D lens would give a refractive outcome of around −2.25 D and a +3.00-D lens would give an outcome between −2.75 D and −3.00 D. After detailed discussion, she strongly preferred +3.00 D. "With the contact lens of +1.75 and my −1.00 myopia, I can read very well, so near −3.00 will be just fine for me." (She was amazingly familiar with the optics.)

Surgery was done in November 2016 (FZ's second monovision-related piggyback IOL in 20+ years). Postoperative uncorrected distance vision was OD 20/20, OS 20/400; Corrected distance vision OD Plano 20/20, OS 20/20 with −2.75. Uncorrected near visions were OD J16 and OS J1+. Stereopsis and contrast sensitivity tests showed significant decreases comparing full monovision with the piggyback with modest monovision prior to piggyback. See ▶ Table 8.1 and ▶ Table 8.2.

Table 8.1 Preoperative and postoperative stereopsis comparison

Stereopsis	
Preoperative	Postoperative
4/9 circles 140 seconds of arc	2/9 circles 400 seconds of arc

Source: Pseudophakic Monovision: A Clinical Guide. Zhang F, Sugar A, Barrett G, ed. 1st Edition. Thieme; 2018.

Table 8.2 Preoperative and postoperative contrast sensitivity comparison

	Contrast sensitivity test results			
	Day		Night	
	Preop	Postop	Preop	Postop
RE	1.35	1.35	1.20	1.20
LE	1.35	1.05	1.35	1.05
BE	1.65	1.50	1.50	1.35

Source: Pseudophakic Monovision: A Clinical Guide. Zhang F, Sugar A, Barrett G, ed. 1st Edition. Thieme; 2018.

Despite the downside from full monovision of 2.75 D, she is very happy with her overall condition and does not have any complaints. (Her husband came to see me later and he wanted me to do the same thing as what I did for his wife.) However, when she was asked if she noted any other differences between pre-piggyback and post-piggyback, she acknowledged that she had to use backup glasses more often for nighttime driving and also had to get "closer" to her computer. That situation fits what we discussed in our previous publication about the Not-Sharply-Focused-Zone in full monovision.[1] She continued to do well in the following years of office visits with no signs of iris transillumination defect or pigmentary glaucoma. The original surgery was more than 2 years before the piggyback surgery; otherwise, IOL exchange might be a better option if we do not have a great piggyback lens.

8.10 Who Can Be Good Candidates for the First Few Cases of Pseudophakic Monovision?

See ▶ Table 8.3.

8.11 Who Should We Avoid for Pseudophakic Monovision?

Avoiding contraindications is one of the three key factors for IOL monovision success. (The other two are preoperative consultation and being able to hit the refractive target with correction of astigmatism.)[1] That also seems to be one of the main

Table 8.3 Candidate selection pearls for beginners' first few pseudophakic monovision

	Good candidates	Try to avoid
Motivation	Hate glasses	Don't mind glasses
Refractive status	Hyperopia	Mild myopia
History	Contact lens or laser vision–induced monovision and happy	Multifocal contact lens and happy
Ocular comorbidities	Healthy eyes	Significant to affect good vision potential especially distance eye
Contraindications	None	See below detailed discussions
Types of monovision	Simple monofocal IOLs	Hybrid or modified monovision, mixed with EDOF or accommodative IOLs
Personality	Easy going	Demanding

reasons why some surgeons are reluctant to initiate intentional IOL monovision, since they do not know what should be avoided (▶ Table 8.4).

8.11.1 Extraocular Muscle (EOM) Related

Patients with noticeable tropias do not have full fusion and should be avoided for pseudophakic monovision. There are some rare exceptions where intentional pseudophakic monovision may correct long-standing stable diplopia taking advantage of neural suppression when there is at least 3D of anisometropia.[27] It is not difficult to understand the fact that significant EOM problems should be avoided for IOL monovision because the anisometropia from monovision will add extra burden to the EOM system.

With a history of diplopia, prism usage, or EOM surgery, diplopia could recur with monovision (contact lens, or laser-assisted in situ keratomileusis (LASIK) or posterior capsular intraocular lens (PCIOL)). Twelve cases were reported with

Table 8.4 Ocular contraindications of IOL monovision

	Contraindications of IOL monovision
EOM-related	Tropia
	≥8 PD phoria
	History of double vision
	History of prism usage
	History of strabismus and/or EOM surgery
	Monofixation syndrome
Non-EOM-related	Unilateral long-standing dense cataract
	Severe maculopathy
	Severe peripheral field loss
	Hemianopia

Abbreviations: EOM, extraocular muscles; IOL, intraocular lens.

the conclusion: "Monovision is successful for the far majority of patients who try it. However, in patients with a previous history of strabismus or those with significant phoria, caution should be used in recommending monovision."[28]

Kushner[17] reported 16 cases of acquired diplopia as "fixation switch diplopia" in patients who had a history of strabismus or amblyopia since childhood. Six out of 16 developed diplopia due to monovision correction because the nonfixating eye was made the fixating eye. In all 16 patients, symptoms were completely eliminated when optical correction was prescribed that restored the preferred eye for fixation. In this nonalternating strabismus situation, with or without amblyopia, these patients may experience diplopia if they fixate with the eye that is not preferred. This has been referred to as "fixation switch diplopia."[17,19,29,30,31] It has been speculated that because the suppression that accompanies strabismus is facultative, suppression may not be present in the usually dominant eye when the nondominant eye is fixing.[19,30]

Monofixation syndrome is a loss of bifixation or foveal fusion resulting in the manifestation of a facultative absolute scotoma in the fovea of the nonfixating eye.[16,32,33] Monofixation syndrome can be primary, without any noticeable etiology, or secondary to small angle strabismus, anisometropia, or a monocular macular lesion. Monofixation syndrome patients can become diplopic following mistakes in prescription of glasses, contact lenses, or IOLs. It can also develop after LASIK.[34] The absence of foveal fusion that characterizes monofixation syndrome can occur in strabismic and orthotropic eyes.[32,33] One-third of monofixation patients show orthophoria with the cover and uncover test.[33] They maintain good peripheral fusion. Two-thirds of monofixation syndrome patients were noted to have amblyopia, but one-third were not amblyopic.[33]

Preoperative examination with a stereopsis test, 4-D base out prism test, and Worth 4-Dot fusion at a distance of 6 meters is helpful in making the diagnosis, although it may not be reliable if the cataract is dense and vision is very poor. In this scenario, the safer way is not to offer monovision. Of note, normal fusion with the Worth 4 Dot test at near does not rule out monofixation because peripheral fusion may still be maintained.[33] Since most of the scotomas of monofixating patients are approximately 3 degrees, most, if not all, monofixation syndrome patients can fuse at 13 inches with the Worth 4 Dot test but are unable to fuse at a distance of 20 feet.[33] If eccentric fixation is present in one eye, the cover and uncover test may not reveal any shift.

One routinely asked question can be helpful: Are you aware of one eye always being weaker than the other eye for your whole life? If the answer is yes, then we should be careful about the decision to offer IOL monovision, although answering "yes" to that question does not necessarily mean that patient is a monofixater. It can be due to refractive errors too. If the patient answers "no," it does not mean there is no problem, since the patient may not be aware of some mild conditions. The challenge is that monofixation syndrome patients are often asymptomatic. Their eyes can be straight or nearly straight, with average fusional vergence amplitudes as bifixaters and appreciation of gross stereopsis and do not get worse as they age.[33] Two cases of monofixation were reported in our previous publication,[1] one with IOL monovision and one with a ReSTOR multifocal IOL clear lens exchange. The diagnosis of monofixation syndrome becomes clinically important when a clinician misses the diagnosis and chooses the nonfixating eye for distance. Fixation switch diplopia can occur as a consequence. Even in conventional monovision, it will have a risk of breaking down the balance of a stable asymptomatic monofixation syndrome due to monovision-induced anisometropia.

For unilateral long-standing dense cataract, especially traumatic cataract, even if the eyes do not seem to have strabismus, they may already have compromised central fusion. If they do have some strabismus, of course, we should not offer IOL monovision, especially crossed IOL monovision. It can be difficult or impossible to accurately evaluate ocular alignment if the strabismus is small in these patients due to poor vision and poor fixation from the dense cataract. The history is the key in this scenario. Surgeons should remain mindful of all contraindications for any surgical procedure, and cataract is not an exception. If preoperative strabismus is noted on examination due to the long-standing unilateral cataract, even if trauma occurred during adulthood, there is a good chance that such a patient will have diplopia after the surgery.[29,30,35] This is possibly due to fusion disruption. Pratt-Johnson[36] reported 24 cases of unilateral long-standing traumatic cataract from 1984 to 1988. All of these 24 cases had unilateral traumatic cataracts and had intractable diplopia after their vision was restored with IOLs or contact lenses to 20/40 or better. None of these 24 cases had a known history of interrupted binocular function prior to their trauma and the average age at trauma was 18 years old (from 6 to 39). There was no central nervous system trauma associated with the ocular trauma. The study noted that the risk of diplopia increased if the interval from cataract formation to vision restoration reached 2.5 years or longer. The authors also noted that these patients typically had secondary strabismus in the injured eye, one year or longer after the injury.

8.11.2 Non-EOM-Related Severe Ocular Comorbidities

Severe ocular comorbidities can cause extensive damage, limiting the possibilities for IOL monovision: significantly compromised central vision as in wet ARMD, diabetic retinopathy or significantly compromised peripheral field as in advanced glaucoma, past panretinal laser photocoagulation and hemianopia should not be considered for IOL monovision. Most patients with mild, and many with some moderate ocular comorbidity, as long as it is stable and not progressive can actually do well with IOL monovision. Some patients with a history of successful contact lens–induced monovision or laser refractive surgery–induced monovision may have a very strong desire to keep their monovision when they are ready for cataract surgery. In these situations, it is reasonable to consider IOL monovision as long as a good preoperative consultation is performed and fully documented in the medical record.

8.12 What Kind of Systemic Conditions Should We Avoid for Monovision Candidates?

Systemic conditions involving EOM function should be avoided for IOL monovision. We may not recognize these problems until years after IOL monovision surgery: They typically do not have the expected glasses independence as we hoped for. This is one of the two most easily missed contraindications. (The other is monofixation.) Ophthalmologists can often miss nonocular situations unless they have a checklist to include systemic evaluation. Parkinson disease, Graves disease, myasthenia gravis, and multiple sclerosis are typical samples. Extraocular muscle function and accommodative convergence can be affected at the onset or during the progress of these diseases.

Meniere disease is likely not an absolute contraindication for IOL monovision, but it can be a reason for caution. The vestibular system includes the parts of the inner ear and brain that process sensory information controlling balance and affecting eye movements. If disease or injury damages these processing areas, vestibular disorders can result. Meniere disease is one of the most commonly diagnosed vestibular disorders. It is probably advisable to avoid IOL monovision for any patient who has had a history of repeated vertigo episodes because those diseases are often chronic in nature. Monovision itself may not necessarily make Meniere disease worse, but an added anisometropic load may make balance and visual system function more complicated and be blamed as the etiology.

8.13 Can Amblyopic Patients Do Well with Pseudophakic Monovision?

Amblyopia and monofixation syndrome can coexist. Patients with amblyopia often relate the diagnosis of "lazy eye" in their history because it is typically remarkable. In amblyopia, where strong ocular dominance occurs, patients tend to suppress information originating from the nondominant eye regardless of its clarity. These patients are not good candidates for monovision. It does not necessarily make the amblyopic eye worse, but from a spectacle independence point of view, it does not work well. In cases of borderline phoria, the extra anisometropic load from monovision can potentially worsen the preexisting balance and may even lead to a manifest deviation.

A Case Report (4): A 61-year-old gentleman with hyperopia OU and a history of amblyopia OD came for clear lens extraction with a strong desire not to wear glasses for far or near. He had no history of extraocular muscle surgery, prism use, or double vision. Preoperative refraction was OD + 5.75 + 0.25 × 039 giving 20/40 and OS + 6.00 sphere giving 20/20 acuity. OS was dominant with the hole-in-card and camera tests. Ocular exam was normal except for a trace ERM OD, but optical coherence tomography (OCT) was unremarkable. The Worth 4 Dot test at near showed 4 dots: 2 green and 2 yellow (not reported as red). Worth 4 Dot test at distance 2 dots: 1 green and 1 yellow. Cover and uncover test at distance with glasses: 4 prism D esophoria in primary gaze, left gaze and right gaze, and right and left head tilt.

Monovision was planned with OD aimed at −1.00 and OS at plano. Surgery was uneventful OU. Three-month later distance vision uncorrected was OD 20/50, OS 20/20, near vision uncorrected OD J5 and OS J3. Corrected distance vision OD −1.25 + 0.50 × 027 20/25 and OS Plano 20/20. He stated that he did not need glasses for far, but needed glasses for arm's length such as using a computer and for all near work as a pharmacist. For convenience, he wore glasses all the time. The fact that the anisometropia was low might also have played some role for his nonoptimal near vision, but uncorrected near vision was J5 OD, which was worse than his J3 OS. Uncorrected near vision would be expected to be better OD than OS if he did not have amblyopia in OD. At his 1-year postoperative visit, his ocular condition was the same. Monovision just did not work out well for his intermediate vision and his near vision. Fortunately, his cover and uncover test was the same with no deterioration at 1-year follow-up. He was not unhappy with wearing the glasses since his overall visual function was much better than prior to the surgery, but we were not satisfied because he came for clear lens exchange paying all the costs in the hope that he would not need glasses postoperatively.

8.14 Must We Correct All Astigmatism for Pseudophakic Monovision?

Significant corneal astigmatism is not a contraindication for IOL monovision, but IOL monovision may not work well if we do not correct it. There is no agreement as to what should be considered a "significant" amount of astigmatism for pseudophakic monovision. Our experience suggests that the maximum astigmatism for the distance eye should be no more than 0.50 D. In the near eye we have more leeway, and monovision often works well even with 1.0 to 1.5 D of uncorrected astigmatism. We are not aware of peer-reviewed studies validating if with-the-rule versus against-the-rule astigmatism may make a significant difference in this regard. Due to angular magnification and the ability to move near targets in and out to the preferred vertex distance, mild residual astigmatism can actually enhance depth of focus.[37,38] Let us think about −2.0 + 1.00 × 90 (same as −1.0 − 1.0 × 180) as the near eye. This patient should be expected to do well if the dominant eye is emmetropic with good distance vision and this near eye will do well without correcting the 1-D cylinder. The near eye has −1.0 D at 90-degree meridian and has −2.0 at 180 degrees, resulting in increased depth of focus.

Similar as "all the astigmatism should be corrected," another myth is spherical aberration (SA) correction. It is clear that correction of positive SA will improve distance vision quality, but for a near eye, leaving some positive SA actually may improve the depth of focus. SN60AT/SA60AT from Alcon and SofPort AO from Bausch Lomb are some of the non-SA correcting lenses.

Eyhance IOL (Johnson & Johnson) is a monofocal lens designed to slightly extend the depth of focus. It does have −0.27 microns SA correction, similar as other Tecnis IOLs, but the new lens has a continuous refractive optical surface that results in a progressive increase in power from the periphery to the center of the lens which will extend the depth of focus.

8.15 Is a History of Oculomotor Palsy a Contraindication for Pseudophakic Monovision?

For patients with a history of a cranial nerve palsy and a short period of double vision, such as third, fourth, or sixth cranial nerve palsies, these may not be absolute contraindications, but we probably should not offer IOL monovision, even when they do not have any manifest residual EOM misalignment. The concerns are mainly twofold: The EOM system may still have some leftover dysfunction and the palsy may recur because of underlying systemic conditions.

8.16 What Are Occupational Concerns for Pseudophakic Monovision?

The profession and avocations of monovision candidates should always be considered. Some professions may require perfect stereovision and we may need to avoid IOL monovision for those patients. One medical-legal case was reported[39] of an airplane accident related to contact lens monovision in a pilot. The practitioner was not aware of the occupation of the patient. Truck drivers, and professional athletes, such as tennis, baseball, and golf players, may not be ideal candidates for full monovision. Specific details should be elicited from each patient.

8.17 What Are the Concerns for Crossed Pseudophakic Monovision?

There are two major concerns if we choose crossed pseudophakic monovision. One to avoid full or complete monovision, with anisometropia around 2 D, and the other is to avoid contraindications as discussed above.

We do sometimes run into situations where crossed IOL monovision is needed, choosing the dominant eye for near and the nondominant eye for far. For example, if you operate on the nondominant eye first, aiming for −1.0 D, but it ends up as −0.25 D with good uncorrected distance vision, then you may need to choose the dominant eye for near as crossed monovision or abandon the original monovision plan. Sometimes a patient may change their mind after the first eye is done and then want to have the unoperated eye to cover whatever the first eye is not able to see clearly without glasses.

Generally speaking, crossed IOL monovision works well in most patients if contraindications are avoided and if anisometropia is at a mini or modest level.[7,15] For minimonovision, the need for a dominance test is almost negligible. With this knowledge and experience, clinicians can double their chance to achieve glasses independence with monovision. The knowledge of crossed monovision can be very helpful for premium IOL patients, such as with EDOF Symfony IOL and Crystalens/Trulign IOLs in case the first operated eye refraction target is missed.

A 14-year conventional versus crossed IOL monovision review study[7] was published in the JCRS in September 2015. For full text, visit the following link: https://www.ncbi.nlm.nih.gov/pubmed/?term=crossed + monovision + Zhang

Generally speaking, we still recommend use of the conventional monovision pattern if possible, since crossed monovision has more contraindications and a higher chance of causing fixation switch diplopia, or disturbing borderline balanced ocular alignment, if we fail to avoid potential contraindications, such as monofixation syndrome, borderline phoria, mild amblyopia, or long-standing unilateral dense cataract.[16,17,19,33] Subtle contraindication can be a challenge. Detailed strategy regarding how to detect subtle contraindication can be found from our previous publication.[1]

8.18 Why Do We Say Monovision Knowledge Is Also Helpful with Premium IOLs?

Integrating IOL monovision into premium IOL practice is very helpful and essential for successful premium refractive cataract surgery. With the introduction of intermediate range IOLs, such as the Crystalens (Bausch & Lomb) and EDOF Symfony (Johnson & Johnson Vision) Vivity lenses

(Alcon), minimonovision seemed to be essential to enhance the near vision eye. We all sometimes miss the first eye refractive target, especially for post corneal laser vision procedures and when the eyes are very short or very long where effective lens position (ELP) is more difficult to predict. Knowing that crossed monovision may do as well as conventional monovision,[7,15] we can feel very comfortable changing the second eye refractive target to still make the patient happy.

8.19 What Is the Concept of Modified IOL Monovision?

We sometimes can run into a situation where one eye had cataract surgery done long ago with a monofocal IOL and with good uncorrected distance vision (UCDVA) or good uncorrected near vision (UCNVA). Traditional pseudophakic monovision has two main concerns: the near vision eye cannot see far clearly without glasses and there is a compromise for fine depth perception. The impact of depth perception on IOL monovision in daily life is almost negligible,[1] but the distance vision of the near vision eye can be an issue for some patients. (See Case Report 1 in this chapter.) What can we do if such a patient does not want traditional pseudophakic monovision? If the pseudophakic eye has good UCDVA, an EDOF Symfony or Vivity lenses aiming for −0.50 D for the second eye may work well: the near eye can also see far well with much better intermediate and near vision than the distance vision eye.

Even for new patients, once the first eye achieves great UCDVA and compromised UCNVA, but they do not want traditional IOL monovision where the near vision eye is not able to see clearly at distance, this combination seems to work well per our limited recent clinical experience. (See the following Case Report 5.) If the pseudophakic eye had good UCNVA at the −1.00 to −1.50 level, a Crystalens or an EDOF Symfony or Vivity lenses aiming at plano also works well. This is what we call "modified or hybrid IOL monovision." MFIOLs also were reported to work well if the pseudophakic eye has a monofocal IOL with good uncorrected distance vision.[40] This is also our anecdotal experience.

We have tried to avoid using MFIOLs in the dominant eye when the nondominant eye has a monofocal IOL for near, because of our impression that the visual system works better when the dominant distance vision eye has better contrast sensitivity and a sharper image. We have an ongoing prospective study to compare vision, stereopsis, and contrast sensitivity among conventional non-monovision IOL, monofocal monovision IOL, and EDOF Symfony IOL patients.

A Case Report (5): A 31-year-old gentleman with congenital posterior polar cataract OU was referred for cataract surgery in April 2018. His vision was good until about 1 year prior to his presentation when he noticed more and more blurry vision, especially for driving. His distance vision was 20/30 with −3.75 + 3.25 × 115 OD and 20/25 with −4.00 + 3.75 × 64 OS. ▶ Fig. 8.7, ▶ Fig. 8.8, and ▶ Fig. 8.9 shows posterior polar

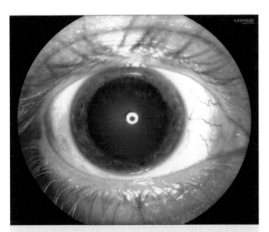

Fig. 8.7 Sharp margin posterior polar cataract OD. (The white dot is a reflection from cornea.)

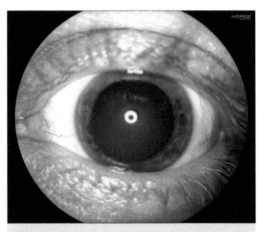

Fig. 8.8 Sharp margin posterior polar cataract OS. (The white dot is a reflection from cornea.)

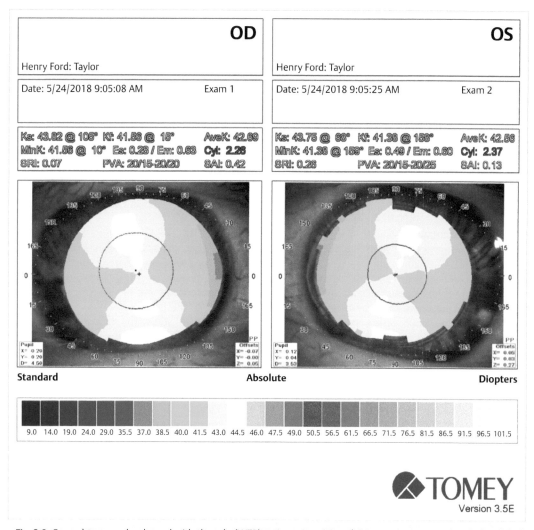

OD

Henry Ford: Taylor

Date: 5/24/2018 9:05:08 AM   Exam 1

Ks: 43.82 @ 105° Kf: 41.56 @ 15°   AveK: 42.69
MinK: 41.56 @ 10° Es: 0.28 / Em: 0.63 Cyl: 2.26
SRI: 0.07   PVA: 20/15-20/20   SAI: 0.42

OS

Henry Ford: Taylor

Date: 5/24/2018 9:05:25 AM   Exam 2

Ks: 43.75 @ 68° Kf: 41.38 @ 158°   AveK: 42.56
MinK: 41.38 @ 158° Es: 0.49 / Em: 0.60 Cyl: 2.37
SRI: 0.28   PVA: 20/15-20/25   SAI: 0.13

Standard   Absolute   Diopters

9.0 14.0 19.0 24.0 29.0 35.5 37.0 38.5 40.0 41.5 43.0 44.5 46.0 47.5 49.0 50.5 56.5 61.5 66.5 71.5 76.5 81.5 86.5 91.5 96.5 101.5

TOMEY
Version 3.5E

Fig. 8.9 Corneal topography showed with-the-rule (WTR) astigmatism OD and OS.

cataract in each eye and corneal topography. OD was his dominant eye with hole-in-card and camera. He desired no glasses for far or near. Good distance vision without glasses was his priority goal. Due to increased risk of posterior capsule rupture from the notoriously fragile posterior polar cataract, he did not want to spend much money for EDOF Symfony lenses (trifocal IOLs were not approved by the FDA in the United States at that time) but he did want to correct astigmatism if possible.

Surgery was done OD in June 2018 without complication with a monofocal toric lens to correct astigmatism. At his 2-week postoperative

visit, UCDVA was 20/20; UCNVA was 20/100. At that time, he complained about difficulty in reading his cell phone with OD alone at 31-year-old. He definitely wanted to have better reading vision and he strongly preferred no glasses for both far and near. He was also a very active hockey player.

We had a lengthy detailed discussion and consultation about what to do for his OS with this active and healthy young gentleman and his wife, who was the manager of our optometry branch in the same building. He did not want to have traditional monofocal IOL monovision due to the downside of compromised uncorrected distance vision of the near vision eye. (Partially influenced by his wife's opinion.) He wanted to have good distance vision and good intermediate vision to cover computer/cell phone and casual reading. He was willing to pay whatever was needed because the first eye went well without posterior capsule rupture. The decision was to use an EDOF Symfony toric lens for OS. The possible side effect of dysphotopsia was fully discussed. OS surgery was done in July 2018 with a ZXT 225 Symfony toric version without complication.

At the 2-month postoperative visit, UCDVA was 20/20^{-2} OD and 20/20^{-2} OS. UCNVA was 20/200 OD and 20/25 OS. He did not have visual problems for driving, watching TV, computer, cell phone, and average size print books. He did not mind using readers for very small print. He did acknowledge the presence of some halo and glare after OS surgery with the Symfony lens, but he did not have much night driving trouble. Early posterior capsular opacification was noticed in his OD due to the lack of capsular polishing intraoperatively because of the fragile posterior polar cataract. Overall, he was very happy, essentially spectacle- and contact lens-free for his daily life. He enjoys his hockey without any depth perception issue (▸ Fig. 8.7, ▸ Fig. 8.8, and ▸ Fig. 8.9).

8.20 Do You Charge Extra for IOL Monovision Patients?

We do not charge extra at our Henry Ford Health System for IOL monovision, but we do have an extra office visit after all the preoperative tests. The main purpose of that visit is to make sure that the patient does not have contraindication for IOL monovision. During the previous office visit, the pupils were dilated when the patients were seated in my examination lane. The cover and uncover test, sometimes 4-D base out prism test if necessary, is best to be performed with undilated pupils. During that office visit, we also analyze all the tests, and detail the patient consultation for the final decision. If astigmatism correction becomes necessary, the cost for LRI/Toric will be billed accordingly. Some of the preoperative tests necessary for IOL monovision are not covered by many insurance companies, such as corneal topography, ocular dominance, cover and uncover test, plus lens tolerance test, etc. Some practices

charge for these tests.[41] You can also consult the Corcoran office at www.corcoranccg.com

References

[1] Zhang F, Sugar A, Barrett GD. Pseudophakic monovision: a clinical guide. New York, NY: Thieme; 2018

[2] ESCRS Clinical Survey 2016. ESCRS. Accessed March 12, 2021. www.eurotimes.org/wp-content/uploads/2017/11/ET22-11_Clinical_Survey_supplement.pdf

[3] ASCRS Database; 2019

[4] Ito M, Shimizu K, Iida Y, Amano R. Five-year clinical study of patients with pseudophakic monovision. J Cataract Refract Surg. 2012; 38(8):1440–1445

[5] Finkelman YM, Ng JQ, Barrett GD. Patient satisfaction and visual function after pseudophakic monovision. J Cataract Refract Surg. 2009; 35(6):998–1002

[6] Zhang F, Sugar A, Jacobsen G, Collins M. Visual function and patient satisfaction: Comparison between bilateral diffractive multifocal intraocular lenses and monovision pseudophakia. J Cataract Refract Surg. 2011; 37(3):446–453

[7] Zhang F, Sugar A, Arbisser L, Jacobsen G, Artico J. Crossed versus conventional pseudophakic monovision: patient satisfaction, visual function, and spectacle independence. J Cataract Refract Surg. 2015; 41(9):1845–1854

[8] Hayashi K, Hayashi H. Stereopsis in bilaterally pseudophakic patients. J Cataract Refract Surg. 2004; 30(7):1466–1470

[9] Gossman M. What intraocular lens would you want in your eyes. EyeWorld 2016;21(7):34. Published July 2016. Accessed March 12, 2021. www.eyeworld.org/what-intraocular-lens-would-you-want-your-eyes

[10] Logothetis HD, Feder RS. Which intraocular lens would ophthalmologists choose for themselves? Eye (Lond). 2019; 33(10):1635–1641

[11] Ito M, Shimizu K, Amano R, Handa T. Assessment of visual performance in pseudophakic monovision. J Cataract Refract Surg. 2009; 35(4):710–714

[12] McDonald JE, Rotramel G. Integrating Monovision into presbyopic intraocular lens surgery. In: Hovanesian JA, ed. Refractive cataract surgery. 2nd ed. Slack Incorporated; 2017:177–188

[13] Jain S, Arora I, Azar DT. Success of monovision in presbyopes: review of the literature and potential applications to refractive surgery. Surv Ophthalmol. 1996; 40(6):491–499

[14] Schor C, Erickson P. Patterns of binocular suppression and accommodation in monovision. Am J Optom Physiol Opt. 1988; 65(11):853–861

[15] Kim J, Shin HJ, Kim HC, Shin KC. Comparison of conventional versus crossed monovision in pseudophakia. Br J Ophthalmol. 2015; 99(3):391–395

[16] Fawcett SL, Herman WK, Alfieri CD, Castleberry KA, Parks MM, Birch EE. Stereoacuity and foveal fusion in adults with long-standing surgical monovision. J AAPOS. 2001; 5(6):342–347

[17] Kushner BJ. Fixation switch diplopia. Arch Ophthalmol. 1995; 113(7):896–899

[18] Parks MM. The monofixation syndrome. Trans Am Ophthalmol Soc. 1969; 67:609–657

[19] Boyd TA, Karas Y, Budd GE, Wyatt HT. Fixation switch diplopia. Can J Ophthalmol. 1974; 9(3):310–315

[20] Evans BJW. Monovision: a review. Ophthalmic Physiol Opt. 2007; 27(5):417–439

[21] Pointer JS. The absence of lateral congruency between sighting dominance and the eye with better visual acuity. Ophthalmic Physiol Opt. 2007; 27(1):106–110

[22] Schwartz R, Yatziv Y. The effect of cataract surgery on ocular dominance. Clin Ophthalmol. 2015; 9:2329–2333

[23] Hayashi K, Ogawa S, Manabe S, Yoshimura K. Binocular visual function of modified pseudophakic monovision. Am J Ophthalmol. 2015; 159(2):232–240

[24] Pardhan S, Gilchrist J. The effect of monocular defocus on binocular contrast sensitivity. Ophthalmic Physiol Opt. 1990; 10(1):33–36

[25] Naeser K, Hjortdal JO, Harris WF. Pseudophakic monovision: optimal distribution of refractions. Acta Ophthalmol. 2014; 92(3):270–275

[26] Duke-Elder S, Abrams D. System of ophthalmology. Vol. 5. C.V. Mosby Co; 1970:505–511

[27] Osher RH, Golnik KC, Barrett G, Shimizu K. Intentional extreme anisometropic pseudophakic monovision: new approach to the cataract patient with longstanding diplopia. J Cataract Refract Surg. 2012; 38(8):1346–1351

[28] Pollard ZF, Greenberg MF, Bordenca M, Elliott J, Hsu V. Strabismus precipitated by monovision. Am J Ophthalmol. 2011; 152(3):479–482

[29] Pratt-Johnson JA, Tilison G. Why does the patient have double vision? Management of strabismus & amblyopia: a practical guide. Thieme Medical Publishers Inc.; 1994:242–246

[30] Pratt-Johnson JA, Wee HS, Ellis S. Suppression associated with esotropia. Can J Ophthalmol. 1967; 2(4):284–291

[31] Richards R. The syndrome of antimetropia and switched fixation in strabismus. Am Orthopt J. 1991; 41:96–101

[32] Weakley DR. The association between anisometropia, amblyopia, and binocularity in the absence of strabismus. Trans Am Ophthalmol Soc. 1999; 97:987–1021

[33] Parks MM. Monovision: The case for two binocular vision systems. The 1999 Gunter K. von Noorden Visiting Professorship Lecture. Binocul Vis Strabismus Q. 2000; 15(1):13–16

[34] Buckley EG. Diplopia after LASIK surgery. In: Balkan RJ, Ellis Jr. G.S., Eustis HS, eds. At the crossings: pediatric ophthalmology and strabismus. Kugler Publications; 2004:55–66

[35] Ruben CM. Unilateral aphakia. Br Orthopt J. 1962; 19:39–60

[36] Pratt-Johnson JA, Tillson G. Intractable diplopia after vision restoration in unilateral cataract. Am J Ophthalmol. 1989; 107(1):23–26

[37] Kieval JZ, Al-Hashimi S, Davidson RS, et al. ASCRS Refractive Cataract Surgery Subcommittee. Prevention and management of refractive prediction errors following cataract surgery. J Cataract Refract Surg. 2020; 46(8):1189–1197

[38] Lindstrom RL. Future looks bright for patients with cataract and their surgeons. Ocular Surgery News. Published January 10, 2021. Accessed March 18, 2021. https://www.healio.com/news/ophthalmology/20210104/future-looks-bright-for-patients-with-cataract-and-their-surgeons

[39] Nakagawara VB, Véronneau SJ. Monovision contact lens use in the aviation environment: a report of a contact lens-related aircraft accident. Optometry. 2000; 71(6):390–395

[40] Ito M, Shimizu K. Pseudophakic monovision. CRSTEurope. Published October 2009. Accessed March 18, 2021. https://crstodayeurope.com/articles/2009-oct/1009_14-php/

[41] McDonald JE, Rotramel G. Integrating monovision into presbyopic intraocular lens surgery. In: Hovanesian JA, ed. Refractive cataract surgery. 2nd ed. Slack Incorporated; 2017:177–188

9 Multifocal Intraocular Lenses

Fuxiang Zhang, Alan Sugar, and Lisa Brothers Arbisser

Abstract

It is not exaggerating to say that the arrival of multifocal intraocular lenses (MFIOLs) was one of the major milestones for refractive cataract surgery. It has helped many patients get rid of their readers, but it has also brought lots of challenges for both patients and surgeons. This chapter will discuss overall patient satisfaction, the main visual and optical tradeoffs of MFIOLs, the strategies used if a patient is not happy with the first eye MFIOL, the impact of aberration profile, central ring size, angle alpha and angle kappa, the neuroadaptation process and reliability, and candidate selections.

Keywords: multifocal IOL, refractive cataract surgery, spherical aberration, angle alpha, angle kappa, dysphotopsia, halo and glare

9.1 What Is the Overall Satisfaction Rate and Spectacle Independence Rate among Patients with Bilateral MFIOL?

The multifocal IOL (MFIOL) is designed with the purpose of improving unaided near vision while minimally impacting distance acuity to reduce overall spectacle dependence. The brain selects the clearest image to process and abhors diplopia, making these strategies tolerable for most. Diffractive technology allows incoming light to split, creating separate distance and near focal points. Because of this separation, patients can see both far and near without conscious awareness of the second image, resulting in a sense of seeing both far and near with high satisfaction for relative spectacle independence.[1,2,3,4] Trifocal lenses have another focus to cover intermediate distance. For example, the AcrySof IQ PanOptix (Alcon) optic diffractive structure divides the incoming light to create a +2.17 D intermediate and a +3.25 D near add power at the IOL plane (representing approximately +1.65 D and +2.35 D at the corneal plane after implantation, respectively, for an average human eye).[5] A 2016 meta-analysis of patients with bilateral multifocal IOLs revealed true spectacle independence in about 80% of patients.[6] Generally speaking, most of these patients are happy or very happy, although some of them do have complaints and the implant explantation rate is not negligible.

9.2 What Are the Main Tradeoffs of MFIOLs and How Do We Decrease the MFIOL Explanation Rate?

- Decreased contrast sensitivity: Diffractive technology inexorably correlates to a loss of some of the light rays, resulting in varying degrees of decreased contrast sensitivity. This is compounded when there is comorbidity already impacting contrast. The diffractive structure causes about 20% light loss with MFIOLs.[7] There is approximately a 30% loss of contrast sensitivity and a decrease of slightly less than one line of best corrected visual acuity (0.1 logMAR) associated with MFIOLs, which is usually from 20/16 to 20/20.[8]
- Dysphotopsia: This is the most common complaint from unhappy patients, especially under low light conditions, much more than decreased contrast, which when symmetric bilaterally is difficult to perceive. Halos/glare and other unwanted photic phenomena have been well documented in the literature, with lots of peer-reviewed studies.
- Increased IOL exchange rate: The number of explanted multifocal IOLs reported through the ASCRS/ESCRS online survey was pretty high, with the vast majority removed because of dysphotopsias.[9] Up to 10% of patients reported that the glare and halos were debilitating, and a varying percentage (up to 7%[10]) of these patients required a lens exchange to correct these symptoms.[1,11] Therefore, our advice is that if a candidate clearly tells you the possibility of IOL exchange is unacceptable, do not choose an MFIOL for that patient. Same day sequential bilateral surgery seems to be becoming more accepted among cataract surgeons, but our concern is that this may not be best for refractive cataract surgery where we often need

to make some adjustment, IOL type as well as IOL power, or even may use different styles of IOLs. (See discussion below.)

- Image gap: There is also an image gap between far and near, which is different from extended depth of focus (EDOF) lenses and trifocal IOLs. The lower add in newer MFIOLs is better in this regard but this worsens the near reading acuity.
- Tradeoff for ophthalmologists: For clarity of retina fundus examination, our impression echoes a study from retina-vitreous surgeons; it is more difficult to view the fundus in patients with MFIOLs than with monofocal IOLs.[12] From that study, we can understand why our patients complain, given that our view from outside to inside mirrors our patients' view from inside to outside. The bottom line is reduced image quality.

Knowing these trade-off features, you will know who to allow to be candidates. Those who hate reading glasses and bifocals are likely to do well, but those for whom night vision is very important, such as taxi and truck drivers, you might counsel with greater caution or better avoid MFIOLs.

9.3 What Should I Do If the Patient Is Not Impressed or Not Happy with the First Eye with an MFIOL?

- Make sure each eye has good potential for MFIOL. Avoid marginal candidates due to comorbidities.
- If the patient is not happy with the first eye outcome, nail down the etiology and fix it before further decisions, including the decision for the second eye.
- Suboptimal vision is often due to missing the refraction target and/or residual astigmatism. Laser vision correction or manual limbal relaxing incision (LRI) may be needed for enhancement. A short period of spectacle or contact lens trial is beneficial to find out the reason why the patient is not impressed or not happy. With the refraction correction, if the patient is still not happy, then enhancement will not help.
- It is relatively easy to find posterior capsular opacification (PCO), cystoid macular edema (CME), etc., but it may be a challenge to find irregular astigmatism and residual refractive abnormally. Refraction and manifest can be critical here.

- If the complaint is mainly about nighttime dysphotopsia with good vision far and near, and if the complaint is mild, then there are two common options. One is to offer the fellow eye with the same company's monofocal IOL aiming for emmetropia. This method may work well, especially if the monofocal IOL eye is the dominant eye. In a modified monovision model, a computer-based simulation study also suggested that this kind of modified monovision combination was doing better than adding spherical aberration to the near eye combination model.[13] The patient may appreciate the MFIOL eye for better reading when compared to the monofocal IOL eye. The other option is to offer the fellow eye the same MFIOL (or with lower add power). Bilateral MFIOL is expected to be better for neuroadaptation. Chair time is needed to explain that the vast majority of the time patients are happier with the MFIOL bilaterally where the brain can more easily tune out noise and tune in the information than with the new visual system in just one eye which invites comparison and delays the process of "neuroadaptation." The trouble however is that there is no guarantee; they might not work, then you are faced with the desire to exchange both lenses!
- If the patient tells you the dysphotopsia is not acceptable, even with great vision and an optimal ocular condition after a few weeks of waiting, do not put the same IOL in the second eye. The only option will likely be explantation, although it does not hurt to postpone the IOL exchange until after the fellow eye receives a monofocal IOL. Sometimes, patients can change their mind after second eye surgery, especially when they realize the better unaided reading from the MFIOL eye.
- Fully explain the consequence of spectacle dependence before IOL exchange.

9.4 What Do the MFIOL Add Powers Mean to You and to Your Patients?

- Not all MFIOLs behave the same way. Different add powers have different near focal lengths. We will not discuss refractive MFIOLs such as the ReZoom which is essentially defunct.

- The ReSTOR (Alcon) aspheric 4.0 lens has a near focus around 33 to 35 cm (about 13–14 inches).
- With the ReSTOR 3.0 lens the near focus is around 44 cm (about 17 inches).
- The newer version ReSTOR +2.5 has the near vision focus around 50 cm (about 20 inches).
- The Tecnis ZMB00 +4.0 (Johnson & Johnson) has the near focus around 35 to 37 cm (14–15 inches).
- The ZLB00 +3.25 near focus is around 44 to 45 cm (about 17–18 inches).
- The ZKB00 +2.75 near focus is around 48 to 50 cm (about 19–20 inches).

Where do these numbers come from? Math formulas do not fit if we use focal length formulas at the IOL plane. As we all know the optic formula:

Near focal length (centimeters) = 100/lens power in diopters.

Apparently, the focal lengths of our MFIOLs given by our manufacturers are not calculated from the IOL plane, but at the spectacle plane. For example, with the ReSTOR 4.0 add, the add power at the IOL plane is 4.0 D. The effective add power of the lens at the spectacle plane is ~3.0 D.

So using our formula below:

$$100/4.0 \text{ D} = 25 \text{ cm}$$

This is calculated at the IOL plane which is not accurate when relating to the visual distance for the patient where the vertex distance must be considered.

If we calculate with the formula using the add power at the spectacle plane it would be:

$$100/3.0 \text{ D} = 33 \text{ cm}$$

The point we want to make here is to let our residents know that we need to be familiar with these approximations, not necessarily to memorize the numbers. Dysphotopsia and contrast loss are a sort of parallel to the add power and that is the reason why lower newer power versions are better tolerated. By the same token, they provide less magnification for near work.

Now, what do these numbers mean to our patients? Consider patient height, arm length, and reading posture habits when choosing add power. Ask the patient to demonstrate his/her reading posture with the desired reading distance. This is one of the most easily missed items, but avoidable if we pay attention to it. If you miss this factor, you may find them not quite happy postoperatively. A fisherman tying flies at dawn will require

a higher add while a musician wanting to see the score at full arm's length as well as the conductor will need a lower add MFIOL. The former needs to know she won't be able to read the computer text on their desktop unless she adjusts the reading distance but the latter won't be able to read fine print. This is why many surgeons choose to mix and match since we have the opportunity to blend bilateral functions.

9.5 Pay Attention to the Aberration Profile

Minimal attention has been paid to aberration profiles for MFIOL patients until the past few years. Patients with significant higher order aberrations (HOA) may be poor candidates for MFIOLs. Studies have shown that spherical aberration has the strongest impact on MFIOL image quality when typical pseudophakic corneal HOAs are present.[14] Higher order aberrations are not currently correctable with glasses while lower order aberrations, such as sphere, cylinder, and prism, are correctable with glasses. Refractive index shaping and refractive indexing are other possible future solutions.

Due to its high refractive power, the cornea is a known primary contributor to HOAs. At a typical 6-mm pupillary diameter, the cornea contributes about +0.274-μm spherical aberration (SA), based on which −0.20 μm spherical correction was built in some of the AcrySof IQ lens series to compensate positive corneal SA.[15] Another study of 228 eyes of 134 patients with refractive surgery and cataract patients with mean age 50 years ±17 (SD) demonstrated that the mean coefficient of the 4th-order spherical aberration (SA) of anterior cornea was 0.281 ± 0.086 μm.[16]

Positive spherical aberrations can compromise retinal image quality and cause glare and halo.[17] The McCormick study[18] also found that symptomatic postoperative laser refractive surgery patients with irregular corneas had higher order aberrations that were 2.3 times greater than asymptomatic postoperative LASIK patients and 3.5 times greater than normal preoperative eyes. Patients above 0.75 μm of higher order aberration are believed to be poor candidates for MFIOLs because they would have an additional reduction in the optical quality of their retinal image.[19] You can use iTrace (Tracey) and Galilei (Ziemer) to measure HOA. The Atlas (Zeiss) topographer also provides this information. Clinically important higher order aberration items include spherical aberration, coma, and trefoil. Our clinical cutoffs for MFIOL are spherical aberration <0.6 and coma <0.3 μm when we use the Atlas topographer (Zeiss).

The evolution of wavefront analysis technology has contributed significantly to the understanding and management of the eye's aberration for planning premium IOLs, but compared to other elements, such as axial length and corneal refractive power measurements, wavefront measurement is still in an early stage. A study by Piccinini et al[20] compared two commonly used devices, a Scheimpflug image system (Pentacam HR) and dual Scheimpflug-Placido imaging system (Galilei G4) with measurement of HOAs in normal eyes (105 eyes of 105 patients). They concluded that the Pentacam HR and the Galilei G4 produced significantly different values for all HOAs evaluated except for spherical aberration; however, correlations between devices were moderate to strong. The lack of optimal agreement between devices could be significant in research reports that use HOAs as endpoint measures for diagnostic or therapeutic purposes. Other studies that evaluated the agreement in HOA measurements between devices based on different technologies also found they are not interchangeable but are often reasonably well correlated.[21,22] The lesson to draw from this is to stick with one technology for this purpose.

Most virgin eyes do not seem to have issues of HOAs in the decision making for premium IOLs. It becomes essential for those patients who have had corneal refractive surgery. See more discussion in Chapter 19, Refractive Cataract Surgery for Patients with History of Keratorefractive Surgery (LASIK/PRK/RK).

9.6 What Does the Center Ring Size Mean?

The diameter of the center ring is also important for patient selection. The ReSTOR (Alcon) + 3.0 has 0.86 mm[23] and + 2.50 has 0.938 mm.[24] The central ring size for the Tecnis ZMB00 + 4.0 is 1.0 mm; ZLB00 + 3.25 is 1.2 mm; and ZKB00 + 2.75 is 1.3 mm. The center optic is largest on the Symfony as 1.6 mm.[25] The size of the central ring is related with the add power which is further related with the number of rings. The higher the add power, the more rings will be needed and the smaller the central ring diameter.[26] A large central ring is more forgiving for borderline angle alpha and

angle kappa. We need to be cautious when we consider MFIOL if the angle alpha or angle kappa is more than 0.5 mm. Nudging the one-piece MFIOL a bit nasally by the end of surgery is believed to be beneficial to better align the optic center of the IOL to the visual axis. From this perspective, an MFIOL with a large central ring size can be more forgiving.

Moshirfar and colleagues suggested that an MFIOL is unacceptable for use if the angle K-value is greater than half of the diameter of the central optical zone.[27] Based on this hypothesis, the ReSTOR (Alcon) would have a tolerance for an angle K-value around 0.4 mm, Tecnis MFIOL (Johnson & Johnson) around 0.5 mm, and FineVision (PhysIOL) around 0.6 mm.[28]

9.7 What Are Angle Alpha and Angle Kappa and How to Measure Them?

The angle between the pupil center and visual axis is called angle kappa, while the angle between the optical center of the cornea and the visual axis is called angle alpha. It can be difficult to physically measure them in a clinical setting as degrees, but some corneal topographers and biometers automatically calculate the angle kappa by software using the distance between the center of the pupil and the center of the Placido ring reflection on the cornea as a chord length.[28] When angle kappa is not automatically measured by automated topography instruments, the distance between the corneal vertex and pupil center (X and Y Cartesian values) can also be used to estimate angle kappa. Pentacam (Oculus, Wetzlar, Germany) and Atlas 9000 (Carl Zeiss Meditec, Jena, Germany) display X–Y Cartesian coordinates between the corneal vertex and pupil center. The cornea vertex is the point of maximum elevation when viewing the target.[29]

The total angle kappa can be mathematically calculated. It is the square root of the sum of the squares of the x and y values (Pythagorean theorem). Clinically, the sum of x and y should be close enough for clinical estimation.[30] Angle alpha and angle kappa were both predominantly located temporal to the visual axis.[31] (See Cartesian point locations in ▶ Fig. 9.1 IOLMaster 700 Px and Py; ▶ Fig. 9.2 Lenstar Pcx and Pcy; ▶ Fig. 9.3 Atlas Pup center ▶ Fig. 9.4, iTrace. Also see schematic

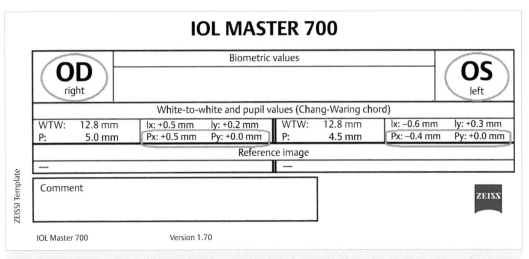

Fig. 9.1 Cartesian point location for angle kappa measurement from IOLMaster 700. Used with permission from Zeiss.

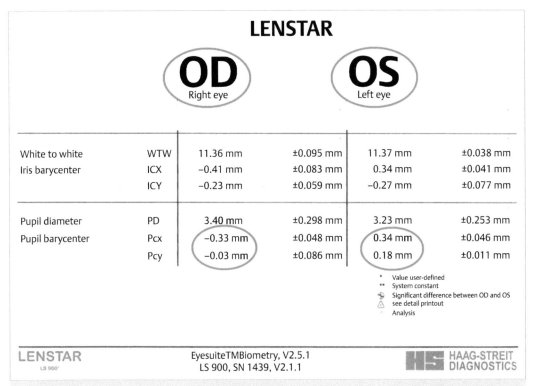

Fig. 9.2 Cartesian point location for angle kappa measurement from LenStar. Used with permission from Haag-Streit.

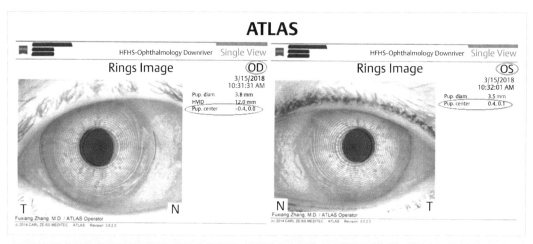

Fig. 9.3 Cartesian point location for angle kappa measurement from Atlas. Used with permission from Zeiss.

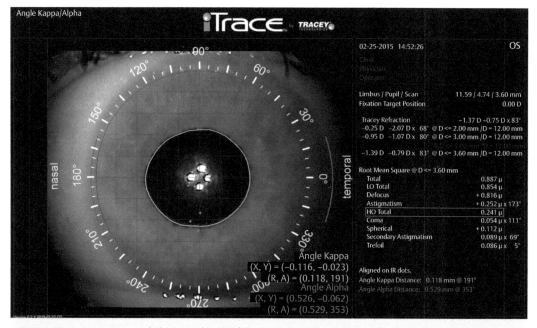

Fig. 9.4 iTrace to measure angle kappa and angle alpha, as well as spherical aberration and coma. Used with permission from iTrace.

drawings in ▶ Fig. 9.5, ▶ Fig. 9.6, ▶ Fig. 9.7, and ▶ Fig. 9.8).

A large angle kappa can lead to suboptimal outcomes and photic phenomena in MFIOL patients.[29,32,33,34] Holladay reported that 0.6 mm or higher will have more chance of subjective complaints of halo and glare even if the MFIOL is centered properly.[30] Donders cited the distribution of angle kappa in the normal population, 5.1 degrees (range from 3.5 to 6.0) in emmetropic eyes, from 6.0 to 9.0 in hyperopic eyes, and averaging approximately 2.0 degrees in myopic eyes.[29] This may explain why hyperopic patients have more asthenopia complaints when reading than

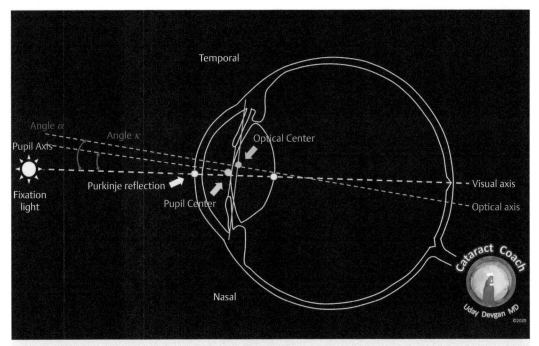

Fig. 9.5 Angle alpha is the distance between the visual axis and the optical center. It is a common practice to nudge a one-piece multifocal intraocular lens (MFIOL) a bit nasally to have the IOL central ring align with the visual axis. Used with permission from Uday Devgan, MD. Image © 2021 by Uday Devgan MD/CataractCoach.com.

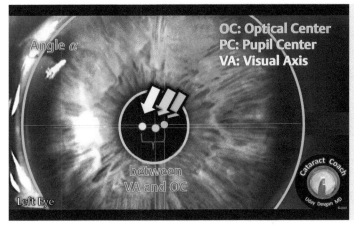

Fig. 9.6 Schematic drawing of angle alpha. Used with permission from Uday Devgan, MD. Image © 2021 by Uday Devgan MD/CataractCoach.com.

myopes in addition to their greater demand for accommodation. Our experiences do not suggest, however, that hyperopic patients are not good candidates for refractive cataract surgery. A study by Qi et al noted more glare and halo in patients implanted with the AT LISA trifocal IOL when angle kappa cord length was greater than 0.4 mm

and visual quality reduction when the cord length was greater than 0.5 mm.[35] It is not hard to understand the rationale, because a large angle kappa means the pupillary axis and visual axis are simply too far apart for comfort.

The measurement of angle alpha may not be as precise, because the limbus is not completely visi-

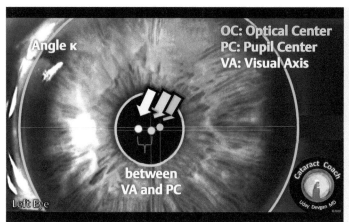

Fig. 9.7 Schematic drawing of angle kappa. Used with permission from Uday Devgan, MD. Image © 2021 by Uday Devgan MD/CataractCoach.com.

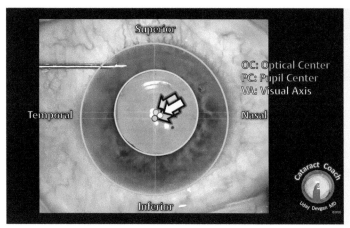

Fig. 9.8 Good candidate for multifocal intraocular lens (MFIOL) because of small angle alpha and small angle kappa. Used with permission from Uday Devgan, MD. Image © 2021 by UdayDevganMD/CataractCoach.com.

bly distinguishable or consistently in most images, but iTrace (Tracey Technologies) and the OPD-III (Marco) are reportedly able to provide a good measurement for angle alpha (▶ Fig. 9.4).

Ideally, the diffractive rings to be concentric with the pupil and lined up with the visual axis so the optic center, the pupil center, and the visual axis are all tightly placed in the same center of the inner ring of the lens optic. Those patients with small angle alpha and angle kappa are better candidates for MFIOL and trifocal IOLs. The ideal location for an IOL in the rare eye with zero angle kappa is to be centered at the visual axis and the pupil center simultaneously. For the average eye however, the optimal placement is centered between the pupil center and the visual axis (▶ Fig. 9.6, ▶ Fig. 9.7, and ▶ Fig. 9.8). This is why

many surgeons routinely nudge the IOL a bit to the nasal side when using a one-piece MFIOL. This is the most commonly used way to have the optic center align with the visual axis. Better centration can be achieved by using the Purkinje reflex to center the capsulorhexis (most reliably with the Zepto Precision Capsule device—Mynosys Cellular Devices, Inc.) while the topical anesthesia patient fixates on the microscope and the surgeon manually positions the suction device accordingly. Femtosecond laser-assisted cataract surgery possibly provides extra value.

Based on 15,127 eyes of 15,127 cataract patients tested by IOLMaster 700 (Carl Zeiss Meditec AG, Germany), a study[31] revealed that the mean angle alpha and angle kappa values were 0.45 ± 0.21 mm and 0.30 ± 0.18 mm, respectively.

(Also see ▸ Fig. 9.6 and ▸ Fig. 9.7 for schematic presentation.) A greater angle alpha or angle kappa was associated with older age, lower corneal power, shorter white-to-white distance, and shallower anterior chamber depth (all $p < 0.05$). Angle alpha correlated positively with angle kappa. With increasing axial length, angle alpha gradually decreased in a nonlinear way and shifted to the nasal side of the visual axis, whereas angle kappa decreased in eyes with axial length <27.5 mm but increased again in eyes with longer axial length.[31]

Optically, pupil is just an aperture which does not always have the correlation with visual axis, meaning angle alpha should have more impact on image quality than angle kappa. Almost all in-the-bag PCIOLs are designed to have symmetric, self-centering haptics that center naturally within the capsular bag. Because of that, preoperative measurement of angle alpha likely will predict postoperative IOL centration relative to the visual axis, assuming that the center of the capsular bag has better correlation with the optic center than the pupil center. A study at Mayo[36] measured 11,871 eyes with iTrace (Tracey Technologies) wavefront aberrometer/corneal topographer angle alpha (both preoperative and pseudophakic) and provided very useful data. For the 3382 unique patients, the mean angle alpha magnitude was 0.44 ± 0.15 mm (median was also 0.44 mm, 25th and 75th percentiles 0.34 mm, 0.53 mm). Angle alpha orientation was predominantly horizontal with a mean of 186 ± 32 degrees of those 3382 right eyes at front-back anterior view. The expected point of IOL centration based on the geometric center of the corneal limbus was temporal to the visual axis in 3212 eyes (95%), nasal in 92 eyes (2.7%), inferior in 56 eyes (1.7%), and superior in 22 eyes (0.6%). The take-home message from this large-scale study is that the estimated IOL position relative to the visual axis is shifted about 0.44 mm temporally in 95% of cataract population eyes and if using 0.5 mm as cutoff limit would potentially exclude 32% of eyes from multifocal IOLs implantation.

In terms of preoperative measurement, there is still a lack of standard measurement of angle kappa. We do not believe it is interchangeable among most measurements. The above two studies[31,36] with large sample cases also suggest that measurements may not be interchangeable.

9.8 How Much Residual Astigmatism Can MFIOLs Tolerate?

Unlike monofocal IOLs, MFIOLs cannot tolerate much residual astigmatism. A study on through-focus image quality showed that MFIOLs had the most severe decline in depth of focus from corneal astigmatism when compared with several other monofocal IOLs.[14] Knowing this, one should not attempt to use MFIOLs if not competent to manage cylinders.

How much postoperative residual astigmatism is acceptable in order to have an MFIOL work? There are lots of studies in the literature in this regard. Berdahl and others stated that if the residual corneal astigmatism in an eye implanted with an MFIOL is more than 0.50 D, it is less likely to meet the expectations in these patients.[37] Per the ASCRS Cataract Clinical committee, "Astigmatism management is vital to the performance of multifocal IOLs. A rule of thumb is that these IOLs perform best with less than three-quarters of a diopter (D) of cylinder. Beyond this, the image may degrade below satisfactory levels to achieve proper visual function."[38] Our experience also suggests the same. A study from Hayashi et al[39] clearly demonstrated the negative impact of astigmatism on MFIOLs; as the simulated astigmatism power increased, the vision in all distances decreased. Based on 17,152 dominant eyes of 17,152 patients, a retrospective study by Schallhorn and associates revealed that compared to eyes with 0.0 D residual astigmatism, the odds of not achieving 20/20 vision in eyes with 0.25- to 0.50-D residual astigmatism increased by a factor of 1.7 and 1.9 ($p < 0.0001$) in monofocal and multifocal IOLs, respectively. For the residual astigmatism 0.75 to 1.00 D, the odds ratio for not achieving 20/20 vision compared to eyes with no astigmatism was 6.1 for monofocal and 6.5 for multifocal IOLs ($p < 0.0001$).[40] The orientation of astigmatism was not a significant predictor in multivariate analysis.

In the presence of regular corneal astigmatism, it is always preferable to use the toric version of the MFIOL, such as ActiveFocus (Alcon) or ZXT serial toric IOLs (Johnson & Johnson). It is true that use of a toric version MFIOL takes a longer OR time to get NRR (No rotation recommended) than a simple LRI, but you will be happier to see the almost forever lasting effect of toricity correction. Consider LRI, either manual or with FLACS, only if astigmatism is less than the lowest toric version of the MFIOL.

9.9 Do You Use ReSTOR and/or Symfony IOLs to Augment Near Vision?

Yes, if one eye is already at plano with a monofocal IOL, we can put an MFIOL or Symfony IOL in the second eye if the patient desires to have better near vision but still wants to have good distance vision. This is the concept of revised or hybrid IOL monovision as we discussed in Chapter 8. Some monofocal IOL monovision patients have complaints of not seeing well for far with the near vision eye.

9.10 If You Are Implanting an MFIOL Bilaterally, Do You Aim for Slightly Different Refractive Targets?

For MFIOLs and trifocal IOLs, usually it is better to target plano in each eye. If you are forced to choose a little minus versus a little plus, it is better to pick a little minus. It is very common to apply mini monovision in bilateral EDOF Symfony IOLs. The nondominant eye target of −0.50 to −0.75 D is well tolerated and helps unaided binocular acuity at near. We don't advise risking −1.0 D or more, as the vision quality of that eye suffers due to the image falling in front of retina due to too much myopic defocus causing more halo. Though the defocus curve in ▶ Fig. 9.9 implies up to 1.50 defocus, and still allows 20/20 acuity, our practical experience says otherwise (▶ Fig. 9.9).

9.11 Is Neuroadaptation Real and How Reliable Is It?

Neuroadaptation is a process in which our brain reacts to a sensory input by adapting to a change, habituating to a foreign stimulus by tuning out the noise and tuning in the useful information. How does the brain react when suddenly experiencing something which is quite different from our "normal pattern" such as the MFIOL handling of light rays? It is very complicated to explore this question, but we have all probably experienced a common phenomenon like background noise or smell which, after a certain period of time, fades into unawareness and is ignored. The young person's nervous system is likely more plastic and adjustable to disturbing sensory inputs than an adult. Neuroadaptation can occur within the visual system as well as in response to visual disturbances. The challenge is the fact that this kind of neuroplasticity decays with aging,[41,42] and we just cannot and should not expect all of our patients will have that capability, especially among perfectionists.

A recent study[43] with functional MRI (fMRI) demonstrated recruitment of visual attentional

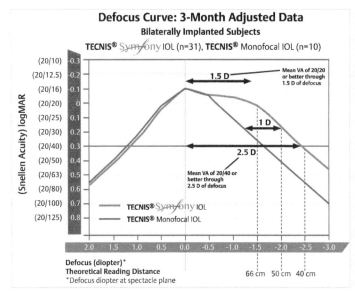

Fig. 9.9 Defocus curve comparison Tecnis Symfony versus Tecnis monofocal intraocular lens (IOL). The Tecnis Symfony IOL has better tolerance than Tecnis monofocal IOL in terms of the level of defocus. Used with permission from Johnson & Johnson Vision.

and procedural learning networks of the human brain. Long-term adaptation/functional plasticity leads to brain activity regularization toward a non-effort pattern by 6 months postoperatively. Those changes were not visible in age-matched and sex-matched control groups. This fMRI adaptation change was associated with an improvement in symptoms, visual acuity, and contrast detection.

Beyond neuroplasticity another explanation for patient acceptance of suboptimal visual phenomena is the obvious fact that the postoperative outcome with any lens is typically better than preoperative cataractous acuity. This does not apply, of course, to clear lens exchange patients.

Luckily, most cataract surgical patients are happy regardless of what kind of IOLs they receive. The nature of humans to tolerate imperfection when the alternative involves risk (IOL exchange) plays a role in ultimate satisfaction as well. For a given patient, it may be hard to tell if it is a real neuro-adaptation or neurosurrender.

9.12 Who Can be Good Candidates for the First Few Cases of MFIOLs?

See ► Table 9.1 and ► Fig. 9.10 and ► Fig. 9.11.

Table 9.1 Candidate selection decision for MFIOLs

	Good candidate	Try to avoid[a]
History	Loved multifocal contact lens	Successful happy LASIK/PRK or contact lens IOL monovision
Lifestyle and occupations	Occasional or rare driving at night	Truck and taxi drivers, pilots
Motivation	Strong desire not to have readers	Readers do not bother me
Personality	Easy going	Hypercritical with type A personality; if s/he already asked dozens of questions in writing on the survey sheet, you know you are dealing with a perfectionist
Refractive status	Hyperopia, never been able to read well without readers	Always had great near vision without any glasses Biometry may not be very accurate for axial length measurement in very long myopic eyes, especially when a staphyloma is present
Distance vision quality	Not critical: "I will be happy as long as I do not have to wear glasses"	Obsessive about crisp distance vision with many pairs of glasses each visit
Ocular surface with Placido images	Clear with smooth rings (► Fig. 9.10)	Severe dry eye, MGD, EBMD, Placido ring not clear with irregular changes (► Fig. 9.11)
Zonules and capsular bag	Healthy	Weak zonules/pseudoexfoliation. May not do well due to IOL shift
Optic nerve	Healthy	Any history of optic nerve disorder will further decrease contrast
Macula	A normal OCT macula is needed	It is not advisable to put MFIOL in a patient with noticeable maculopathy
Astigmatism	Less than 0.50 D	0.50 D or more unless correctable; irregular astigmatism
Spherical aberration	<0.6 μm	0.6 μm or more

(*Continued*)

Table 9.1 (*Continued*) Candidate selection decision for MFIOLs

	Good candidate	Try to avoid[a]
Coma	<0.3 µm	0.3 µm or more
Mesopic pupil size	3–5 mm	2.5 mm or less may be too small to have good reading vision; 5.5 mm or more will have more chance of glare/halo
Angle Kappa	<0.6 mm	0.6 mm or more
Angle Alpha	<0.6 mm	0.6 mm or more

Abbreviations: EBMD, epithelial basement membrane dystrophy; IOL, intraocular lens; MFIOL, multifocal intraocular lens; MGD, meibomian gland dysfunction; OCT, optical coherence tomography.
[a] Some of the contents in this column under "Try to Avoid" belong to contraindications, not just to avoid for the first few patients for residents and beginners.

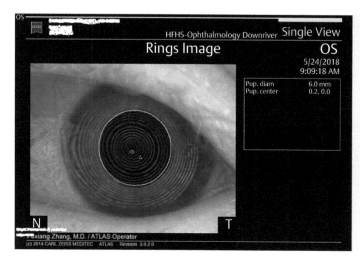

Fig. 9.10 Clean and regular Placido image rings. Good candidate for premium intraocular lens (IOL).

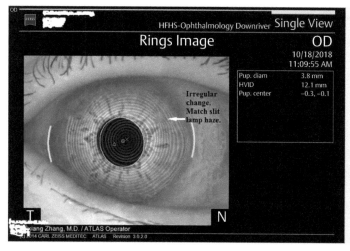

Fig. 9.11 Irregular changes as noted with *white arrow* on Placido ring image. Not good candidate for multifocal intraocular lens (MFIOL).

References

[1] Wilkins MR, Allan BD, Rubin GS, et al. Moorfields IOL Study Group. Randomized trial of multifocal intraocular lenses versus monovision after bilateral cataract surgery. Ophthalmology. 2013; 120(12):2449–2455.e1

[2] Zhang F, Sugar A, Jacobsen G, Collins M. Visual function and patient satisfaction: comparison between bilateral diffractive multifocal intraocular lenses and monovision pseudophakia. J Cataract Refract Surg. 2011; 37(3):446–453

[3] Labiris G, Giarmoukakis A, Patsiamanidi M, Papadopoulos Z, Kozobolis VP. Mini-monovision versus multifocal intraocular lens implantation. J Cataract Refract Surg. 2015; 41(1):53–57

[4] Packer M, Chu YR, Waltz KL, et al. Evaluation of the aspheric tecnis multifocal intraocular lens: one-year results from the first cohort of the food and drug administration clinical trial. Am J Ophthalmol. 2010; 149(4):577–584.e1

[5] Summary of Safety and Effectiveness Data (SSED). U.S. Food and Drug Administration. PMA P040020/S087. https://www.accessdata.fda.gov/cdrh_docs/pdf4/P040020S087B.pdf

[6] Greenstein S, Pineda R, II. The quest for spectacle independence: a comparison of multifocal intraocular lens implants and pseudophakic monovision for patients with presbyopia. Semin Ophthalmol. 2017; 32(1):111–115

[7] Findl O. Intraocular lens materials and design. In: Colvard DM, ed. Achieving excellence in cataract surgery: a step-by-step approach. Self-Published; 2009:95–108

[8] Holladay JT. Multifocal IOLs: patient selection and optical performance. Healio: Ocular Surgery News. Published online January 31, 2017. Published in print February 10, 2017. Accessed January 5, 2021. https://www.healio.com/news/ophthalmology/20170125/multifocal-iols-patient-selection-and-optical-performance

[9] Chang DH. Interview: low-add multifocal and extended depth-of-focus IOLs. Cataract 360. 2016; 1(4):11–14

[10] Kim EJ, Sajjad A, Montes de Oca I, et al. Refractive outcomes after multifocal intraocular lens exchange. J Cataract Refract Surg. 2017; 43(6):761–766

[11] de Vries NE, Webers CA, Touwslager WR, et al. Dissatisfaction after implantation of multifocal intraocular lenses. J Cataract Refract Surg. 2011; 37(5):859–865

[12] Bhavsar AR. Do multifocal optics compromise retinal treatment? In: Chang DF, ed. Mastering refractive IOLs. Slack Incorporated; 2008:866–869

[13] de Gracia P. Optical properties of monovision corrections using multifocal designs for near vision. J Cataract Refract Surg. 2016; 42(10):1501–1510

[14] Zheleznyak L, Kim MJ, MacRae S, Yoon G. Impact of corneal aberrations on through-focus image quality of presbyopia-correcting intraocular lenses using an adaptive optics bench system. J Cataract Refract Surg. 2012; 38(10):1724–1733

[15] Karakelle M. The science behind the AcrySof IQ. Cataract Refract Surg Today. 2018:4–5

[16] Wang L, Dai E, Koch DD, Nathoo A. Optical aberrations of the human anterior cornea. J Cataract Refract Surg. 2003; 29(8):1514–1521

[17] Holladay JT, Piers PA, Koranyi G, van der Mooren M, Norrby NE. A new intraocular lens design to reduce spherical aberration of pseudophakic eyes. J Refract Surg. 2002; 18(6):683–691

[18] McCormick GJ, Porter J, Cox IG, MacRae S. Higher-order aberrations in eyes with irregular corneas after laser refractive surgery. Ophthalmology. 2005; 112(10):1699–1709

[19] Holladay JT. Small aperture IOLs will be helpful in patients with significant corneal higher-order aberrations. Ocular Surgical News. 2018:32–33

[20] Piccinini AL, Golan O, Hafezi F, Randleman JB. Higher-order aberration measurements: comparison between Scheimpflug and dual Scheimpflug-Placido technology in normal eyes. J Cataract Refract Surg. 2019; 45(4):490–494

[21] Xu Z, Hua Y, Qiu W, Li G, Wu Q. Precision and agreement of higher order aberrations measured with ray tracing and Hartmann-Shack aberrometers. BMC Ophthalmol. 2018; 18(1):18

[22] Hao J, Li L, Tian F, Zhang H. Comparison of two types of visual quality analyzer for the measurement of high order aberrations. Int J Ophthalmol. 2016; 9(2):292–297

[23] Fisher BL. Presbyopia-correcting intraocular lenses in cataract surgery: a focus on ReSTOR intraocular lenses. US Ophthalmic Rev. 2011; 4(1):44–48

[24] Hovanesian JA. The family of AcrySof IQ IOLs helps us customize the approach to vision correction. Cataract Refractive Surgery Today. Accessed April 29, 2021. https://crstoday.com/articles/my-journey-to-activefocus-optical-design-2019-jan/the-family-of-acrysof-iq-iols-helps-us-customize-the-approach-to-vision-correction-2/

[25] Millán MS, Vega F. Extended depth of focus intraocular lens: Chromatic performance. Biomed Opt Express. 2017; 8(9):4294–4309

[26] Cohen AL. Diffractive bifocal lens designs. Optom Vis Sci. 1993; 70(6):461–468

[27] Moshirfar M, Hoggan RN, Muthappan V. Angle Kappa and its importance in refractive surgery. Oman J Ophthalmol. 2013; 6(3):151–158

[28] Garzón N, García-Montero M, López-Artero E, et al. Influence of angle κ on visual and refractive outcomes after implantation of a diffractive trifocal intraocular lens. J Cataract Refract Surg. 2020; 46(5):721–727

[29] Park CY, Oh SY, Chuck RS. Measurement of angle kappa and centration in refractive surgery. Curr Opin Ophthalmol. 2012; 23(4):269–275

[30] Holladay JT. Premium IOL centration and patient suitability. Healio: Ocular Surgery News. Published online July 8, 2016. Published in print July 10, 2016. Accessed January 6, 2021. https://www.healio.com/news/ophthalmology/20160708/premium-iol-centration-and-patient-suitability

[31] Meng J, Du Y, Wei L, et al. Distribution of angle alpha and angle kappa in a population with cataract in Shanghai. J Cataract Refract Surg. Published ahead of print online November 19, 2020. DOI: 10.1097/j.jcrs.0000000000000490

[32] Sachdev GS, Sachdev M. Optimizing outcomes with multifocal intraocular lenses. Indian J Ophthalmol. 2017; 65(12):1294–1300

[33] Karhanová M, Marešová K, Pluháček F, Mlčák P, Vláčil O, Šín M. [The importance of angle kappa for centration of multifocal intraocular lenses]. Cesk Slov Oftalmol. 2013; 69(2):64–68

[34] Prakash G, Prakash DR, Agarwal A, Kumar DA, Agarwal A, Jacob S. Predictive factor and kappa angle analysis for visual satisfactions in patients with multifocal IOL implantation. Eye (Lond). 2011; 25(9):1187–1193

[35] Qi Y, Lin J, Leng L, et al. Role of angle κ in visual quality in patients with a trifocal diffractive intraocular lens. J Cataract Refract Surg. 2018; 44(8):949–954

[36] Mahr MA, Simpson MJ, Erie JC. Angle alpha orientation and magnitude distribution in a cataract surgery population. J Cataract Refract Surg. 2020; 46(3):372–377

[37] Berdahl JP, Hardten DR, Kramer BA, Potvin R. Effect of astigmatism on visual acuity after multifocal versus monofocal intraocular lens implantation. J Cataract Refract Surg. 2018; 44(10):1192–1197

[38] Braga-Mele R, Chang D, Dewey S, et al. ASCRS Cataract Clinical Committee. Multifocal intraocular lenses: relative indications and contraindications for implantation. J Cataract Refract Surg. 2014; 40(2):313–322

[39] Hayashi K, Manabe S, Yoshida M, Hayashi H. Effect of astigmatism on visual acuity in eyes with a diffractive multifocal intraocular lens. J Cataract Refract Surg. 2010; 36(8):1323–1329

[40] Schallhorn S, Hettinger KA, Pelouskova M, et al. Effect of residual astigmatism on uncorrected visual acuity and patient satisfaction in pseudophakic patients. J Cataract Refract Surg. Published ahead of print online December 18, 2020. DOI: 10.1097/j.jcrs.0000000000000560

[41] Kershner RM. Neuroadaptation. In: Chang DF, ed. Mastering refractive IOLs: the art and science. Thorofare, NJ: SLACK, Inc.; 2008:302–304

[42] Alió JL, Pikkel J. Neuroadaptation. In: Alió JL, Pikkel J, eds. Multifocal intraocular lenses: the art and practice. Cham: Springer; 2014:47–52

[43] Rosa AM, Miranda AC, Patrício MM, et al. Functional magnetic resonance imaging to assess neuroadaptation to multifocal intraocular lenses. J Cataract Refract Surg. 20 17; 43 (10):1287–1296

10 Accommodating Intraocular Lenses

Fuxiang Zhang, Alan Sugar, and Lisa Brothers Arbisser

Abstract

Crystalens and Trulign lenses are the only FDA-approved accommodating intraocular lenses (IOLs) in the United States. This chapter discusses their unique role in the refractive cataract surgery spectrum and also the possible reasons why there are some variations of refractive outcomes. Necessary surgical steps to improve success rate are reviewed. Pearls and pitfalls, clinical features, as well as candidate selections are discussed.

Keywords: crystalens, Trulign, accommodating IOL, refractive cataract surgery

10.1 Introduction

Currently the Crystalens and its toric version Trulign (Bausch & Lomb, Inc., Rochester, New York) are the only intraocular lenses (IOLs) approved by the FDA as accommodating IOLs. The third-generation advanced optics (AO) model has an aspheric design. Astigmatism correction is integral to the Trulign lens; otherwise, the two lenses share similar characteristics in terms of appearance, structure, and mechanism (▶ Fig. 10.1 and ▶ Fig. 10.2).

10.2 Do Crystalens and Trulign Still Have Any Roles in Refractive Cataract Surgery?

Since the availability of newer premium IOLs, such as the extended depth of focus (EDOF) and trifocal, the Crystalens and Trulign lenses have become less popular.[1] A 2018 survey[2] in *Review of Ophthalmology* noted a very low market share for the Crystalens: the Technis Symfony IOL (Johnson & Johnson) captured the largest share at 23%, the AcrySof aspheric ReSTOR 2.5 D was at 22%, the AcrySof aspheric ReSTOR 3 D at 8%. The market share of the Crystalens AO was the least at 3%. Since the FDA approval of the PanOptix trifocal (Alcon, Fort Worth, Texas) in August 2019, we expect that the Crystalens market share has declined further. The availability of Tecnis Eyhance lenses (Johnson & Johnson) and the Vivity EDOF lenses (Alcon) will lower the market share of Crytalens further due to less side effects and better predictability.

There are still some candidates for these lenses. They are good for those patients hoping for some degree of spectacle independence but who have comorbidities that decrease contrast sensitivity. If a patient has a large angle kappa or angle alpha, you may wish to avoid a multifocal IOL and the monofocal Crystalens can be an option. Because of the design, the Trulign lens has great rotational stability. Those patients in our office who had a Crystalens implanted in one eye opted for it in the second eye.

One study demonstrated the fact that patient satisfaction for the Crystalens equaled that for a multifocal IOL in 5-year clinical follow-up.[3] Another randomized study[4] consisting of 32 patients with the Crystalens HD and 32 patients with the Tecnis ZCBOO (Johnson & Johnson) aspherical monofocal lenses at the 3-month follow-up was performed at St. Thomas Hospital in London. They looked at IOL movement, depth of focus, intermediate and distance vision, objective refraction, and pupil size at distance and near fixation at the 3-month follow-up visits. There was no statistically significant difference in distance vision, but the Crystalens group did show better near and intermediate acuities ($p < .001$). The effect however was not directly linked to IOL movement but was at least partly due to depth of focus possibly associated with "accommodative arching," a term developed to explain this effect.

10.3 Why Is Crystalens Not That Popular Anymore?

The current generation of accommodating IOLs in the United States provides far and intermediate vision, but near vision is limited. In theory, different from EDOF, multifocal IOLs (MFIOLs), and trifocal IOLs, an accommodating IOL should demonstrate one of the following features to achieve refractive power change: movement of the IOL, or increased curvature of the IOL, increased thickness of the IOL, increased separation of the optics of a dual optic IOL.[5] In Crystalens and Trulign lenses, the joints between the optic and the haptics should remain flexible, allowing the optic to move slightly forward upon contraction of the ciliary muscle. Upon typical

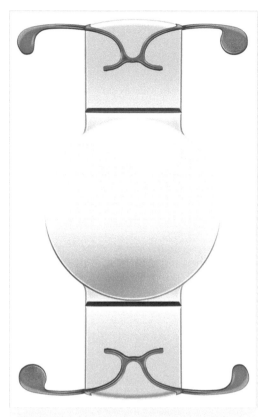

Fig. 10.1 Crystalens. Used with permission from Bausch + Lomb.

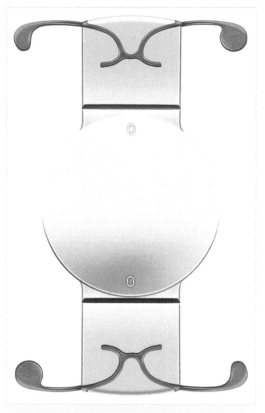

Fig. 10.2 Trulign lens. Used with permission from Bausch + Lomb.

capsular fibrosis, however, the joints will more likely become fixed. This is what we see at the slit lamp a few months postoperatively.

Studies have noted that the current generation of accommodating IOLs in the United States and several other single-optic presbyopia-correcting IOLs may be providing improved intermediate or near vision predominantly through pseudo accommodative mechanisms.[6,7] Studies with the laser ray tracing aberrometer, UBM, and three-dimensional OCT have demonstrated a significant percentage of paradoxical posterior optic movement during accommodative effort.[7,8]

We have implanted all of the different versions and three generations of Crystalens and Trulign lens in the past. Our personal impression echoes the studies mentioned above in terms of their predictability and durability, although most of our patients with Crystalens and Trulign lenses are still happy with reasonable spectacle independence, which we believe may be due to the mini-monovision we intentionally employ. We have seen noticeable variations in terms of outcome. Many patients can have good uncorrected distance vision and great uncorrected near vision, but some patients could hardly show much advantage in uncorrected near vision. An unanswered question is whether that is mainly due to the accommodating mechanism or mainly due to the mini-monovision mechanism. A very commonly used pattern for Crystalens and Trulign lenses is to aim the nondominant eye at −0.50 to −0.75 D. As we all know, when we use this mini-monovision with conventional monofocal IOLs, we still can get a reasonable percentage of patients to achieve spectacle independence. Based on our 10-year conventional monofocal IOL monovision with de-identified survey summary, the mini-monovision group (-0.50 to -0.75 D) had 36.2% complete spectacle freedom. It would be interesting to have a study comparing Crystalens and conventional monofocal IOL mini-monovision to find out if there is a statistical difference favoring the Crystalens in terms of uncorrected near visual acuity (UNVA) and spectacle independence when the nondominant eyes of both groups is aimed at the same mini-monovision level. We could have done a study to compare the two groups, but the sample size for the accommodating IOL group would not have been large enough to generate any meaningful statistical data.

It has however been shown that the bag size is not always proportional to the axial length or white to white. The overall length of the current AO1UV is 11.50 mm and AO2UV is 12.00 mm. The relationship of bag size and the lens size can impact the clinical outcome. This may be a reason for the variable outcomes that most surgeons experience. In a hyperopic small bag, the implant can vault more posteriorly causing a hyperopic shift while with a myopic large bag, the implant may not vault much causing relative myopic shift.

10.4 Crystalens Is Monofocal IOL, Why Is the Pupil Size Still Important?

The diameter of the Crystalens is smaller than that of most conventional monofocal IOLs, 5 mm versus 6 mm. That design alone may be helpful to increase uncorrected near vision, but the downside of a small optic is that it may not work well for patients with large pupils. This can also affect nighttime driving. One of our Crystalens patients needed an IOL exchange for this reason; he was doing well without any complaints after IOL exchange to a conventional 6-mm monofocal IOL. We postulate that this might be due to the hinged plate-haptic- to -optic junction not being well covered by his large pupil because the Crystalens was perfectly positioned without any visible tilt or decentration. A scotopic pupil size should ideally be measured preoperatively before deciding on this lens.

10.5 Why Do We Recommend Laser Created Capsulorhexis for Crystalens?

A well-centered and round rhexis is necessary for Crystalens and Trulign lenses. The femtosecond laser has a unique role in this regard. There is no consensus in terms of the size of capsulorhexis. The size of the optic in both Crystalens and Trulign lens is 5.0 mm. Many surgeons believe a 5- to 6-mm rhexis works better,[9] leaving the haptic-optic junction uncovered by the capsule will have better accommodating movement, while others advocate less than 5 mm, creating better optic coverage and good centration with less chance of posterior capsular fibrosis and less chance of optic tilt.

10.6 What Are the Other Techniques Important for the Crystalens Besides Accurate Rhexis?

- Capsular polishing is necessary, not just for the posterior capsule, but the anterior capsule leaf as well. A well-polished capsule (360 degrees) will decrease the risk of postoperative capsular fibrosis and contraction. One of the severe complications unique to Crystalens is the "Z-Syndrome." When asymmetric capsular fibrosis and contraction happen, depending on the position of the capsule edge, it can cause one plate haptic to move anteriorly and one posteriorly. Mild forms of Z-syndrome can be managed with the ND:YAG laser, but severe cases typically need explantation as severe astigmatism results if we do not do anything. When you learn to polish both through the paracentesis and main incision to achieve the full circle goal you will be amazed at the bulk of cells that remain on the capsule even after thorough irrigation and aspiration and low suction vacuum of the capsule (▶ Fig. 10.3).
- Different from other types of IOLs, which can be more forgiving, the Crystalens must be fully and evenly placed in the bag without tucking it or significant complications will occur. Once it is in

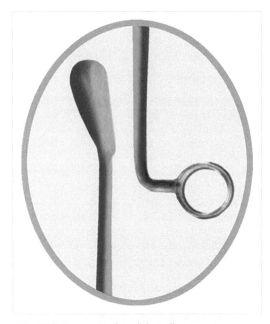

Fig. 10.3 Singer capsule polisher, allows access through a paracentesis as well. Used with permission from Epsilon USA.

the bag, it is recommended to fully turn the implant 360 degrees to make sure all the haptic parts are inside the bag and centrally sited. All the viscoelastic should be fully aspirated out including that behind the lens, and the optic should be pressed against the posterior capsule so the lens is in a posteriorly vaulted position. This requires that the incision, which is slightly larger than for other foldable IOLs, be secure before the ophthalmic viscosugical devices (OVD) is removed so that, upon complete OVD evacuation, the chamber will not shallow intraoperatively with subsequent forward bowing of the Crystalens optic. Look twice to be sure the lens is posteriorly vaulted at the end of the case.

- It is critical to have a perfect wound structure with no postoperative leaking; otherwise, the posteriorly vaulted implant may undergo a forward positional shift. Some surgeons routinely place a stitch to close the wound for all Crystalenses, but if the incision is well structured with a tunnel, a stitch is usually not necessary. If the phaco incision is 2.2 mm, it will need to be enlarged prior to the insertion. A 2.75-mm incision does not need incision enlargement. The round tip of the haptic should be at the right side and the oval tip at the left side during insertion to make sure that the IOL is not inserted backwards. (See ▶ Fig. 10.1 and ▶ Fig. 10.2.)
- Some surgeons routinely use a capsular tension ring (CTR) and they believe it is the only way to prevent unpredictable refractive outcomes. To our knowledge, there has been no study validating this option.
- There is great controversy regarding the efficacy of postoperative atropine usage. The purpose is to atropinize the ciliary muscle to prevent accommodation so that the Crystalens can remain in a posterior vaulted position in the immediate postoperative period until it had settled in and started to fibrose to the capsular bag. Based on our literature search, including our librarian's formal search, we could not find peer-reviewed studies in this regard.
- Explantation almost always requires leaving the haptics in place. It is best to perform anterior optic capture from the sulcus using a three-piece lens, with a larger optic if the continuous curvilinear capsulorhexis (CCC) is large when exchanging a Crystalens to prevent the remaining haptics from exiting the bag or causing the new lens to tilt in the postoperative period. As most of these patients with unacceptable results have had an ND:YAG laser posterior capsulotomy, these exchanges can present significant challenges.

10.7 Who Can be the First Few Candidates of Crystalens for the Beginners?

See ▶ Table 10.1.

Table 10.1 Candidate selection decision for Crystalens

	Good candidate	Try to avoid
Vision requirement	Distance and intermediate vision; Computer and digital reading vision	Small print book reading vision
Ocular surface with Placido images	Clean with smooth rings	Not clean, with irregular changes
Astigmatism level	<2.0 D	2.0 D or more The highest Trulign is 2.75 D, corneal plane is <2.0 D
Mesopic pupil size	<5 mm	5 mm or more
Capsule and zonules	Healthy	Compromised capsule and/or zonules, such as pseudoexfoliation and history of trauma should be contraindications
Optic nerve and macula	Healthy	Mild disease is ok Significant case will not have good vision potential
Laser considerations	Cooperative and expected to be able to lay flat with normal head position and reasonable size lid aperture	Nervous, small lid aperture, neck problem to have normal head position, unable to lay flat, deep eye socket, too small cornea diameter

References

[1] Monthly Pulse. Current and future IOL choices. EyeWorld. 2018; 23(3):106–108

[2] Bethke W. Surgeons share their views on IOLs. Review of Ophthalmology. Published January 10, 2018. Accessed on April 26, 2020. https://www.reviewofophthalmology.com/article/surgeons-share-their-views-on-iols

[3] Hovanesian JA. Patient-reported outcomes of multifocal and accommodating intraocular lenses: analysis of 117 patients 2–10 years after surgery. Clin Ophthalmol. 2018; 12:2297–2304

[4] Dhital A, Spalton DJ, Gala KB. Comparison of near vision, intraocular lens movement, and depth of focus with accommodating and monofocal intraocular lenses. J Cataract Refract Surg. 2013; 39(12):1872–1878

[5] Glasser A, Hilmantel G, Calogero D, et al. Special report: American Academy of Ophthalmology Task Force recommendations for test methods to assess accommodation produced by intraocular lenses. Ophthalmology. 2017; 124(1): 134–139

[6] Pérez-Merino P, Birkenfeld J, Dorronsoro C, et al. Aberrometry in patients implanted with accommodative intraocular lenses. Am J Ophthalmol. 2014; 157(5):1077–1089

[7] Pepose JS, Burke J, Qazi MA. Benefits and barriers of accommodating intraocular lenses. Curr Opin Ophthalmol. 2017; 28(1):3–8

[8] Marcos S, Ortiz S, Pérez-Merino P, Birkenfeld J, Durán S, Jiménez-Alfaro I. Three-dimensional evaluation of accommodating intraocular lens shift and alignment in vivo. Ophthalmology. 2014; 121(1):45–55

[9] Weinstock RJ. Accommodating implants: The Cyrstalens. In: Hovanesian JA, ed. Refractive cataract surgery. 2nd ed. SLACK, Inc.; 2017:199–212

11 Extended Depth-of-Focus Intraocular Lenses

Fuxiang Zhang, Alan Sugar, and Lisa Brothers Arbisser

Abstract

We can view the extended depth-of-focus (EDOF) intraocular lenses (IOLs) as having characteristics that lie between traditional monofocal IOLs and the various multifocal intraocular lenses (MFIOLs), such as the Symfony IOL (Johnson & Johnson Vision). EDOF technology has an extended far focus area which reaches to the intermediate distance, providing comparable distance vision over a continuous range of focus, rather than distinct foci with blur in between as diffractive multifocal technology offers. It attempts to bridge the gap between the two and find a sweet spot balancing distance vision quality, unaided intermediate/near vision, degree of loss of contrast sensitivity, as well as the downsides of dysphotopsias. The hallmark of EDOF is the ability to provide better unaided intermediate distance vision enabling social and digital reading such as the dashboard, computer/template, and cell phone so essential in modern society. Unfortunately, patients with bilateral EDOF lenses usually need magnification for small print reading but the technology has its unique and important role within the full spectrum of refractive cataract surgery at the time of this writing. This chapter will briefly discuss different EDOF lenses, with emphasis on Symfony and Vivity lenses, basic optic designs, candidate selection, and analysis of visual disturbances, and will offer pearls for enhancing near reading capacity.

Keywords: extended depth-of-focus lenses, EDOF, refractive cataract surgery, Symfony IOL, Vivity, IC-8 pinhole lenses, Mini Well, AT LARA

11.1 How Can We Define an IOL as an EDOF IOL?

The following list is from the American Academy of Ophthalmology (AAO) extended depth-of-focus (EDOF) study criteria[1]:

- The EDOF group should have >100 patients and the control group should be similar for comparisons.
- The EDOF intraocular lenses (IOLs) should provide equivalent monocular mean best-corrected distance visual acuity to the monofocal IOLs as determined by a noninferiority analysis with a noninferiority margin of 0.1 logMAR.
- An EDOF IOL should have a statistically significant improved distance-corrected intermediate vision (DCIVA) at 66 centimeters at 6 months in photopic condition when compared with a monofocal IOL control group, with 50% of these eyes achieving monocular DCIVA of better than or equal to logMAR 0.2 (20/30).
- The monocular depth of focus for the EDOF eyes needs to be at least 0.5 D greater than the depth of focus for the monofocal IOL controls at logMAR 0.2 (20/30).

Interestingly, there is no criterion regarding visual disturbances for EDOF IOL criteria from the AAO.

11.2 What Are the Main EDOF IOLs on the Market?

There are currently at least five types of EDOF IOLs. In this chapter, we are going to focus on the Symfony EDOF (Johnson & Johnson Vision) and Vivity EDOF IOLs (Alcon). The IC-8 IOL will be discussed in Chapter 14 and the other two IOLs are not FDA approved in the United States as of this writing.

- The IC-8 is small-aperture one-piece hydrophobic acrylic posterior chamber IOL (AcuFocus Inc., Irvine, California). The small-aperture design blocks *unfocused* peripheral light rays via its 3.23-mm-wide opaque mask while allowing central and paracentral light rays through its 1.36-mm central aperture.[2] This unique design theoretically should work well for those patients whose cornea has significant irregular astigmatism such as s/p radial keratotomy (RK), corneal transplant, etc. The IC-8 lens is typically implanted in a nondominant eye while the dominant eye receives a traditional monofocal IOL aiming for emmetropia. See details in Chapter 14.
- Mini Well (SIFI MedTech Srl) is considered to be a refractive EDOF lens with asphericity manipulations in three zones[3]: a central zone with positive spherical aberration (SA), a middle

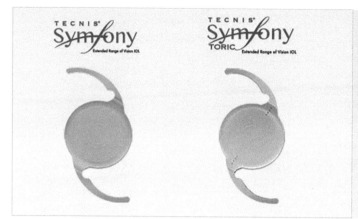

Fig. 11.1 Symfony extended depth-of-focus (EDOF; Johnson & Johnson Vision): On the left is Symfony ZXR00 aspherical version; on the right is the Symfony ZXT Toric version. Used with permission from Johnson & Johnson Vision.

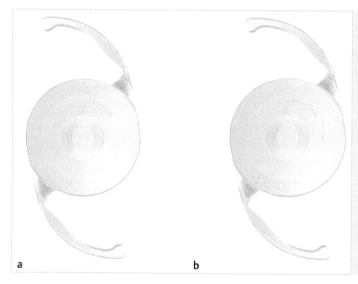

Fig. 11.2 AcrySof® IQ Vivity extended depth-of-focus (EDOF) intraocular lens (IOL) (Alcon). Used with permission from Alcon. On the left is aspherical version (**a**) and on the right is toric version (**b**). Used with permission from Alcon.

zone with negative SA, and an outer monofocal zone.

- The AT LARA is another diffractive design EDOF (Carl Zeiss Meditec AG) lens as a one-piece hydrophilic acrylic IOL. It is a plate-haptic design which may have rotational stability concerns as we experienced from the Staar plate-haptic Toric IOL design.
- Symfony IOL (Johnson & Johnson Vision) (▶ Fig. 11.1): Together with aberration compensation and enhancement of contrast sensitivity (CS), the Symfony lens provides a far focus corresponding to a base power of the refractive carrier lens and an intermediate focus

corresponding to a diffractive power of +1.75 D add, where a difference between the base power and the add power defines an extended depth of focus.[4] The Symfony lens and a conventional multifocal intraocular lens (MFIOL), such as the same company's ZKB00 with +2.75 D add, have the common context of a refractive carrier with aspherical −0.27 μm SA, but diffractive saw-tooth pattern of echelettes engraved on the posterior surface is different.

- AcrySof IQ Vivity IOL (Alcon Surgical, Inc.) (▶ Fig. 11.2a and b): The AcrySof IQ Vivity IOL is a one-piece, hydrophobic aspheric posterior chamber IOL with blue-light filter and ultraviolet protection. It was approved by the FDA in February 2020[5] but was not fully commercially available until Spring of 2021 in the United States. The Vivity lens is a non-diffractive EDOF IOL with wavefront-shaping technology. It has a slight plateau (1 μm high) on the central 2.2-mm optic, which creates a two-surface transition (X-WAVE) that causes a "stretch and shift" of the wavefront.[6,7] As a result, there is no light split and less risk of dysphotopsia. Given the fact that the lens is non diffractive, angle kappa may not be as much of a concern as it is for diffractive multifocal IOLs.[7] The FDA bench data also suggest that Vivity is very tolerant of decentrations and tilt.[8] Because of this X-Wave technology, simultaneous surface transitions create a continuous extended focal range to cover intermediate vision and even some near vision. The anterior surface of the AcrySof IQ Vivity IOL is designed with −0.2 μm SA, identical to the aspheric AcrySof IQ Monofocal IOL (SN60WF).[7]

11.3 When Should a Beginner of Refractive Cataract Surgery Start Using the Symfony or the Vivity IOLs?

Most Symfony IOL patients are aware of the presence of visual disturbances, especially in low light conditions, but the severity is usually less than that of an MFIOL.[9,10] The explantation rate of the Symfony EDOF IOLs should be expected to be much lower than that of traditional MFIOLs, although a literature and google search in collaboration with our health systems library yielded no results for data on the explantation rate of Symfony EDOF IOLs. Symfony EDOF IOLs also have better tolerability of postoperative residual astigmatism.[11,12] From this perspective, the Symfony EDOF IOL can be a good IOL choice for beginners who are already comfortable with astigmatism correction such as toric IOLs and manual/laser-created limbal relaxing incisions (LRI) but have not started MFIOL or trifocal IOLs. Early reports for the Vivity are also promising,[7,8] but our personal limited experience is not enough to offer meaningful advice, as of this writing, in terms of tolerability to preexisting comorbidities and postoperative suboptimal conditions, such as residual astigmatism.

11.4 How Do Symfony IOLs Manage Aberrations to Enhance Vision Quality?

11.4.1 Spherical Aberration (SA)

Studies have revealed that the young human crystalline lens has negative SA at about the same level as the positive SA from the cornea.[13,14] As we age, our total SA increases, mainly from the aging crystalline lens shape change as lens fibers continue to grow and compact.[13,14] There is no doubt that the human cornea has positive SA, although different studies reached different conclusions in terms of whether corneal SA increases with age.[14,15,16,17,18] Corneal SA has been shown to increase as corneal astigmatism increases.[19]

Due to its high refractive power, the cornea is a known primary contributor to higher order aberrations (HOAs). At a typical 6-mm pupillary diameter, the cornea contributes about +0.274 μm SA.[14] Another study of 228 eyes of 134 patients with refractive surgery and cataract patients with mean age 50 years ±17 (SD) demonstrated mean SA of the anterior cornea of +0.281 ± 0.086 μm.[16] Positive SAs can compromise retinal image quality and cause glare and halo.[20]

A laboratory study[21] noted that overall the Symfony IOL showed a tendency to perform better with the ISO2 model cornea (with +0.28 SA in the ISO2 model cornea) at all pupil sizes than another EDOF lens, AT LARA IOL (Zeiss, Germany), because of the built-in negative SA component (▸ Fig. 11.3a and b).

Currently, Symfony lenses have a fixed negative SA (a built-in −0.27 μm) to compensate for the positive SA of the average cornea. The anterior surface of the AcrySof IQ Vivity IOL is designed with −0.2 μm SA, identical to the aspheric AcrySof IQ Monofocal IOL (SN60WF).[7] If the amount of built-in negative SA power could be customized for each individual eye, it would likely yield even better results. An early study in Germany with the Invidua-aA (Humanoptics AG) IOL has already proven that this approach is possible and promising.[22]

11.4.2 Chromatic Aberration

Multiple wavelengths of the visible spectrum will focus at different points resulting in chromatic aberration (▸ Fig. 11.3b). The aspherical anterior surface is designed to compensate for positive

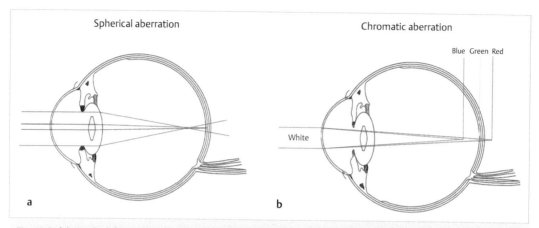

Fig. 11.3 (a) On the left is spherical aberration. Peripheral rays overrefract compared to central light rays. **(b)** On the right is chromatic aberration. Light with different wavelengths has different focal lengths.

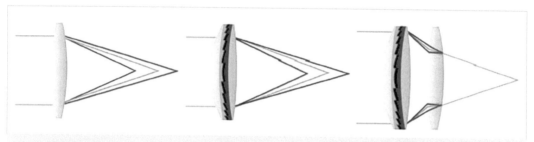

Fig. 11.4 Specific design to compensate chromatic aberration by the Symfony lens. Used with permission from Johnson & Johnson Vision.

corneal SA and the posterior diffractive profile of the Symfony lens is designed to compensate for chromatic aberration.[23] While it is relatively familiar to cataract surgeons with a built-in −0.27 μm to compensate corneal positive SA, the Symfony EDOF lens has a much more sophisticated design mechanism to mitigate the impact of achromatic aberration by engineering delicate echelette shape, direction, and height to compensate for chromatic aberration and then to increase image contrast.[23,24,25] This specific design was the key to making red light bend more and blue light bend less, thereby decreasing chromatic aberration (▶ Fig. 11.4). One study[3] found that the Symfony EDOF lens had better resistance to chromatic aberration due to its diffractive design echelettes than the refractive design of the Mini Well EDOF lens.

11.4.3 Contrast Sensitivity (CS)

We would expect the CS of the Symfony EDOF lens to not be as good as that of the same company's monofocal IOLs,[26] but studies seemed to show a better CS than with other premium lenses, including trifocal IOLs.[26] A nonrandomized prospective study was done in Italy with 120 eyes of 60 patients undergoing cataract surgery with bilateral implantation of three different IOLs: Symfony (40 eyes), PanOptix (40 eyes), and AT LISA (40 eyes). Visual results, photopic and mesopic CS, binocular reading skills (MNREAD charts), and patient satisfaction were evaluated 3 months after surgery. The Tecnis Symfony IOL provided significantly better photopic and mesopic CS outcomes compared to both PanOptix (Alcon) and AT LISA (Zeiss) trifocals ($p < 0.001$).[27] Better CS was also

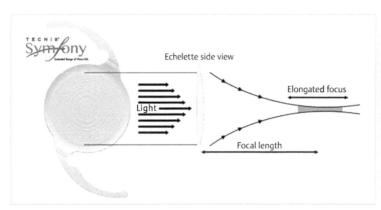

Fig. 11.5 Extended depth-of-focus (EDOF) Symfony lens with elongated focus. Used with permission from Johnson & Johnson Vision.

reported in Symfony patients than in PanOptix patients in another study.[28]

11.4.4 Extended Depth of Focus

In addition to aberration correction, the diffractive optic design also elongates the depth of focus.[25] Because of the diffractive optic component, some scholars consider Symfony EDOF as "Hybrid MF diffractive/EDOF IOL," rather than pure EDOF IOL.[29] Compared to MFIOL (Tecnis ZMB and ZLB), Trifocals Finevision (PhysiIOL) and AT LISA (Zeiss), and EDOF Mini Well (SIFI MedTech), a study in Spain[30] suggested that the Symfony EDOF IOL group had better subjective as well as objective depth of focus, with $p < 0.001$ (▶ Fig. 11.5).

Many studies have shown great outcomes for Symfony lenses.[12,31,32,33] According to the monthly Pulse survey from EyeWorld (2018), the EDOF lens became the most popular choice for presbyopia management in the adult cataract patient population while the current accommodating IOL (Crystalens) was the least favored.[34] About 28% of responders chose EDOF IOLs "For presbyopic correction in my patients" while about 18% chose IOL monovision. This was the first time, to our knowledge, premium IOLs surpassed monofocal IOL monovision among cataract surgeons who were surveyed. This popularity/preference has already changed, however, since the arrival of trifocal lenses. See Chapter 12 "Trifocal IOLs."

11.5 Can the Symfony Lens Tolerate More Residual Astigmatism?

Due to the elongated focus, the EDOF should have better tolerance to residual spherical equivalent

(SE) and astigmatism when compared to traditional MFIOLs and trifocal IOLs.

A prospective, comparative, interventional, single-center study in Italy included 80 eyes of patients with implantation of four different IOLs: AcrySof ReSTOR+2.5 D (20 eyes), AcrySof ReSTOR+3.0 D (20 eyes), AcrySof PanOptix (20 eyes) (Alcon), and Tecnis Symfony ZRX00 (Abbott Medical Optics, now Johnson and Johnson) (20 eyes). Patients were followed up for 3 months after surgery. With mild added negative cylinders, AcrySof ReSTOR+2.5 D and Symfony IOLs maintained the baseline uncorrected visual acuity, while it was mildly reduced with AcrySof ReSTOR+3.0 D and PanOptix IOLs. With moderate induced cylinders, the Tecnis Symfony IOL maintained good visual acuity satisfaction. PanOptix IOL was the IOL most affected by the induced astigmatism with regard to dissatisfaction and visual acuity. The highest tolerance to the astigmatic distortion and blur induced with a −1.50 D cylinder was obtained with the Symfony group. The Symfony group showed less dissatisfaction and less reduction of visual acuity than the other groups. The authors concluded that simulated residual cylinders after the implantation of the Symfony EDOF IOL up to 1.0 D have a very mild and not clinically relevant impact on visual acuity or patient satisfaction.[11] This may reduce the necessity for refractive enhancement with this lens.

Another study, in France, found that residual cylinder up to 0.75 D had a very mild impact on monocular and binocular vision with this lens.[12] Symfony EDOF lenses have also been reported to have better tolerance to SE error when compared to monofocal implants.[35]

We would still recommend that astigmatism be aggressively treated in the same way as for

MFIOLs and trifocals, because we have noted that among those patients who have complained of dysphotopsia or who are not really impressed with the clinical outcome, their corneal topographies often show some residual astigmatism.

11.6 Between Symfony EDOF and PanOptix Trifocal IOL, Which Is More Forgiving from the Patient Satisfaction Perspective? Which IOL Should I Use First if I Have Never Implanted a Presbyopia-Correcting IOL?

The Symfony EDOF (J&J) is not going to provide as good uncorrected near vision (UNVA) as the PanOptix lens (Alcon). Despite this, Symfony lenses may be more forgiving for the following reasons:

- From a material perspective, the high reflectance, glistening, and chromatic aberration, they all can lead to image quality issues for PanOptix.[36]
- The Symfony EDOF lens has a single wide peak in the defocus curve versus multiple peaks for a trifocal lens. It is more forgiving if you miss the emmetropic refractive target as well as astigmatism correction in an EDOF lens.
- The Symfony EDOF lens has lower diffractive add power, so dysphotopsia should be less significant.
- The Symfony EDOF lens has a larger inner central ring (1.6 mm),[23] bigger than most traditional diffractive optics. So it is more forgiving in terms of angle alpha/angle kappa and decentration.

11.7 Can Post Corneal Refractive Surgery Patients be Good Candidates for Symfony EDOF IOLs?

This will depend on the patient's ocular conditions, especially corneal topography/aberration profile, expectation/personality, and the surgeon's surgical track record with regard to being able to hit the refractive target.

Postrefractive surgery patients are among the most highly motivated, but they need to be treated conservatively. A study in Portugal[32] consisting of 22 patients and 44 eyes in each group demonstrated the suitability and success of the Symfony lens in post myopic laser-assisted in situ keratomileusis (LASIK) patients with comparable uncorrected distance vision (UDVA) but statistically significantly better binocular uncorrected intermediate and binocular uncorrected near vision; and similar CS when compared with the same company's monofocal ZCB00 IOL patients. Subjective complaints of mild halo were equal (13.6%) but mild glare was more prevalent in the Symfony group (22.7%) than the ZCB00 group (9.1%).

Our experience with Symfony EDOF lenses in patients with a history of myopic LASIK has been mixed, mainly depending on their corneal curvature: doing very well with healthy corneas but not so well with preexisting corneal irregularities. Coma and SA are significant factors to evaluate. Hyperopic LASIK may not do well due to the increased negative SA because the EDOF Symfony lens is designed to compensate for positive corneal aberration, thereby compounding the preexisting aberration. It is better to quantitatively measure the amount of SA in these patients. In low amounts of hyperopic LASIK correction with minimal induced negative SA, these patients tolerate the EDOF lens well.

For post-RK patients, with few incisions (4–6), and regular, stable Ks, we have found success with monofocal toric lenses. We have not used the EDOF lens in post-RK patients mainly due to frequently present high levels of coma. EDOF lenses have however been reported by others to be successful in post-RK patients.[37,38] One study at Thompson Vision noted that at final follow-up, 15 of 24 eyes (62.5%) were at or within 0.5 D of target refraction, while 20 of 24 eyes (83.3%) were at or within 1.0 D. In total, 79% of eyes (19 of 24) had UCVA of 20/40 or better at distance. In the survey, 78% of patients reported satisfaction with their vision after surgery and 44% of patients reported being spectacle free for all tasks.[38]

11.8 What Should You Tell Your Patients If Asked "Will I Need Reading Glasses after My Cataract Surgery If I Have Symfony Implants"?

A study by Kohnen and colleagues noted that of 26 patients with bilateral Symfony EDOF lenses, spectacle independence was achieved in 100% for distance and intermediate vision but only 71% of patients were spectacle free for near tasks.[39] In a comparative study between 25 patients with bilateral EDOF Symfony and 23 patients with "blended" multifocal technology (ReStor +2.5/+3.25 Alcon), while distance and near vision were similar in both groups, intermediate vision was better in the EDOF IOL cohort.[40] Another study from Norway of the EDOF toric version in 30 patients aiming for emmetropia showed that half of the patients never needed glasses; 86%, 96%, and 64% of patients were totally spectacle independent for distance, intermediate, and near visual tasks, respectively.[9] Ninety-three percent of those patients with Tecnis Symfony IOLs were reported to be spectacle independent at near when the nondominant eyes were targeted at −0.50 D as micromonovision.[41]

Our clinical experience shows very good patient satisfaction for distance and intermediate visual quality and acceptable near vision. What we typically tell our patients in this regard is that they can expect great distance and intermediate vision, and fair near vision. Basically, they are likely to achieve good digital and social vision without spectacles, for driving, watching TV, GPS, computer, and cell phones, but reading small print, especially for a long duration, likely will need readers. Combined with minimonovision (−0.50 D in one eye and emmetropia in the fellow eye) we usually expect satisfactory spectacle independence for most of our patients except for reading small print, which is consistent with a published study in Europe.[24] We have been able to expect no need for glasses for casual reading and computer/cell phone use. While we have not done a survey in terms of spectacle independence, our anecdotal experience suggests that about 50% of bilateral Symfony EDOF have achieved total glasses independence when we aimed one eye for emmetropia and one eye for −0.50.

11.9 Which Eye Should be Done First?

For minimonovision with anisometropia between 0.50 and 0.75 D, both conventional and crossed monovision work well.[42] So, we really do not need to worry about which eye is operated on first as long as the patient does not have a history of diplopia, extraocular muscle surgery, amblyopia,

monofixation, or significant ocular comorbidities. This allows us to choose the eye with the most visually significant cataract to operate first; most often a good idea from both the patient's and the surgeon's perspective.

11.10 Minimonovision Is Helpful, But How Much Defocus Can We Allow?

Symfony EDOF lenses have low add power and they usually need minimonovision to sufficiently enhance near vision. In a study of 411 bilateral Symfony IOL patients in Europe reported by Cochener et al[24] it was noted that when comparing monovision (nondominant eye aiming at −0.50 to −0.75 D, 112 patients) with the nonmonovision group (bilaterally emmetropia 299 patients), the monovision group did much better with improvement in UNVA ($p = 0.01$), UIVA ($p = 0.003$), and near spectacle independence and satisfaction. A US study reached similar conclusions: the monovision group did much better at UNVA while binocular UDVA and UIVA were similar.[43]

The question is how much defocus can be tolerated? The Tecnis Symfony defocus curve below shows that distance vision can still be 20/20 even when the defocus is −1.5 D (▶ Fig. 11.6) but the tradeoff is that image quality on the retina will decrease and more dysphotopsia will occur when defocus increases. Our advice is not to aim for more than −0.75 D for the Symfony lens. For the distance eye, emmetropia or near emmetropia at < −0.25 D will provide the best outcome.[44] If you really want to get as close to plano as possible, you can choose the least plus side to make close to plano rather than the least minus side.

An early clinical report by Cathleen McCabe, MD, for the Vivity lens suggested the sweet spot is around −0.50 D for the nondominant eye.[8]

11.11 If We Mix and Match IOL Types, What Should We Avoid?

As you now know, the Symfony EDOF is good for UDVA and UIVA, but UNVA is often limited. That seems to be the main reason to consider a mix-and-match strategy. Although we try to use the same family of IOLs, this does not seem to be critical. We have implanted a PanOptix trifocal IOL (Alcon) in those patients who had Symfony EDOF

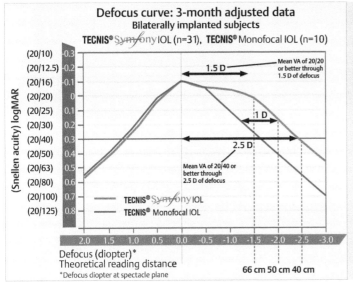

Defocus curve: 3-month adjusted data
Bilaterally implanted subjects
TECNIS® Symfony IOL (n=31), TECNIS® Monofocal IOL (n=10)

Fig. 11.6 Defocus curve comparison of Tecnis Symfony versus Tecnis monofocal intraocular lens (IOL). The Tecnis Symfony IOL has better tolerance than Tecnis monofocal IOL in terms of the level of defocus. Used with permission from Johnson & Johnson Vision.

lens in one eye in the past and the clinical outcome was excellent. It is advisable to choose the same color IOLs because some patients may notice a color difference when comparing eyes with one blue filtering chromophore and one UV blocking-only lens. It is probably acceptable to have a Symfony EDOF lens in the dominant eye while the nondominant eye has a traditional monofocal IOL because the Symfony EDOF has good CS which is close to or at the "same level" compared to that of the same company's monofocal IOL.[45] The general guideline is to have a better CS lens in the dominant eye and the higher add lens in the nondominant eye. It is advisable not to choose an MFIOL or a trifocal IOL in the dominant eye while a monofocal IOL is chosen for the nondominant eye aiming for myopia because the image quality of an MFIOL or a trifocal IOL is usually not as good as the image quality of a monofocal IOL.

11.12 How Significant Will Dysphotopsia be in a Typical Symfony EDOF Patient?

Although optically it uses a distinctly different mechanism, functionally the Symfony EDOF works like a 1.75 D add multifocal IOL. There are studies that noted less photic phenomena in Symfony EDOF patients than in multifocal IOL patients.[9,10] ▶ Fig. 11.7 models the severity of dysphotopsia,

but it may have a potential bias as this information is from the Symfony IOL manufacturer.

Our experience suggests that most patients acknowledge the presence of night vision dysphotopsia "starburst" or "spider web glare," especially when there is residual refractive error, but very few actually complain about these problems. We have not had any single Symfony lens explantation due to dysphotopsia as of now. Most of our Symfony patients, would say "none" when we asked them "is there any problem for your vision?" If we asked them, "Do you see halo and glare at nighttime driving?", then most of them would answer "yes, but it does not bother me." The bottom line is that patients who choose any modern IOL intended to provide broad range of vision given today's technology are accepting a tradeoff between quality and convenience of vision. We can strike the right balance with currently available lenses if we are meticulous about refractive outcomes for most patients most of the time. This is why honest discussion with realistic goals has such great importance. We can only hope this Faustian bargain will become less of an issue as technology advances.

11.13 What Is Your Strategy in Terms of "Under Promise and Over Deliver"?

List all existing ocular pathologies at the decision-making office visit. We should tell the patient the

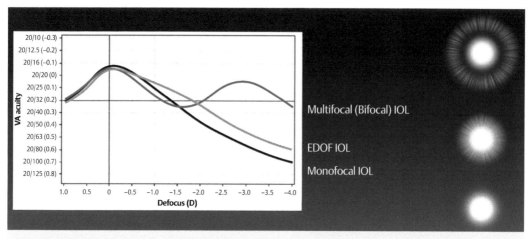

Fig. 11.7 Dysphotopsia severity from Symfony extended depth-of-focus (EDOF) lenses is between monofocal intraocular lens (IOL) and multifocal IOL (MFIOL) of the same company. Used with permission from Johnson & Johnson Vision.

potential negative impact from ocular comorbidities before the surgery, not after. This fully detailed examination will help you to evaluate the patient and help the patient to have realistic expectations. We do let our patients know all the available options, pros and cons and cost, but usually the surgeon will give only one or two preferred options and let the patient make the final decision. Honestly explain the main downsides of the specific IOL or modality you plan to use. *Never exaggerate the pros and mitigate the cons to achieve a high conversion rate for any premium IOLs.* In cases of reluctant patients, it is better to exclude rather than to include. Most patients with bilateral EDOF likely will have good distance and intermediate vision. They seem to do well with digital reading but may need help for book reading. Approximately 50% or more of our bilateral EDOF patients do not need any readers if the non-dominant eye is aimed at minimonovision at −0.50 to −0.75 D range. We routinely tell our patients that they may need readers for book print reading. If they end up not needing any readers, they will be happier. Tell every patient that they will experience some night vision phenomena. The reality is that most of them do not even mention it to us if we do not specifically ask. It should also be explained that even with perfect outcomes, we are not able to make the vision as great as when they were age 18.

11.14 How Does the Visual Performance of the AcrySof Vivity IOL Compare with the AcrySof IQ Monofocal IOL?

In terms of the visual performance, in the US clinical study, the AcrySof® IQ Vivity IOL was found to provide an extended range of focus (>0.5 D) compared with the AcrySof® IQ Monofocal IOL at 0.2 logMAR at 6 months, with superior best-corrected intermediate and near visual acuity, and noninferior best-corrected distance visual acuity.[7] In the FDA study,[5] subjects had their cataracts removed and replaced with either the AcrySof IQ Vivity IOL or a monofocal IOL. Six months after surgery, corrected distance vision (CDVA) was 20/25 or better for 89% (95/107) with the AcrySof IQ Vivity IOL, compared to 94% (104/113) with the control IOL. Distance corrected Intermediate vision was 20/25 or better for 37% (40/107) of subjects with the AcrySof IQ Vivity IOL, compared to 9% (10/113) with a monofocal SN60WF IOL. Distance corrected near vision was acceptable (20/40 or better) for 40% (43/107) of subjects with the AcrySof IQ Vivity IOL, compared to 12% (13/113) for subjects with a monofocal SN60WF IOL group. The binocular defocus curves 6 months after implantation in the outside-the-US trial group were similar to those of the US group.[46]

The Vivity lens seemed to have a large plateau of 20/20 from +0.50 to −0.50 on the binocular defocus curve. Per Cathleen McCabe, MD, who was part of the FDA clinical trial, Vivity provides a flexible and forgiving plateau of targeting for postoperative refractive error. Because of that forgiveness around plano, Vivity patients had slightly better uncorrected distance visual acuity than monofocal patients,[8] although the FDA study suggested slightly better CDVA at 6 months follow-up in the monofocal IOL group.[5]

11.15 What Specific Attention Do We Need to Have with Vivity Lenses?

- As of now, the lens is available only in powers of +15 D to +25 D in 0.5 D increments. For high myopic or high hyperopic eyes, we are not able to use this lens.
- Alcon recommends targeting emmetropia to slight myopia.[7] Minimonovision (−0.5 D) was noted to do better to enhance near vision.[8]
- It has been reported to do well in eyes with comorbidities,[8] but there is not currently much data to support this claim.
- There is a small elevation on the anterior optical surface. While aberrometers may be able to characterize the refractive status of these patients, aberrometers without enough sampling resolution to resolve subtle surface

changes may not reliably detect the depth-of-focus–extending surface elements.[7]

11.16 Who May be Good Candidates for the First Few Cases of Symfony or Vivity Lenses?

Essentially this is the same cohort of patients as is appropriate for MFIOLs and trifocal IOLs, despite the greater forgiveness of Symfony (Johnson & Johnson) and Vivity (Alcon) for imperfect refractive outcome, residual astigmatism, and lens position. Some believe that mild macular changes or early glaucoma without obvious field loss are not as significant a problem as for traditional MFIOLs. In an EyeWorld survey, 40% of responders would consider an EDOF Symfony IOL for their early/mild glaucoma patients.[34] We recommend that even in mild and moderate glaucoma, we should still do a 10–2 visual field test to make sure there is no early central fixation involvement. Subtle central scotoma is more common than we have thought, and a 24–2 Humphrey visual field can be completely normal.[47] Due to the larger size of the central ring of the Symfony lens (1.6 mm),[23] and nondiffractive optic in Vivity, it is more forgiving than MFIOLs and trifocals in terms of angle kappa and angle alpha. All agree we should still avoid patients who have significant corneal SA and coma (▶ Table 11.1).

Table 11.1 Candidate selection decision for Symfony and Vivity IOLs

	Good candidate	Try to avoid
Lifestyle and occupations	Occasional or rare driving at night for Symfony lens	Truck and taxi drivers, pilots for Symfony lens
Vision requirement	Distance vision, intermediate vision, computer and digital reading	Strong demand for good small print book reading vision
Refractive category	Hyperopia	Mild myopia often not impressed by EDOF lenses for uncorrected near vision
Ocular surgical history	No	s/p laser vision correction LASIK/PRK/RK
Ocular surface with Placido images	Clean with smooth rings	With irregular changes Poor tear film EBMD Fuchs' dystrophy

(Continued)

Table 11.1 (*Continued*) Candidate selection decision for Symfony and Vivity IOLs

	Good candidate	Try to avoid
Zonules	Healthy	Weak zonules such as pseudoexfoliation which may lead to IOL shift later
Macula	Healthy. Minimal abnormality seems to be ok, but should be approached with care Prefer not to have any diabetic retinopathy	Moderate maculopathy Any microaneurysm and hemorrhage in central macula or any active diabetic macular edema should be considered as contraindications
Glaucoma	Mild glaucoma with no field loss and expectation of stability	Unstable IOP control, or with field loss Poor ocular surface due to antiglaucoma drops should be considered as contraindications
Optic nerve	Healthy	History of optic neuropathy
Axial length	Normal range	Extreme length, especially very short eyes, ELP will be more critical and harder to hit refractive target and make the overall outcome less predictable
Personality	Easy going	Demanding

Abbreviations: EBMD, epithelial basement membrane dystrophy; EDOF, extended depth of focus; ELP, effective lens position; IOL, intraocular lens; IOP, intraocular pressure; LASIK, laser-assisted in situ keratomileusis; PRK, photorefractive keratectomy; RK, radial keratotomy.

References

[1] MacRae S, Holladay JT, Glasser A, et al. Special report: American Academy of Ophthalmology Task Force consensus statement for extended depth of focus intraocular lenses. Ophthalmology. 2017; 124(1):139–141

[2] Kohnen T, Suryakumar R. Extended depth-of-focus technology in intraocular lenses. J Cataract Refract Surg. 2020; 46(2):298–304

[3] Lee Y, Łabuz G, Son HS, Yildirim TM, Khoramnia R, Auffarth GU. Assessment of the image quality of extended depth-of-focus intraocular lens models in polychromatic light. J Cataract Refract Surg. 2020; 46(1):108–115

[4] Weeber HA. Inventor; AMO Groningen BV, assignee. Multiring lens, systems and methods for extended depth of focus. US Patent 2014/0168602 A1. June 19, 2014

[5] AcrySof™ IQ Vivity™ Extended Vision Intraocular Lens (IOL) (Model DFT015), AcrySof™ IQ Vivity™ Toric Extended Vision IOLs (DFT315, DFT415, DFT515), AcrySof™ IQ Vivity™ Extended Vision UV Absorbing IOL (DAT015), and AcrySof™ IQ Vivity™ Toric Extended Vision UV Absorbing IOLs (DAT315, DAT415, DAT515)—P930014/S126. U.S Food & Drug Administration. Current as of March 12, 2020. https://www.fda.gov/medical-devices/recently-approved-devices/acrysoftm-iq-vivitytm-extended-vision-intraocular-lens-iol-model-dft015-acrysoftm-iq-vivitytm-toric. Accessed May 12, 2021

[6] Kohnen T. Nondiffractive wavefront-shaping extended range-of-vision intraocular lens. J Cataract Refract Surg. 2020; 46(9):1312–1313

[7] AcrySof® IQ Vivity™ IOL FAQs. Alcon. 2020

[8] Leonard C. IOL review: 2021 newcomers. Rev Ophthalmol. 2021:38–44

[9] Gundersen KG. Rotational stability and visual performance 3 months after bilateral implantation of a new toric extended range of vision intraocular lens. Clin Ophthalmol. 2018; 12:1269–1278

[10] Coassin M, Di Zazzo A, Antonini M, Gaudenzi D, Gallo Afflitto G, Kohnen T. Extended depth-of-focus intraocular lenses: power calculation and outcomes. J Cataract Refract Surg. 2020; 46(11):1554–1560

[11] Carones F. Residual astigmatism threshold and patient satisfaction with bifocal, trifocal and extended range of vision intraocular lenses (IOLs). Open J Ophthalmol. 2017; 7(1):1–7

[12] Cochener B. Tecnis Symfony intraocular lens with a "sweet spot" for tolerance to postoperative residual refractive errors. Open J Ophthalmol. 2017; 7(1):14–20

[13] Smith G, Cox MJ, Calver R, Garner LF. The spherical aberration of the crystalline lens of the human eye. Vision Res. 2001; 41(2):235–243

[14] Karakelle M. The science behind the AcrySof IQ. Cataract & Refractive Surgery Today. Published May 2018. https://crstoday.com/articles/the-blueprint-for-exceptional-image-quality/the-science-behind-the-acrysof-iq-iol/. Accessed May 12, 2021

[15] Yuan L, Bao Y. [Analysis of the corneal spherical aberration in people with senile cataract]. Zhonghua Yan Ke Za Zhi. 2014; 50(2):100–104

[16] Wang L, Dai E, Koch DD, Nathoo A. Optical aberrations of the human anterior cornea. J Cataract Refract Surg. 2003; 29(8):1514–1521

[17] Oshika T, Klyce SD, Applegate RA, Howland HC. Changes in corneal wavefront aberrations with aging. Invest Ophthalmol Vis Sci. 1999; 40(7):1351–1355

[18] Guirao A, Redondo M, Artal P. Optical aberrations of the human cornea as a function of age. J Opt Soc Am A Opt Image Sci Vis. 2000; 17(10):1697–1702

[19] Labuz G, Khoramnia R, Auffarth GU. Corneal spherical aberration in an elderly population with high astigmatism. Paper presented at 2020 ASCRS Virtual Annual Meeting. May 16–17, 2020

[20] Holladay JT, Piers PA, Koranyi G, van der Mooren M, Norrby NE. A new intraocular lens design to reduce spherical aberration of pseudophakic eyes. J Refract Surg. 2002; 18(6):683–691

[21] Chae SH, Son HS, Khoramnia R, Lee KH, Choi CY. Laboratory evaluation of the optical properties of two extended-depth-of-focus intraocular lenses. BMC Ophthalmol. 2020; 20(1):53

[22] Schrecker J, Langenbucher A, Seitz B, Eppig T. First results with a new intraocular lens design for the individual correction of spherical aberration. J Cataract Refract Surg. 2018; 44(10):1211–1219

[23] Millán MS, Vega F. Extended depth of focus intraocular lens: chromatic performance. Biomed Opt Express. 2017; 8 (9):4294–4309

[24] Cochener B, Concerto Study Group. Clinical outcomes of a new extended range of vision intraocular lens: International Multicenter Concerto Study. J Cataract Refract Surg. 2016; 42(9):1268–1275

[25] Weeber HA, Meijer ST, Piers PA. Extending the range of vision using diffractive intraocular lens technology. J Cataract Refract Surg. 2015; 41(12):2746–2754

[26] Holladay J. Our refractive IOL armamentarium, more choices than ever. 20/Happy in 20 webinar. August 29, 2020. https://ascrs.org/20happy/agenda/our-refractive-iol-armamentarium

[27] Mencucci R, Favuzza E, Caporossi O, Savastano A, Rizzo S. Comparative analysis of visual outcomes, reading skills, contrast sensitivity, and patient satisfaction with two models of trifocal diffractive intraocular lenses and an extended range of vision intraocular lens. Graefes Arch Clin Exp Ophthalmol. 2018; 256(10):1913–1922

[28] Escandón-García S, Ribeiro FJ, McAlinden C, Queirós A, González-Méijome JM. Through-focus vision performance and light disturbances of 3 new intraocular lenses for presbyopia correction. J Ophthalmol. 2018; 2018:6165493

[29] Alió JL, Kanclerz P. Extended depth-of-field IOLs: clarification of current nomenclature. Ophthalmology Times. 2020; 45(18):33–35

[30] Palomino-Bautista C, Sánchez-Jean R, Carmona-González D, Piñero DP, Molina-Martín A. Subjective and objective depth of field measures in pseudophakic eyes: comparison between extended depth of focus, trifocal and bifocal intraocular lenses. Int Ophthalmol. 2020; 40(2):351–359

[31] Pedrotti E, Bruni E, Bonacci E, Badalamenti R, Mastropasqua R, Marchini G. Comparative analysis of the clinical outcomes with a monofocal and an extended range of vision intraocular lens. J Refract Surg. 2016; 32(7):436–442

[32] Ferreira TB, Pinheiro J, Zabala L, Ribeiro FJ. Comparative analysis of clinical outcomes of a monofocal and an extended-range-of-vision intraocular lens in eyes with previous myopic laser in situ keratomileusis. J Cataract Refract Surg. 2018; 44(2):149–155

[33] Pilger D, Homburg D, Brockmann T, Torun N, Bertelmann E, von Sonnleithner C. Clinical outcome and higher order aberrations after bilateral implantation of an extended depth of focus intraocular lens. Eur J Ophthalmol. 2018; 28 (4):425–432

[34] EyeWorld Monthly Pulse Survey. Current and future IOL choices. EyeWorld. 2018; 23(3):106–108

[35] Son HS, Kim SH, Auffarth GU, Choi CY. Prospective comparative study of tolerance to refractive errors after implantation of extended depth of focus and monofocal intraocular lenses with identical aspheric platform in Korean population. BMC Ophthalmol. 2019; 19(1):187

[36] Chang D. Tips for success with trifocal lenses. Rev Ophthalmol. 2020; XXVII(10):54–56

[37] Waring GO IV. EDOF lenses in post-refractive eyes. Ocular Surgery News. 2018:19

[38] Baartman BJ, Karpuk K, Eichhorn B, et al. Extended depth of focus lens implantation after radial keratotomy. Clin Ophthalmol. 2019; 13:1401–1408

[39] Kohnen T, Böhm M, Hemkeppler E, et al. Visual performance of an extended depth of focus intraocular lens for treatment selection. Eye (Lond). 2019; 33(10):1556–1563

[40] Hammond MD, Potvin R. Visual outcomes, visual quality and patient satisfaction: comparing a blended bifocal approach to bilateral extended depth of focus intraocular lens implantation. Clin Ophthalmol. 2019; 13:2325–2332

[41] Hogarty DT, Russell DJ, Ward BM, Dewhurst N, Burt P. Comparing visual acuity, range of vision and spectacle independence in the extended range of vision and monofocal intraocular lens. Clin Exp Ophthalmol. 2018; 46(8):854–860

[42] Zhang F, Sugar A, Arbisser L, Jacobsen G, Artico J. Crossed versus conventional pseudophakic monovision: patient satisfaction, visual function, and spectacle independence. J Cataract Refract Surg. 2015; 41(9):1845–1854

[43] Sandoval HP, Lane S, Slade S, Potvin R, Donnenfeld ED, Solomon KD. Extended depth-of-focus toric intraocular lens targeted for binocular emmetropia or slight myopia in the nondominant eye: Visual and refractive clinical outcomes. J Cataract Refract Surg. 2019; 45(10):1398–1403

[44] Jackson MA, Edmiston AM, Bedi R. Optimum refractive target in patients with bilateral implantation of extended depth of focus intraocular lenses. Clin Ophthalmol. 2020; 14:455–462

[45] Nivean M, Nivean PD, Reddy JK, et al. Performance of a new-generation extended depth of focus intraocular lens: a prospective comparative study. Asia Pac J Ophthalmol (Phila). 2019; 8(4):285–289

[46] Varma D. Presbyopia-correcting IOL with nondiffractive design offers gains. Ophthalmology Times. 2021:26

[47] Hangai M, Ikeda HO, Akagi T, Yoshimura N. Paracentral scotoma in glaucoma detected by 10-2 but not by 24-2 perimetry. Jpn J Ophthalmol. 2014; 58(2):188–196

12 Trifocal Intraocular Lenses

Fuxiang Zhang, Alan Sugar, and Lisa Brothers Arbisser

Abstract

The FDA approved the first trifocal intraocular lens (IOL) implant PanOptix (Alcon) in the United States in 2019. The domestic literature appears to be consistent with the international data: the trifocal lens is gaining more popularity mainly due to the coverage of intermediate distance when compared with traditional multifocal IOLs and better near vision when compared with the extended depth of focus (EDOF) IOLs. Should a beginner use PanOptix as his/her first premium IOL because of that? This chapter will review and discuss PanOptix's basic design characteristics, main advantages and disadvantages, patients' satisfaction and complaints, the main differences between traditional multifocal/Symfony EDOF lenses and PanOptix, and a candidate selection checklist for residents and beginners. The goal of this chapter is to help beginners understand the role/position of this trifocal lens within the refractive cataract surgery spectrum.

Keywords: trifocal lenses, trifocal IOL, PanOptix, refractive cataract surgery, multiple focal IOL, EDOF, Symfony IOL

12.1 What Are the Main Trifocal IOLs on the Market?

There are at least three trifocal intraocular lens (IOLs) currently popularly used outside of the United States: PanOptix (Alcon, Fort Worth, Texas), AT LISA (Carl Zeiss Meditec, Jena, Germany), and FineVision (PhysIOL, Liège, Belgium). FineVision and AT LISA trifocal IOLs were introduced in 2010 and 2012, respectively.[1] The AcrySof IQ PanOptix Model TFNT00 was first launched in Europe in 2015,[1] and in the United States in the Fall of 2019.[2] Unlike traditional trifocal IOLs that usually have an intermediate focal point of 80 cm, the PanOptix IOL is designed to have an intermediate focal point of 60 cm (arms-length), a more natural and comfortable working distance to perform functional tasks on computers, laptops, and mobiles, among others.

Many peer-reviewed studies, mainly in Europe, in the past few years demonstrated that, generally speaking, the PanOptix IOLs (Alcon) appeared to have at least as good as, or usually, better performance in terms of uncorrected visual acuity for distance, intermediate and near, optical performance, contrast sensitivity, spectacle independence, and patient satisfaction than FineVision (PhysIOL/BVI) and AT LISA (Zeiss) trifocal IOLs.[1,3,4,5,6] Because of these studies and the fact that PanOptix is the only trifocal IOL with FDA approval in the United States, in this chapter, we will discuss Alcon's trifocal PanOptix only (▶ Fig. 12.1, ▶ Fig. 12.2, and ▶ Fig. 12.3).

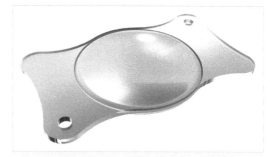

Fig. 12.1 Trifocal lens AT LISA. The AT LISA IOL discussed in this chapter is not available in all markets. Used with permission from Zeiss.

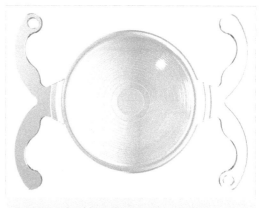

Fig. 12.2 Trifocal lens, Fine Vision. Used with permission from PhysIOL/BVI.

12.2 Is PanOptix Trifocal (Alcon) the Most Popular Presbyopia Correcting IOL in the United States?

Trifocal IOLs have been dominant in the European market in the past few years. The main reason why trifocal IOLs are the most popular presbyopia lenses in Europe is that they are believed to provide good near, intermediate, and distance vision.[7,8,9,10] Based on ESCRS surveys, currently trifocal IOLs have been the most popular option among cataract surgeons, followed by extended depth of focus (EDOF) IOLs, while multifocal IOLs

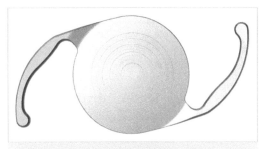

Fig. 12.3 Trifocal lens, PanOptix. Used with permission from Alcon.

have gradually become less popular.[7,11,12] ▶ Fig. 12.4 is the summary comparison based on European Society of Cataract & Refractive Surgeons (ESCRS) clinical surveys in 2017,[13] 2018,[12] and 2019.[14]

Based on the 2019 American Society of Cataract & Refractive Surgeons (ASCRS) clinical survey, the Symfony EDOF (Johnson & Johnson) was the most popular presbyopia correction IOL with 72.6% while the PanOptix (Alcon) was used by only 1.2% (among the American responders only) due to the lag of the FDA's approval date.[15] Growing popularity has been noted in the United States. In a 2021 survey by *Review of Ophthalmology*, 67% of the responders chose nontoric Trifocal PanOptix IOLs (Alcon) while 30% chose nontoric Symfony EDOF ZXROO (Johnson & Johnson). This survey's scope was much smaller than those of ASCRS and ESCRS; only 9% of the 12,258 recipients on *Review*'s email list opened the message and 75 surgeons took the survey.[16]

12.3 What Are the Basic Design Characteristics for the PanOptix?

PanOptix was already available in more than 70 countries prior to the approval by FDA on August 26, 2019.[2] The optic consists of a proprietary high

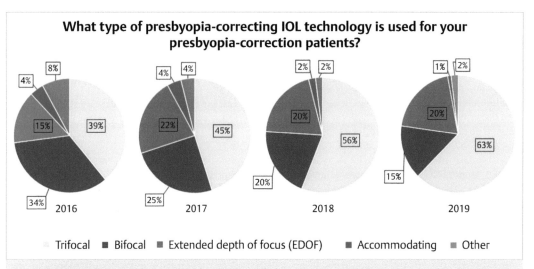

Fig. 12.4 Presbyopia-correcting intraocular lens (IOL) trend in European countries from 2016 to 2019. Data from the European Society of Cataract & Refractive Society Clinical Trends Survey from 2016 to 2019. Used with permission from European Society of Cataract & Refractive Society.

refractive index hydrophobic acrylic material in *spherical* model TFNT00 and toric models. The optic is 6.0 mm in diameter and the lens has an overall diameter of 13.0 mm. The optic diffractive structure is in the central 4.5 mm portion of the optic (the periphery is monofocal) and divides the incoming light to create a +2.17 D intermediate and a +3.25 D near add power at the IOL plane (representing approximately +1.65 D and +2.35 D at the corneal plane after implantation, respectively, for an average human eye).[2] Light is split to 3 foci (distance, intermediate at 60 cm, and near at 40 cm). This light energy is distributed 25% each for near and intermediate and 50% for distance vision,[1] with a 12% light loss when pupil size is at 3 mm.[17,] The anterior surface is designed with negative spherical aberration −0.10 μm[1] to compensate for the positive spherical aberration of the cornea.

12.4 What Are the Highlights of the National Study Based on Which FDA Approved the PanOptix?

A prospective, 6-month, 12 clinical site study in the United States, which was bilateral, non-randomized, vision-assessor masked, and parallel-group study, was designed to evaluate trifocal AcrySof IQ PanOptix and monofocal SN60AT lenses with a total of 250 enrolled subjects (125 bilaterally implanted subjects in each arm). Statistical analysis consisted of the final 129 TFNT00 study patients and 114 SN60AT control patients.[2] This study was also presented at 2020 ASCRS by Cionni et al,[20] and published in the February 2021 issue of *Ophthalmology*.[18] This study was designed to evaluate the effectiveness and safety of AcrySof IQ PanOptix trifocal IOLs in providing a range of vision (distance, intermediate, and near) as compared to a standard monofocal IOL, the AcrySof Monofocal IOL Model SN60AT. Of note, we believe that in this study, SN60WF as control would have been more comparable because the SN60WF also has an aspherical optic while the SN60AT is a spherical IOL.[19] We know that spherical aberration also has an impact on the visual quality.

This lens mitigates the effects of presbyopia by providing improved intermediate and near visual acuity while maintaining comparable distance visual acuity with a reduced need for eyeglasses, compared to the monofocal IOL. The binocular contrast sensitivity results were slightly reduced for the PanOptix IOL compared to the monofocal control IOL. However, the differences were not clinically meaningful. Overall, this study not only showed excellent spectacle independence and patient satisfaction with the PanOptix lens but also revealed the noticeable or significant downsides.

12.5 What Are the Main Complaints from Patients Who Have PanOptix?

The main complaints from PanOptix patients are not slightly compromised distance vision or contrast sensitivity, but are night visual dysphotopsias: glare, halo, and starbursts. That is similar to what we have noted in our multifocal IOL patients. How severe are they? Here is the summary based on the study[2] from which FDA approved the trifocal (▶ Table 12.1).

12.5.1 Do Those Dysphotopsias Really Bother These Patients?

See ▶ Table 12.2.

The highest rate of most bothersome reports ("Bothered Very Much") at 6 months was for starburst at 4.8%, halo 2.4%, and glare 1.6% for the PanOptix Trifocal IOL. There was one explant of the IOL due dissatisfaction with the level of vision, which was determined to be related to the optical properties of the IOL.[2]

12.6 What Is the Satisfaction Rate from Those Patients Who Had Bilateral PanOptix?

See ▶ Table 12.3.

The impressive positive finding was that 95.3% of the PanOptix patients were satisfied (21.3%) or very satisfied (74.0%), 99.2% would like to have the lens again, and 98.4% would refer it to their family and friends.

In addition to this FDA study,[2] studies presented at ASCRS in 2020 also showed excellent outcomes.[21,22,23] They had extremely high patient satisfaction and excellent vision. Even with mild to moderate halos, these patients would still choose the same lens again and were very happy with their results.

Table 12.1 PanOptix and monofocal control group visual disturbance, severity[2]

		n^a	None (%)	A little (%)	Mild (%)	Moderate (%)	Severe (%)
Glare	PanOptix	126	49.2	7.9	21.4	18.3	3.2
	SN60AT	111	67.6	3.6	13.5	13.5	1.8
Halo	PanOptix	127	36.2	9.4	18.9	22.8	12.6
	SN60AT	110	77.3	7.3	8.2	6.4	0.9
Star-Burst	PanOptix	125	44.0	2.4	10.4	27.2	16.0
	SN60AT	109	73.4	8.3	9.2	7.3	1.8

[a] PanOptix total $n = 129$, SN60AT total $n = 114$. "n" as actual number of patients for each specific question. Percentage calculated as 100%.

Table 12.2 PanOptix and monofocal intraocular lens (IOL) control group visual disturbance, bothersomeness[2]

		n^a	Not experienced or not bothered at all (%)	A little bit (%)	Some-what (%)	Quite a bit	Very much (%)
Glare	PanOptix	126	54.8	18.3	18.3	7.1	1.6
	SN60AT	111	69.4	15.3	8.1	6.3	0.9
Halo	PanOptix	127	51.2	21.3	16.5	8.7	2.4
	SN60AT	110	83.6	10.9	3.6	0.9	0.9
Star-Burst	PanOptix	125	55.2	16.8	16.0	7.2	4.8
	SN60AT	109	79.8	10.1	8.3	0.9	0.9

[a] PanOptix total $n = 129$, SN60AT total $n = 114$. "n" as actual number of patients for each specific question. Percentage calculated as 100%.

12.7 If a Patient Can Use Either a Traditional MFIOL or PanOptix, Which One Would You Choose?

There is not much advantage to use MFIOLs if the patient is a good candidate for PanOptix. Before trifocal IOL availability, we often implanted an EDOF IOL or a lower add multifocal in the dominant eye, and a higher add bifocal in the nondominant eye in an attempt to get all three distances. When a multifocal IOL is the option, use of a trifocal is our recommendation. We do not see a place for bifocals anymore. A trifocal offers everything a bifocal can plus the intermediate vision at no extra expense or downside. We had quite a few patients with successful bilateral MFIOL, but they had to sit closer to their computer due to compromised intermediate vision. With the trifocal IOLs, we can aim both eyes at plano without mini-monovision or mixing and matching different IOLs. Binocular summation is a visual reward for patients and one that we compromise to some degree when each eye is focused differently.

What is more, PanOptix actually should be more forgiving in terms of patient pupil size. The PanOptix has a larger (4.5 mm) diffractive zone than ReSTOR (3.6 mm).[24,25] The central optic

Table 12.3 Patient satisfaction rate for PanOptix and monofocal intraocular lens (IOL) control group[2]

Question	Response	PanOptix	SN60AT
In the past 7 days, how satisfied were you with your vision?	Total patient number	127	110
	Very dissatisfied	1.6%	0%
	Dissatisfied	1.6%	2.7%
	Neither satisfied nor dissatisfied	1.6%	6.4%
	Satisfied	21.3%	30.9%
	Very satisfied	74.0%	60.0%
Given your vision today, if you had to do it all over, would you have the same lenses implanted again?	Total patient number	127	111
	No	0.8%	12.6%
	Yes	**99.2%**	87.4%
Given your vision today, would you recommend the lenses you had implanted to your family or friends?	Total patient number	127	110
	No	1.6%	4.5%
	Yes	**98.4%**	95.5%

of the PanOptix is slightly larger (1.164 mm) than previous bifocal diffractive IOLs. This makes the PanOptix lens less pupil dependent and more forgiving from angle kappa and angle alpha perspectives.

Trifocal IOLs also save our preoperative patient consultation time because we do not have to spend time explaining possible mix-and-match strategies any more.

12.8 What Are the Main Components You Convey to Prospective Candidates for Trifocal IOLs?

First, we need to make sure that a patient is a good candidate for trifocal implants, without significant ocular comorbidities, with a strong desire for spectacle freedom and does not drive a lot at night. Based on our track record, We tell patients that 8 or 9 out of 10 of our premium IOL patients will be happy or very happy with what they choose and what they pay. Contrast sensitivity is slightly decreased for trifocal IOLs when compared with monofocal IOLs, but this is usually

not noticeable and clinically does not seem to be important. We typically do not even bring it up for discussion. We do fully discuss the presence of night dysphotopsias in detail and emphasize the fact that with presbyopia correcting IOLs, everything is a compromise. We are not able to restore the vision of our youth. By providing improved intermediate and near visual acuity, while maintaining comparable distance visual acuity with a reduced need for eyeglasses, most of our patients do not complain of mild dysphotopsias.

12.9 In Terms of Photic Phenomena and Patient Satisfaction, Which One Is Better, PanOptix or Symfony?

A study presented at 2020 ASCRS[26] compared the visual outcomes and quality of the PanOptix with the Symfony EDOF ($n = 60$ patients, 120 eyes, 30 patients in each group). At 3-month follow-up, the trifocal group had significantly better near visual acuity than the EDOF group ($p = 0.03$). The defocus curve showed the trifocal IOL had better intermediate/near performance than the EDOF group. The total higher order aberrations and contrast sensitivity were not significantly different. The QoV questionnaire results showed no differences in dysphotopsias between the two groups.

A good and thorough review[1] done by Sudhir et al did not suggest a noticeable consistent difference between the two IOLs. The authors did a literature search in the PubMed database to identify studies that have assessed the visual and other clinical outcomes. Twelve studies were included in that review article. The contrast sensitivity (CS) under both photopic and mesopic conditions was similar between the PanOptix and the Symfony EDOF IOL and was found to be within the normal range expected for the age group. Perception of halos and difficulty in night driving were the most common visual disturbances reported. However, the majority of patients reported that the visual side effects had no impact on their satisfaction. High patient satisfaction was reported with PanOptix and Symfony patients and there were no reports of patients opting for lens exchange due to photic phenomena in any of the studies.

A nonrandomized prospective study in Italy looked at bilateral implantation of three different IOLs in 60 patients: Symfony ($n = 20$), PanOptix ($n = 20$), and AT LISA ($n = 20$). Visual results, photopic and mesopic CS, binocular reading skills (MNREAD charts), and patient satisfaction were evaluated 3 months after surgery. The Symfony IOL provided significantly better photopic and mesopic contrast sensitivity outcomes than both PanOptix and AT LISA trifocals ($p < 0.001$).[27] PanOptix provided better visual acuity at 60 cm than the other two IOLs; similarly, at 80 cm, Symfony was significantly better than the other two IOLs. The near vision was better with PanOptix than with AT LISA; both IOLs showed significantly better near vision than Symfony. Halos and glare were less in the Symfony group than in PanOptix group, 70% versus 50%.

One presentation at the 2020 ASCRS 20/Happy conference suggests that Symfony EDOF patients have less dysphotopsias and better contrast compared with PanOptix patients.[28] Our limited experience is consistent with this presentation in terms of dysphotopsias. If the uncorrected near visual acuity (UNVA) is very important to a patient's lifestyle and desire, use PanOptix rather than Symfony.

12.10 Are There Any Advantages to Using Symfony EDOF versus PanOptix? Which One Is Easier for a Beginner?

Our impressions of contrast sensitivity and patient satisfaction are very similar between these two lenses. The major difference is the near vision, where PanOptix has much better UNVA than Symfony. If distance and intermediate vision dominate a patient's lifestyle and hobbies, we would still consider bilateral Symfony EDOF lenses rather than trifocal IOLs. On the other hand, if UNVA is very important to the patient, then we will recommend PanOptix.

A prospective, comparative, single center study in Italy suggested better tolerance of interventional induced astigmatism in Symfony EDOF lens patients than in PanOptix patients. The Symfony IOL showed less dissatisfaction and less reduction of visual acuity than the PanOptix IOL. The authors concluded that simulated residual cylinders after the implantation of the Symfony IOL up to 1.0 D have a very mild and not clinically relevant impact on visual acuity or satisfaction.[29]

There was a prospective study in Korea showing that residual refractive error was better tolerated in patients with an EDOF IOL compared with a monofocal IOL of the same design.[30] This is likely due to the diffractive optical design maintaining higher levels of visual acuity at a wider dioptric range of defocus.

Our limited experience suggested that Symfony EDOF has a larger landing zone than PanOptix in terms of hitting the refractive target, meeting patient satisfaction, and mitigating complaints. Symfony EDOF IOLs seem to have less dysphotopsias than PanOptix. We believe that it is easier for beginners to start with a Symfony EDOF rather than a PanOptix. For beginners, except monofocal IOLs, Symfony EDOF IOLs are likely the most forgiving premium IOLs at this time.

12.11 Why Do You Have Your PanOptix Trifocal Patients Come Back for Biometry rather than Do the Measurements on the Same Day?

We have all premium IOL patients, not only trifocal IOL patients, come back to do biometry and other tests. The time to make the decision to have a conventional IOL or premium IOL is at the end of the office visit when eye drops have been applied, pupils dilated, and intraocular pressure (IOP) checked. We cannot expect to have very accurate measurements in this situation.[31] Plus, during busy office flow, it is hard to have two technicians do careful and unrushed measurements. Some practices do biometry tests prior to eye drops for those cataract evaluation patients on the same day as office visits.

12.12 What Is the Number One Reason for an Unhappy Patient in Each Category of Refractive Cataract Surgery?

- Multifocal and trifocal IOL: Halo and glare with nighttime driving. Complaints of decreased contrast are fewer.
- EDOF: Same as MFIOL and trifocal, especially in younger patients, but seem fewer and less severe in intensity. Reading power can also be an issue, but if we use mini-monovision, it is typically acceptable.
- Crystalens: Near reading power.
- Pseudophakic monovision: Distance vision is not as good in the near eye when is compared with the distance vision of the distance eye.
- Patients with a history of corneal refractive surgery: Not being able to hit the exact refractive target, especially for those who had a an enhancement procedure after the original LASIK/PRK.

12.13 Why Do You Exclude Patients with Cornea Guttata for Your Trifocal IOLs?

The corneal endothelium is a single cell layer and typically not repairable. Literature has indicated that guttae alone, without visible corneal edema, can cause glare, halo, and decreased contrast.[32] Dysphotopsias are the number 1 reason for patient complaints from diffractive optical design IOLs. According to the Swedish National Cataract Registry between 2010 and 2012 ($n = 276,363$ patients), there is a 68-fold increased risk for corneal transplantation after phacoemulsification in patients with cornea guttata compared with those without.[33] A large study ($n = 33,741$ patients) also concluded that cornea guttata alone without corneal edema was significantly associated with a poorer visual acuity and a worse self-assessed visual function after cataract surgery.[34] What is more, cornea guttata is a progressive disease and aging is one of the main etiologies, among other factors, such as female gender, thinning cornea, inflammation, trauma, and smoking.[34] For these reasons, it is recommended that we exclude those patients with easily noticeable guttae as premium IOL candidates.

12.14 Who Can be Good Candidates for the First Few Cases of Trifocal IOLs?

See ▶ Table 12.4.

Table 12.4 Trifocal candidate selection checklist for beginners

	Good candidates	Try to avoid
Desire	Strong desire for spectacle freedom	Readers do not bother them
Refractive status	Hyperopia	Mild to moderate myopia typically have great near vision without glasses and hard to impress them with postop UNVA
Ocular surgical history	No laser vision correction	S/P LASIK/PRK/RK
Astigmatism	No astigmatism for the first few cases; Regular astigmatism correctable with LRI or toric version	Any significant irregular astigmatism should be considered as contraindications

(*Continued*)

Table 12.4 (*Continued*) Trifocal candidate selection checklist for beginners

	Good candidates	Try to avoid
Placido Ring images	Clear	With irregularities, especially in the central area
Tear film and ocular surface	Good tear film	Dry eyes and/or with significant MGD
Corneal epithelium and stroma	Clear	EBMD and Fuchs dystrophy
Anterior chamber depth and axial length	Within normal range	Extremity length eyes will have more challenges for ELP and hard to hit refractive target
Pupil	Well-dilated pupil	Poorly dilated pupil or possible cases of intraoperative floppy iris syndrome (IFIS)
Mesopic pupil size	3–5 mm	2.5 mm or less may be too small to have good reading vision; 5.5 mm or more will have more chance of glare
Spherical aberration	<0.6 μm	0.6 μm or more
Coma	<0.3 μm	0.3 μm or more
Angle Kappa	<0.6 mm	0.6 mm or more
Cataract	Moderate	Very dense or other high-risk cataracts
Other ocular Comorbidities	Health macula with normal OCT	Any noticeable macular degeneration or diabetic retinopathy, glaucoma with field loss or poorly controlled IOP
Laser AK if considered	Cooperative and expected to be able to lay flat with normal head position and reasonable size of lid aperture	Nervous, small lid aperture, neck problem to have normal head position, unable to lay flat, deep eye socket, too small cornea diameter
Personality	Easy going; accept some halo and glare	Perfectionist

Abbreviations: EBMD, epithelial basement membrane dystrophy; ELP, effective lens position; IOP, intraocular pressure; MFIOL, multifocal intraocular lens; MGD, meibomian gland dysfunction; OCT, optical coherence tomography; UNVA, uncorrected near visual acuity.

References

[1] Sudhir RR, Dey A, Bhattacharrya S, Bahulayan A. AcrySof IQ PanOptix intraocular lens versus extended depth of focus intraocular lens and trifocal intraocular lens: a clinical overview. Asia Pac J Ophthalmol (Phila). 2019; 8(4):335–349

[2] Summary of Safety and Effectiveness Data (SSED): AcrySof® IQ PanOptix ® Trifocal Intraocular Lens (Model TFNT00) AcrySof® IQ PanOptix ® Toric Trifocal Intraocular Lens (Model TFNT30, TFNT40, TFNT50, TFNT60). United States Food and Drug Administration. Approved August 26, 2019. PMA P040020/S087. Accessed April 30, 2021

[3] Malyugin BE, Sobolev NP, Fomina OV, Belokopytov AV. [Comparative analysis of the functional results after implantation of various diffractive trifocal intraocular lenses]. Vestn Oftalmol. 2020; 136(1):80–89

[4] Ribeiro FJ, Ferreira TB. Comparison of visual and refractive outcomes of 2 trifocal intraocular lenses. J Cataract Refract Surg. 2020; 46(5):694–699

[5] Carson D, Xu Z, Alexander E, Choi M, Zhao Z, Hong X. Optical bench performance of 3 trifocal intraocular lenses. J Cataract Refract Surg. 2016; 42(9):1361–1367

[6] Lapid-Gortzak R, Bhatt U, Sanchez JG, et al. Multicenter visual outcomes comparison of 2 trifocal presbyopia-correcting IOLs: 6-month postoperative results. J Cataract Refract Surg. 2020; 46(11):1534–1542

[7] Alió J. Trifocal IOLs: Presbyopia and astigmatism treatment options. EuroTimes. 2019 Suppl Strategies for success with toric & presbyopia correcting IOLs:3–4

[8] Martínez de Carneros-Llorente A, Martínez de Carneros A, Martínez de Carneros-Llorente P, Jiménez-Alfaro I. Comparison of visual quality and subjective outcomes among 3 trifocal intraocular lenses and 1 bifocal intraocular lens. J Cataract Refract Surg. 2019; 45(5):587–594

[9] Cochener B, Boutillier G, Lamard M, Auberger-Zagnoli C. A comparative evaluation of a new generation of diffractive trifocal and extended depth of focus intraocular lenses. J Refract Surg. 2018; 34(8):507–514

[10] Escandón-García S, Ribeiro FJ, McAlinden C, Queirós A, González-Méijome JM. Through-focus vision performance and light disturbances of 3 new intraocular lenses for presbyopia correction. J Ophthalmol. 2018; 2018:6165493

[11] Lindstrom RL. Lens replacement surgery poised to become most successful refractive procedure. Ocular Surgery News. 2018:3

[12] Morselli S. Precise preoperative planning optimizes premium IOL outcomes. EuroTimes. 2019 Suppl Strategies for success with toric & presbyopia correcting IOLs:1–2

[13] ESCRS 2017 Clinical trends survey. EuroTimes. Accessed April 30, 2021. https://www.eurotimes.org/escrs-2017-clinical-trends-survey-results/

[14] ESCRS 2019 Clinical trends survey. EuroTimes. Accessed April 30, 2021. https://www.eurotimes.org/escrs-2019-clinical-trends-survey-results/

[15] ASCRS. 2019 Clinical survey. ASCRS Database.

[16] Bethke W. IOL survey: new lenses turn surgeons' heads. Rev Ophthalmol 2021;40–42

[17] Kohnen T. Trifocal IOLs—PanOptix. Our refractive IOL armamentarium, more choices than ever. ASCRS 20/Happy in 2020 webinar. August 29, 2020. https://ascrs.org/20 happy/agenda/our-refractive-iol-armamentarium

[18] Cionni RJ, Maxwell WA, Modi SS. Non-randomized prospective assessment of efficacy and safety of a new trifocal IOL presented at 2020 ASCRS Virtual Annual Meeting. May 16, 2020

[19] Modi S, Lehmann R, Maxwell A, et al. Visual and patient-reported outcomes of a diffractive trifocal intraocular lens compared with those of a monofocal intraocular lens. Ophthalmology. 2021; 128(2):197–207

[20] Zhang F. Re: Modi et al.: Visual and patient-reported outcomes of a diffractive trifocal intraocular lens compared with those of a monofocal intraocular lens. Ophthalmology. 2021;128:197–207). Ophthalmology. Published online 2021:S0161–6420(21)00212–8

[21] Hovanesian JA, Quentin A, Jones M. The PanOptix trifocal IOL: a study of patient satisfaction, visual disturbances, and uncorrected visual performance. Paper presented at 2020 ASCRS Virtual Annual Meeting. May 16–17, 2020. https://ascrs.org/clinical-education/presbyopia/2020-pod-sps-108–60552-the-panoptix-trifocal-iol-a-study-of-patient-satisfaction-visual

[22] Rowen SL, Raoof D. Early real world outcomes of the first U.S. approved trifocal IOL. Paper presented at: 2020 ASCRS Virtual Annual Meeting. May 16, 2020. https://ascrs.org/clinical-education/presbyopia/2020-pod-sps-108–64008-early-real-world-outcomes-of-the-first-us-approved-trifocal-iol

[23] Blehm CG, Potvin R. Evaluation of spectacle independence after bilateral implantation of a trifocal intraocular lens. ASCRS May 16, 2020

[24] Kohnen T. First implantation of a diffractive quadrafocal (trifocal) intraocular lens. J Cataract Refract Surg. 2015; 41(10):2330–2332

[25] Fisher BL. Presbyopia-correcting intraocular lenses in cataract surgery: a focus on RESTOR Intraocular Lenses. US Ophthalmic Rev. 2011; 4(1):44–48

[26] Ramamurthy S, Sachdev GS, Dandapani R. Comparison of visual outcomes and internal aberrations following implantation of diffractive trifocal & extended depth of focus IOLs. Presented at: 2020 ASCRS Virtual Annual Meeting. May 16, 2020

[27] Mencucci R, Favuzza E, Caporossi O, Savastano A, Rizzo S. Comparative analysis of visual outcomes, reading skills, contrast sensitivity, and patient satisfaction with two models of trifocal diffractive intraocular lenses and an extended range of vision intraocular lens. Graefes Arch Clin Exp Ophthalmol. 2018; 256(10):1913–1922

[28] Berdahl J. Our refractive IOL armamentarium, more choices than ever. ASCRS 20/Happy in 20 webinar. August 29, 2020

[29] Carones F. Residual astigmatism threshold and patient satisfaction with bifocal, trifocal and extended range of vision intraocular lenses (IOLs). Open J Ophthalmol. 2017; 7(1):1–7

[30] Son HS, Kim SH, Auffarth GU, Choi CY. Prospective comparative study of tolerance to refractive errors after implantation of extended depth of focus and monofocal intraocular lenses with identical aspheric platform in Korean population. BMC Ophthalmol. 2019; 19(1):187

[31] Kieval JZ, Al-Hashimi S, Davidson RS, et al. ASCRS Refractive Cataract Surgery Subcommittee. Prevention and management of refractive prediction errors following cataract surgery. J Cataract Refract Surg. 2020; 46(8):1189–1197

[32] Price FW, Jr, Feng MT. Impact of corneal guttata on cataract surgery results. J Cataract Refract Surg. 2019; 45(11):1692

[33] Viberg A, Samolov B, Claesson Armitage M, Behndig A, Byström B. Incidence of corneal transplantation after phacoemulsification in patients with corneal guttata: a registry-based cohort study. J Cataract Refract Surg. 2020; 46(7):961–966

[34] Viberg A, Liv P, Behndig A, Lundström M, Byström B. The impact of corneal guttata on the results of cataract surgery. J Cataract Refract Surg. 2019; 45(6):803–809

13 The Light-Adjustable Lens

H. Burkhard Dick and Ronald D. Gerste

Abstract

The light-adjustable lens (LAL) is a technology that allows postoperative adjustment for refractive errors up to approximately 2.5 diopters (D) of both sphere and cylinder. It requires cooperative and understanding patients who are highly motivated, since strict adherence to postoperative guideline of UV protection is essential. Long-term follow-up has demonstrated high refractive stability with no clinically significant changes noted to the cornea or the macula from the repeated UV exposures. Based on our long-term experience, the LAL technology is a safe and efficient method to achieve good visual results and high patient satisfaction.

Keywords: cataract surgery, corneal endothelium, hyperopia, light-adjustable lens (LAL), macular thickness, myopia, postoperative refraction, refractive stability, UV exposure

Currently, cataract surgery has in almost all cases become refractive surgery. It might even be stated that cataract surgery has evolved into the most frequently performed technique of refractive surgery. Gone are the days when patients were satisfied with a reasonable postoperative visual acuity provided by whatever kind of glasses they had to wear to achieve that visual function. "Spectacle-independence" is what counts these days, patients (mostly in wealthy countries, as there is still no sufficient infrastructure to treat all cataracts in some poorer regions) often demand 20/20 vision without glasses, at least for distance vision; the most discerning will opt for intraocular lenses (IOLs) that promise good visual acuity also for intermediate and near vision.

Patient expectation is one thing, real-world outcomes are another. In a study published about 20 years ago, 72.3% of all eyes that underwent cataract surgery and implantation of a monofocal IOL were within ±1 diopter (D) of emmetropia[1]; the majority of the patients required spectacles for optimal distance vision. In a more recent study from Denmark, 12% of the operated eyes missed their target refraction by 1.0 D or more.[2] It seems that patients can be so determined to do without glasses after cataract surgery that many who would need a postoperative additional correction refuse to wear them, as a Swedish study had demonstrated: in this cohort reported by Farhoudi et al, almost 50% of patients with both spherical and cylindrical refractive errors of more than 1 D after the operation did not obtain the new distance spectacles they would have needed to attain full visual acuity.[3]

There are numerous reasons why postoperative refraction can turn out to be less than perfect. There are inherent limitations to the accuracy of preoperative biometry as well as to the precision of the IOL power calculation which has a certain potential for refractive surprises. Corneal topography can be misjudged and, for instance, posterior corneal astigmatism underestimated. There can be problems with the IOL position like suboptimal centration, longitudinal shift, and—extremely important in toric IOLs—rotation. Wound healing can influence postoperative refraction by, for instance, causing surgically induced astigmatism (SIA).[4,5] Among all the uncertainness, effective lens position (ELP) is likely the most unpredictable one.

A development that further has to be taken into account: many patients who have undergone corneal refractive surgery in their younger years and thereby have demonstrated an ardent desire for spectacle-independence are now reaching the age at which cataract surgery often becomes necessary. These former refractive patients are coming with an altered cornea in an eye for which cataract surgery might be the last refractive surgical opportunity. IOL power determination has proven particularly challenging and sometimes unreliable in these eyes. Individuals with a history of laser refractive surgery are therefore at an increased risk of marked residual refractive error after IOL implantation.[6]

A number of technologies have been developed to allow postoperative adjustment of the refractive power of an already implanted IOL. Some of these adjustments are part of an invasive procedure, and some are noninvasive. A noninvasive, nonsurgical option to correct postoperative residual refractive errors and to achieve refractive stability over time has been offered in our clinic for more than 10 years now. It is the LAL, the light-adjustable lens (RxSight, Aliso Viejo, CA) which uses profiled doses of ultraviolet light to adjust residual refractive errors after cataract surgery (▶ Fig. 13.1). This technology received CE market approval in Europe in 2007; in the United States approval by the FDA was granted in November 2017. The LAL can be used to correct postoperative myopia, hyperopia, astigmatism, asphericity, and presbyopia.

The LAL is based on the inclusion of a proprietary photoreactive silicone macromer within a medical-grade silicone polymer matrix (▶ Fig. 13.2). Selective irradiation of the implanted LAL using a digital light delivery device to deliver targeted doses of spatially profiled UV light (365 nm) produces modifications in the IOL curvature, resulting in a predictable spherical and/or cylindrical power change postoperatively (▶ Fig. 13.3). For example, an UV irradiation of the central segment of the LAL is performed in cases of hyperopic correction, while to treat residual postoperative myopia, the peripheral portions of the LAL optic are irradiated. Following myopic treatment, the silicone macromers from the untreated central portion of the optic diffuse outward, resulting in central flattening and a reduction in IOL power. Astigmatism can be treated with a special illumination profile; the exact algorithms, however, are not publicly available at this time based on the manufacturer's restriction. Treating

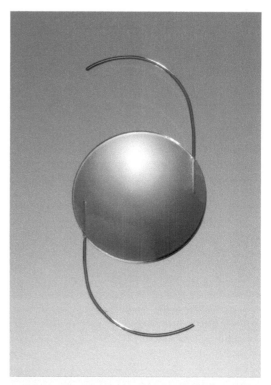

Fig. 13.1 Overview of the light-adjustable intraocular lens (IOL), which is a three-piece, foldable silicone lens with modified C-haptics.

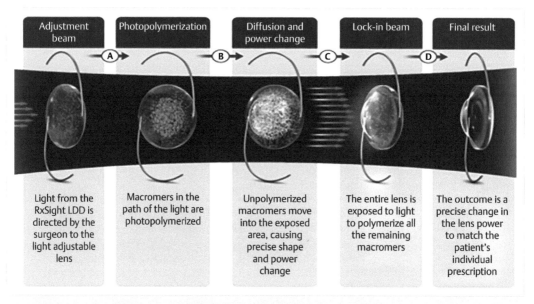

Adjustment beam	Photopolymerization	Diffusion and power change	Lock-in beam	Final result
Light from the RxSight LDD is directed by the surgeon to the light adjustable lens	Macromers in the path of the light are photopolymerized	Unpolymerized macromers move into the exposed area, causing precise shape and power change	The entire lens is exposed to light to polymerize all the remaining macromers	The outcome is a precise change in the lens power to match the patient's individual prescription

Fig. 13.2 Mechanism of action using spatially profiled ultraviolet (UV) light (365 nm).

irregular astigmatism is possible and has been done by us in a small controlled evaluation but is currently not commercially available for clinical use. For that, a major controlled approval study would be necessary. The LAL optic has a thin posterior layer, which contains a higher concentration of UV absorber than the photoreactive lens bulk material to protect the retina from UV-light exposure during adjustment and lock-in of the IOL's power.[7] We have not observed a higher incidence of PCO. Being a three-piece IOL with sharp edges, the LAL is reminiscent of the Tecnis silicone lens which proved to be superior in PCO prevention to many other designs. We have also placed the LAL in Berger's space resulting in an immediate final positioning of the lens.

After a period of postoperative refractive stabilization, typically up to 14 to 21 days, the patient returns for examination and for determining the postoperative refraction by the surgeon who will then decide whether adjustment in spherical and/or cylindrical power is required. To achieve target refraction, sometimes two of these "fine-tuning" sessions are required (▶ Fig. 13.4). If the desired refractive state has been achieved, a final lock-in is performed to permanently fix the refractive power of the lens. During lock-in all remaining monomers are completely polymerized. A special illumination profile is being used which allows lock-in even in eyes with a small pupil. This lock-in does not affect the final dioptric power of the LAL. It is extremely important that the patient wears UV protection glasses until the day of this final lock-in to protect the eye from any ambient UV exposure which could lead to uncontrolled polymerization of the IOL.[8,9,10] If a patient has a significant UV exposure prior to the final lock-in, it would be the result of patient nonadherence. One would expect to have enough monomers left to do a rescue procedure; otherwise the accidental exposure would lead to myopization and additional aberrations. Doing corneal correction could be an option. In an extreme case, exchanging the IOL could be considered.

The LAL is a three-piece, foldable silicone lens with modified C-haptics. It has a sharp-edged design and is biconvex with an optic of 6.0 mm diameter. The LAL is available with a refractive power from 10.0 to 30.0 D in 0.5- to 1.0-D increments. Its implantation is performed during standard phacoemulsification. After pharmacological mydriasis, a clear corneal incision using a 2.75-mm steel keratome (Alcon Laboratories, Inc., Fort Worth, Texas) is made. Two-side port incisions are performed. After instillation of the ophthalmic viscosurgical device (OVD; sodium hyaluronate 1.0%, like Healon, Johnson & Johnson

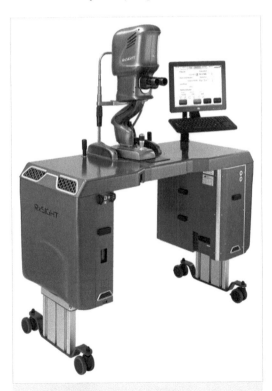

Fig. 13.3 Light delivery device (LDD).

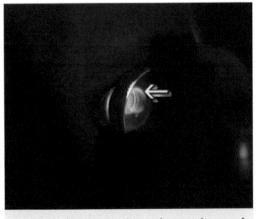

Fig. 13.4 Light treatment (*arrow* shows to the area of light application) using the light delivery device (LDD) and a contact glass.

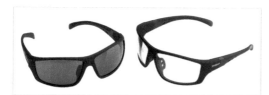

Fig. 13.5 Spectacles for ultraviolet (UV) light protection, also available as bifocal glasses.

Vision, Santa Ana, California) into the anterior chamber, a continuous curvilinear anterior capsulorhexis between 4.5 mm and 5.5 mm is created. Phacoemulsification with the stop-and-chop technique (Stellaris, Bausch & Lomb, Rochester, New York) is performed, and residual cortex is removed with irrigation/aspiration (I/A). During the operation, light in the operating room is dimmed as much as possible. The LAL is taken out of its light-shielding casing only immediately before the implantation. Then the LAL is implanted in the capsular bag by using a 2.75-mm injector system and the OVD is removed. The eye is immediately covered with a patch. Postoperatively, standard treatment with topical antibiotic and steroid eyedrops is applied: four times daily for the first week, then tapered over 6 weeks. The advice to the patient to wear UV-blocking spectacles at all times during daylight hours until the final lock-in treatment is completed needs to be expressed rather too often than not often enough (▶ Fig. 13.5).

The adjustment is performed using an array of micromirrors to create the spatially resolved irradiation profile to correct residual refractive error. That refractive error can amount to about 2.5 D of sphere (hyperopia or myopia) and/or cylinder, and will be corrected by adjusting the refractive power according to the patient's needs and expectations before the final lock-in takes place. The first adjustment is done about 10 days after cataract surgery—it is often the only one: in our patients, there was an average of 1.6 adjustments necessary.

Our clinic was one of the first to implant the LAL and may currently be the one with the most experience worldwide (more than 600 LAL implantations until 12/2020). Therefore, we can with confidence judge the efficacy as well as the safety of this technology—and, in short, both are excellent. There is a wide range of refractive errors and clinical situations that we have successfully treated with the LAL, from spherical and spherocylindrical errors to asphericity, in postcorneal refractive surgery eyes, in long as well as in short eyes. It turned out to be possible with this technique to customize a near addition and to create adjustable (mini-)monovision. It is a technology that has not yet reached the end of its development—and thus further options and wider indications can be expected.

The refractive stability is superb. In a cohort of 122 eyes, over a follow-up of 18 months, the refractive change one-and-a-half years after the final lock-in was on average a minuscule, clinically completely irrelevant –0.02 D. The deviation from target correction was in general extremely small: 98% of eyes were within ±0.5 D, 100% within ±1.0 D of target refraction. All these eyes achieved an uncorrected visual acuity (UCVA) of 20/25 or better, 89% achieved 20/20, and 25% achieved 25/20.[8] These results were confirmed over a much longer time period. In a group of 93 eyes, uncorrected distance visual acuity 1 year after surgery was 0.2 logMAR, and 7 years after surgery it was 0.28 logMAR. There was a minor change in corrected distance visual acuity (CDVA) from 0.07 logMAR 1 year after surgery to 0.12 logMAR 7 years postoperatively. Refraction was also stable. The refraction after 1 year was 0.04 D and after 7 years 0.23 D (n = 93). The average central corneal thickness remained unchanged from 550 μm preoperatively to 555 μm after 1 year (n = 53) and 553 μm after 7 years (n = 54).[11]

Even in challenging eyes, the refractive and visual success rate is high. In 15 eyes with high axial hyperopia (less than 22.20 mm), 100% achieved UCVA of 20/30 or better after final lock-in; 67% achieved 20/25 or better and 27% had a UCVA of 20/20 or better. Eighty-six percent (86%) of these eyes were within 0.5 D and 100% within 1.0 D of target refraction.[12] In high axial myopia (greater than 24.5 mm), 95% of eyes were within 0.5 D and 100% were within 1.0 D of target refraction.[13]

Speaking of corneal thickness: we could demonstrate that the different steps taken like irradiation for adjustment and lock-in do not cause damage to the cornea. Not only was corneal thickness in 122 eyes basically unchanged after 1 year as mentioned above, but endothelial cell loss was in accordance with what is reported in the literature after phacoemulsification and IOL implantation in general. Two weeks after surgery and before adjustment there was 6.91% endothelial cell loss and 12 months after lock-in it amounted to 6.57%. This leads to the conclusion that the UV light exposure for adjustment and lock-in procedures does not add to the endothelial damage caused by cataract surgery.[14] The same high safety-profile could be established vis-a-vis another highly sensitive cell layer: the macula. Thickness measurements performed by OCT preoperatively and repeatedly over 1 year after final lock-in revealed no influence on the incidence of macular edema and showed that the UV exposure did not cause any changes in the macular layers.[15]

Common mistakes that are made in connection with the LAL are generally linked to the refraction. Careful refractive techniques need to be employed and the resulting refraction should demonstrate the expected improvement in uncorrected visual acuity. For complex cases, such as post-RK eyes, care must be taken that a stable refraction has been reached, which may require additional observation time. This can be much different from individual to individual, so there is no general rule or recommendation. This point has to be discussed preoperatively with the patient and he or she will decide whether the procedure under these circumstances is really an option. Usually one can expect to wait at least 1 to 3 months.

Adjusting the IOL power postoperatively is an emerging technology with some fascinating developments, made necessary not the least by the aforementioned residual refractive errors after cataract surgery. Compared with other options of changing an IOL's refractive power, the LAL has the undeniable advantage of a noninvasive power adjustment. That is also the case in two other IOL designs that have been created for power adjustment: neither the magnetically adjustable IOL nor the liquid crystal intraocular adaptive lens that is shaped by wireless control requires any secondary surgical procedures.

In contrast, a number of evolving or already clinically introduced options require another operation like multicomponent IOLs, mechanically adjustable IOLs, and the repeatedly adjustable IOLs.

The LAL does not require the surgeon to deviate from his or her technique and offers the highly demanding patient a good chance, in fact almost a guarantee, to achieve full uncorrected distance visual acuity. It is certainly not recommended in patients who seem incapable of adherence to the treatment regimen, in particular to wearing UV protection most of the time until lock-in. It is an option for cooperative individuals as well as, for example, patients after previous keratorefractive procedures. LAL implantation means an increased work-load for the surgeon—who will be rewarded by extremely satisfied patients.

You may wonder, what are the patient satisfaction differences between LAL patents versus diffractive optic IOLs, such as multifocal IOLs (MFIOLs) and trifocal IOLs? At the time of this writing, there are no controlled trials on patient satisfaction after LAL implantation compared to MIOLs and trifocal lenses. In general, patient satisfaction among LAL patients is extremely high, not in the least since the results are almost "Lasik-like." In our experience, the LAL always delivers while among the MIOL patients there are now and then individuals who express some disappointment. A major factor for this is the ease and convenience of the procedures like the fine-tuning and the final lock-in. In comparison, any "touch up" on an MIOL is regarded as a second operation and might convey the feeling that things have somehow gone wrong. With the LAL, the subsequent procedures are from the very beginning a part of the treatment plan.

Another common concern for LAL is about the refractive stability in the first postoperative 2 to 3 weeks in terms of wound healing and adjustment performance during this time frame. In general, we have no concerns. The reason is that following modern sutureless minimal-incision cataract surgery, wound healing is quite rapid and adjustment is possible, maybe even advisable, at an earlier point in time than recommended in the protocols. Only in cases of severe edema or similar conditions will we be reluctant with adjustments. Our experience of more than 12 years with this technology clearly points toward the benefits of an early adjustment.

References

[1] Murphy C, Tuft SJ, Minassian DC. Refractive error and visual outcome after cataract extraction. J Cataract Refract Surg. 2002; 28(1):62–66

[2] Ostri C, Holfort SK, Fich MS, Riise P. Automated refraction is stable 1 week after uncomplicated cataract surgery. Acta Ophthalmol. 2018; 96(2):149–153

[3] Farhoudi DB, Behndig A, Montan P, Lundström M, Zetterström C, Kugelberg M. Spectacle use after routine cataract surgery: a study from the Swedish National Cataract Register. Acta Ophthalmol. 2018; 96(3):283–287

[4] Fernández J, Rodríguez-Vallejo M, Martínez J, Tauste A, Piñero DP. Prediction of surgically induced astigmatism in manual and femtosecond laser-assisted clear corneal incisions. Eur J Ophthalmol. 2018; 28(4):398–405

[5] Koch DD, Wang L. Surgically induced astigmatism. J Refract Surg. 2015; 31(8):565

[6] Brierley L. Refractive results after implantation of a light-adjustable intraocular lens in postrefractive surgery cataract patients. Ophthalmology. 2013; 120(10):1968–1972

[7] Ford J, Werner L, Mamalis N. Adjustable intraocular lens power technology. J Cataract Refract Surg. 2014; 40(7):1205–1223

[8] Hengerer FH, Dick HB, Conrad-Hengerer I. Clinical evaluation of an ultraviolet light adjustable intraocular lens implanted after cataract removal: eighteen months follow-up. Ophthalmology. 2011; 118(12):2382–2388

[9] Hengerer FH, Mellein AC, Buchner SE, Dick HB. [The light-adjustable lens. Principles and clinical application]. [Article in German]. Ophthalmologe. 2009; 106(3):260–264

[10] Hengerer FH, Conrad-Hengerer I, Buchner SE, Dick HB. Evaluation of the Calhoun Vision UV Light Adjustable Lens implanted following cataract removal. J Refract Surg. 2010; 26 (10):716–721

[11] Schojai M, Schultz T, Schulze K, Hengerer FH, Dick HB. Long-term follow-up and clinical evaluation of the light-adjustable intraocular lens implanted after cataract removal: 7-year results. J Cataract Refract Surg. 2020; 46 (1):8–13

[12] Hengerer FH, Hütz WW, Dick HB, Conrad-Hengerer I. Combined correction of axial hyperopia and astigmatism using the light adjustable intraocular lens. Ophthalmology. 2011; 118(7):1236–1241

[13] Hengerer FH, Hütz WW, Dick HB, Conrad-Hengerer I. Combined correction of sphere and astigmatism using the light-adjustable intraocular lens in eyes with axial myopia. J Cataract Refract Surg. 2011; 37(2):317–323

[14] Hengerer FH, Dick HB, Buchwald S, Hütz WW, Conrad-Hengerer I. Evaluation of corneal endothelial cell loss and corneal thickness after cataract removal with light-adjustable intraocular lens implantation: 12-month follow-up. J Cataract Refract Surg. 2011; 37(12):2095–2100

[15] Hengerer FH, Müller M, Dick HB, Conrad-Hengerer I. Clinical evaluation of macular thickness changes in cataract surgery using a Light-Adjustable intraocular lens. J Refract Surg. 2016; 32(4):250–254

14 The Small-Aperture Lens

H. Burkhard Dick and Ronald D. Gerste

Abstract

Small-aperture optics provides a physiologic solution to the problem of presbyopia that affects more than one billion people worldwide. Such an IOL, like the IC-8 (AcuFocus, Inc., California) provides the patient with an extended depth of focus and reduces optical aberrations from peripheral light rays. Its implantation is no more challenging for the cataract surgeon than any other IOL; it also provides a remarkable tolerance for residual refractive errors, particularly for astigmatism.

Keywords: astigmatism, cataract, cataract surgery, IC-8, intraocular lens, phacoemulsification, presbyopia, small-aperture lens, Xtrafocus

More than 400 years ago, Christoph Scheiner, who was both a cleric in Southern Germany and a scientist, made a remarkable observation which he described in his correspondence to other learned minds: if one looks through a very small hole, vision becomes sharper. Even an eye with "weakness" (by later generations called: myopia) might suddenly distinguish objects farther away though at the price of reduced light perception. Channeling light through a small hole eliminates, as Scheiner hypothesized, stray light and unfocused light from the periphery and sharpens vision. This principle of providing an extended depth of focus nowadays is known as the pinhole or small-aperture effect. It is at work in contact lenses, implants, and intraocular lenses (IOLs), but also in the normal eye: with a small pupil, it is primarily the paraxial light rays that reach the retina while light rays from the more aberrated peripheral cornea are filtered out.

The pinhole principle has been used for some time to treat presbyopia. The irreversible loss of the accommodative amplitude of the eye is an inevitable fate for each and every person and the only way not to become presbyopic is not an attractive option, by dying young. In the year 2020 an estimated 1.37 billion people were presbyopic[1] (though in that year people were concerned with quite a different health issue). Presbyopia is a visual defect that is associated with a substantial reduction in health-related quality of life.[2] Correcting presbyopia has been described as the final frontier in refractive surgery—and rightly so. It poses challenges and it seems doubtful if we will ever have a solution that fits all, providing perfect or even good vision for short, intermediate, and far distance to patients, no matter whether they undergo an intervention primarily for an existing cataract or because they demand independence from glasses as their pinnacle of visual comfort and visual quality of life.

Using a small-aperture device to correct presbyopia is a concept that was first introduced in corneal refractive surgery and has proven successful,[3] though not without complications,[4] and has been described elsewhere in this book. In cataract surgery, such a corneal inlay can also be an option for already pseudophakic patients who desire spectacle independence.[5]

The principle of small-aperture optics used in the corneal inlay can also be applied to an IOL—as in the IC-8 lens (AcuFocus, Inc., Irvine, California), a 1-piece hydrophobic acrylic posterior chamber monofocal small-aperture IOL with an optic that contains an embedded filter with a 1.36-mm central aperture (▶ Fig. 14.1). The filter, which creates a small aperture within the lens, is made from polyvinylidene difluoride and carbon nanoparticles and contains 3200 microperforations. The IC-8 IOL is usually implanted monocularly (into the capsular bag) with a target refraction between −0.75 and −1.00 D (▶ Fig. 14.2). The fellow eye usually receives an aspheric monofocal or monofocal toric IOL.[6]

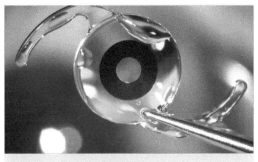

Fig. 14.1 Intraoperative overview of the IC-8 (view through a surgical microscope).

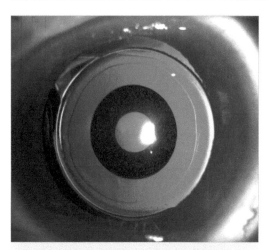

Fig. 14.2 Well-centered IC-8 intraocular lens (IOL) in the capsular bag postoperatively (slit lamp photograph).

Implantation of the IC-8 IOL does not differ from normal cataract surgery (**Video 14.1**). In all of our cases, topical anesthesia is administered three times, and pharmacologic mydriasis is induced. Two side-port paracenteses are performed. Next, the anterior chamber is filled with an ophthalmic viscosurgical device (OVD) and capsulorhexis, hydrodissection, and hydrodelineation are performed. A clear corneal incision of up to 3.5 mm (as of the date of this publication) in width is made. Phacoemulsification of the nucleus is performed using the Stellaris (Bausch & Lomb, Inc.) phacoemulsification machine. After aspiration of the nucleus, the residual cortex is removed with irrigation/aspiration, and the small-aperture lens is implanted just like any other IOL in the capsular bag using the injection system provided by the manufacturer. Finally, after OVD removal, corneal wounds are closed, if needed, with a balanced salt solution for watertightness, and antibiotic and steroidal ointment are applied.[7]

In an international multicenter study, the small-aperture IOL was implanted in 105 patients. The results can only be described as encouraging: At 6 months, the uncorrected distance (UDVA), intermediate (UIVA), and near visual acuities (UNVA) in eyes with the small-aperture IOL were 20/23, 20/24, and 20/30, respectively. Ninety-nine percent, 95%, and 79% of patients achieved 20/32 or better binocular UDVA, UIVA, and UNVA,

respectively. The mean binocular uncorrected visual acuities were unchanged between all postoperative visits. The satisfaction rate among patients was high. Almost 85% said they are now never or only occasionally using spectacles since implantation of the IC-8 IOL; only 6.7% were wearing glasses most of the time. Asked if they would undergo the procedure again, 95% answered in the affirmative.[8]

Ironically, a main side effect is the lens' success: we had patients receiving the IC-8 monolaterally who were so satisfied that they demanded the IC-8 for their second eye. It works and usually patients do not notice effects of this binocular summation. But still, if the patients cover one eye, they might experience a slight degree of vision loss in the dark or at dusk. The patients do usually not report problems with peripheral vision and if they describe a slightly darker perception, it generally happens only in the first postoperative stage. On the contrary, as Pablo Artal has shown, patients with small-aperture optics exhibit an enhanced brightness perception in this eye which is probably attributable to a neural adaptation process.[9]

In one of our studies, macular edema was the most common side effect, occurring in 1.8%; in the control group receiving a monofocal IOL, however, it was also exactly 1.8%.

The IC-8 is often implanted in eyes with a certain refractive history, such as after keratorefractive procedures. These eyes are, as is widely known, a problem for biometry. Explantation can become necessary if there is a significant refractive error. I recall just one such case; there was definitely no explantation in normal eyes.

In a study with a limited group of patients (11 eyes), Ang demonstrated the good tolerance to astigmatic defocus. A visual acuity of 20/25 was maintained with up to 1.50 D of astigmatism. More so, 10 out of 11 eyes had a visual acuity of 20/40 or better with 2.50 D defocus. This is remarkable since residual or induced astigmatism after cataract surgery tends to be difficult to control because it is often induced by the corneal incision and/or a postoperative tilt or rotation of an implanted IOL.[10] Ang's results are in accordance with our own observation that subjects with 1.50 D of astigmatism or less can achieve a visual acuity with the IC-8 IOL of 20/22 while those with a higher residual astigmatism still achieve 20/38 vision (▶ Fig. 14.3).[8]

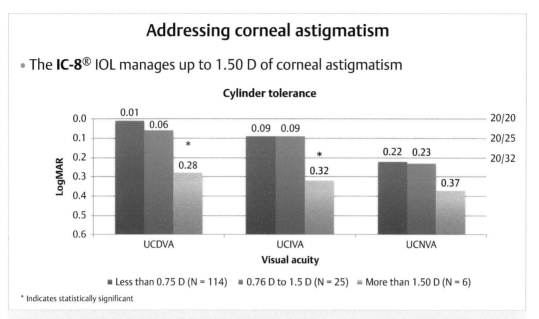

Fig. 14.3 Cylinder tolerance of the IC-8 intraocular lens (IOL) (three groups: group 1 with cylinder <0.75 D, group 2 with cylinder between 0.76 and 1.5 D, group 3 with cylinder >1.5 D) for uncorrected distance visual acuity (UCDVA), uncorrected intermediate near visual acuity (UCIVA), and uncorrected near visual acuity (UCNVA). Data from the European postmarket study.

More than half of the patients implanted with the IC-8 IOL will enjoy complete spectacle independence, as Hooshmand et al have demonstrated in a series of 126 patients, of whom 98% achieved an uncorrected distance visual acuity of 6/9, 94% an uncorrected intermediate visual acuity of 6/12, and 91% an uncorrected near visual acuity of 6/12. Those who still had to resort to spectacles in this group did so only for specific tasks like near-vision hobbies and reading under less than perfect light conditions.[11] After having implanted the IC-8 IOL in a significant number of patients in one eye, we evaluated the clinical outcomes of binocular implantation in a small group ($n = 6$). This resulted in an extended depth of focus and better intermediate as well as near vision; monocular implantation, however, led to higher overall patient satisfaction, which may be influenced by the slightly higher symptom score for halos in the bilateral group.[12]

Shajari et al reported on use of the IC-8 IOL in a series of patients presenting with severe corneal irregularities.[13] In this prospective, nonrandomized interventional case series the IC-8 IOL was implanted in 17 eyes of 17 patients presenting with corneal irregularities due to keratoconus, previous penetrating keratoplasty, postradial keratotomy, or scarring after ocular trauma. Eleven eyes had clear lenses, three had early cataracts, and three had advanced cataract. All patients gained best-corrected distance vision improvement from 0.37 ± 0.09 to 0.19 ± 0.06 logMAR. UDVA, UIVA, and UNVA significantly improved in 100%, 88%, and 88% of IC-8 IOL treated eyes. Further, patients reported improved ability to function in bright and dim light conditions after surgery. This study indicates an additional, unique benefit of the small aperture's ability to filter out the negative effects of severe corneal irregularities while improving vision from far through intermediate and near.

A question quite naturally arises when ophthalmologists implant a lens containing a small aperture in the center that filters out peripheral light from entering the eye: how about the reverse, will

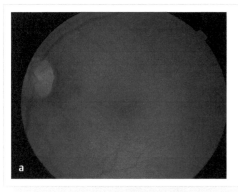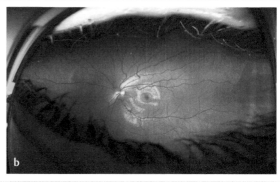

Fig. 14.4 (a) Photography of the retinal fundus through an IC-8 intraocular lens (IOL). (b) Fundus photography through an IC-8 (without pupil dilation) using the wide-angle Optos Daytona photography device.

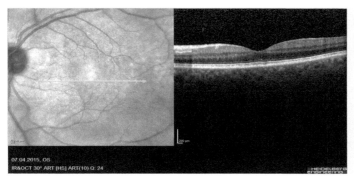

Fig. 14.5 Spectral domain optical coherence tomography (OCT) after IC-8 implantation.

it impact the eye care provider's ability to take a look at the posterior segment, to visualize the retina? This is a particularly crucial issue in patients with additional posterior segment pathology like diabetic retinopathy or disease of the macula. In our experience, the small-aperture lens does not pose a major obstacle to retinal diagnostics (▶ Fig. 14.4a, b, ▶ Fig. 14.5, and ▶ Fig. 14.6) and nor to retina surgery (▶ Fig. 14.7). We have been able to perform epiretinal membrane peel and pars plana vitrectomy for diabetic retinopathy. Yet, it has to be acknowledged that performing these procedures is not as easy as it would be with an ordinary monofocal IOL; but any experienced posterior segment surgeon should be able to perform these interventions after some adjustments (▶ Fig. 14.8a–d).

While our clinical experience with small-aperture IOL optics is based on the IC-8 IOL, it

should be mentioned that there is another product on the market employing the pinhole principle. It is, however, not an IOL since the device, the XtraFocus Pinhole Implant (Morcher, Stuttgart, Germany), does not have any refractive power. It is rather a diaphragm to be placed in the sulcus of pseudophakic eyes, that is, in patients who have severe corneal alterations or irregularities and are dissatisfied with their vision. It is a device made of a black hydrophobic acrylic material with an overall diameter of 14 mm and 6 mm occlusive portion with a central aperture of 1.3 mm. It has an optic–haptic angulation of 14 degrees to prevent iris chafing and a concave–convex design to prevent contact with the primary IOL already implanted in the capsular bag.[14]

The XtraFocus (Morcher) and Sulcoflex IOLs (Rayner) use a different approach, an add-on IOL

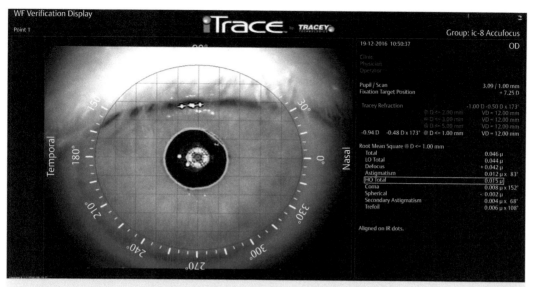

Fig. 14.6 Ocular aberrometry through an IC-8 intraocular lens (IOL) (iTrace).

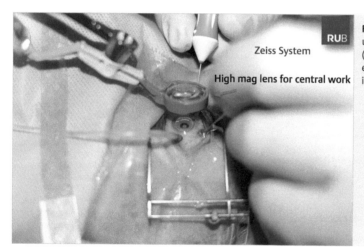

Fig. 14.7 23 G pars plana vitrectomy using the ReSight visualization device (Zeiss, Oberkochen, Germany) in an eye after IC-8 intraocular lens (IOL) implantation (side view).

for eyes that are already pseudophakic and usually have severe corneal problems or other conditions. The Xtrafocus' central aperture is smaller (1.3 mm) than the aperture of the IC-8 (1.6 mm) and there is no opening in the periphery; thus the visual field with an XtraFocus can be expected to be somewhat limited.

As always in refractive surgery, careful patient selection is key to success and mutual satisfaction. Patients should also be counseled on lifestyle and vision requirements to manage their expectations after surgery appropriately. Patients who require intermediate and near vision and patients with irregular pupils because of iris trauma or with abnormal corneas after keratorefractive procedure are definitely good candidates for the small-aperture IOL.

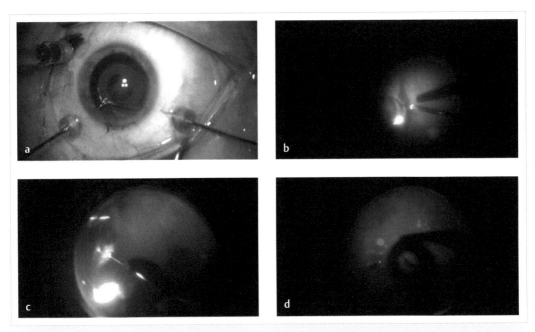

Fig. 14.8 23 G pars plana vitrectomy for the treatment of a pseudophakic retinal detachment (IC-8 in the capsular bag; view through the operating surgical microscope). **(a)** Anterior vitrectomy. **(b)** Central epimacular vitrectomy. **(c)** External indentation for peripheral vitrectomy and shaving. **(d)** Peripheral laser photocoagulation.

References

[1] Holden BA, Fricke TR, Ho SM, et al. Global vision impairment due to uncorrected presbyopia. Arch Ophthalmol. 2008; 126(12):1731–1739

[2] McDonnell PJ, Lee P, Spritzer K, Lindblad AS, Hays RD. Associations of presbyopia with vision-targeted health-related quality of life. Arch Ophthalmol. 2003; 121(11): 1577–1581

[3] Vukich JA, Durrie DS, Pepose JS, Thompson V, van de Pol C, Lin L. Evaluation of the small-aperture intracorneal inlay: three-year results from the cohort of the U.S. Food and Drug Administration clinical trial. J Cataract Refract Surg. 2018; 44(5):541–556

[4] Moarefi MA, Bafna S, Wiley W. A review of presbyopia treatment with corneal inlays. Ophthalmol Ther. 2017; 6 (1):55–65

[5] Elling M, Schojai M, Schultz T, Hauschild S, Dick HB. Implantation of a corneal inlay in pseudophakic eyes: a prospective comparative clinical trial. J Refract Surg. 2018; 34 (11):746–750

[6] Dick HB. Small-aperture strategies for the correction of presbyopia. Curr Opin Ophthalmol. 2019; 30(4):236–242

[7] Schojai M, Schultz T, Jerke C, Böcker J, Dick HB. Visual performance comparison of 2 extended depth-of-focus intraocular lenses. J Cataract Refract Surg. 2020; 46(3): 388–393

[8] Dick HB, Piovella M, Vukich J, Vilupuru S, Lin L, Clinical Investigators. Prospective multicenter trial of a small-aperture intraocular lens in cataract surgery. J Cataract Refract Surg. 2017; 43(7):956–968

[9] Manzanera S, Webb K, Artal P. Adaptation to brightness perception in patients implanted with a small aperture. Am J Ophthalmol. 2019; 197:36–44

[10] Ang RE. Small-aperture intraocular lens tolerance to induced astigmatism. Clin Ophthalmol. 2018; 12:1659–1664

[11] Hooshmand J, Allen P, Huynh T, et al. Small aperture IC-8 intraocular lens in cataract patients: achieving extended depth of focus through small aperture optics. Eye (Lond). 2019; 33(7):1096–1103

[12] Dick HB, Elling M, Schultz T. Binocular and monocular implantation of small-aperture intraocular lenses in cataract surgery. J Refract Surg. 2018; 34(9):629–631

[13] Shajari M, Mackert MJ, Langer J, et al. Safety and efficacy of a small-aperture capsular bag-fixated intraocular lens in eyes with severe corneal irregularities. J Cataract Refract Surg. 2020; 46(2):188–192

[14] Srinivasan S. Small aperture intraocular lenses: the new kids on the block. J Cataract Refract Surg. 2018; 44(8):927–928

15 Ocular Comorbidities and Refractive Cataract Surgery

Fuxiang Zhang, Alan Sugar, and Lisa Brothers Arbisser

Abstract

Ocular comorbidity is an important factor to consider when we plan which intraocular lens (IOL) to use. Generally speaking, this decision involves monofocal IOLs versus multifocal IOLs and conventional cataract surgery versus refractive cataract surgery. Monofocal IOLs, including monofocal toric IOLs are more often encouraged than multifocal IOLs simply because monofocal IOLs have better contrast sensitivity. With many IOLs options for us to select from, the goal of this chapter is not to suggest a rule, but to show our residents, fellows, and beginners what will be the preferred way to meet our patients' desires and to make our patients happy with acceptable long-term outcomes. We cautiously predict that monofocal IOLs with some real accommodating function or with extended depth of focus will be more favored than diffractive optic IOLs as a future trend because of image quality and more tolerability to ocular comorbidities which are very common among elderly patients. This chapter will use a case report format rather than questions and answers.

Keywords: refractive cataract surgery, ocular comorbidity, pseudophakic monovision, toric IOL, extended depth of focus IOL, multifocal IOL

Ocular surface diseases, age-related macular degeneration, epiretinal membrane, diabetic retinopathy, glaucoma, and some other ocular pathologies usually get worse with increasing age. They can occur prior to cataract surgery as well as after cataract surgery. Recent data based on more than half a million registered surgical cases from EUREQUO[1] reported that a coexisting ocular comorbidity was present in about 30% of patients having cataract surgery. Many of these patients with multiple ocular diseases still have a strong desire for glasses independence, typical motivated cases being those with a history of previous refractive corneal surgery. It is the job of cataract surgeons to make a decision in terms of who are reasonable candidates and which modality would be the best possible for each of them. It is also our job to educate these patients in terms of realistic expectations and potential worsening processes.

Two principles are important to consider:

First is the impact of loss of contrast and increased positive dysphotopsias due to the choice of IOL: monofocal versus multifocal. The monofocal optic has no adverse impact or much less negative impact on the quality of the image compared with a diffractive multifocal optic. Likely most refractive cataract surgeons have seen many patients with significantly deteriorated maculopathy and then unacceptable outcomes years after the original cataract surgery and wished to replace the existing multifocal IOL (MFIOL) with a monofocal IOL.

Second, is the pathology is stable versus progressive? For example, diabetic macular edema is much more likely to be progressive/dynamic than well-controlled mild glaucoma.

There are a growing number of surgeons who use some premium IOLs for patients with imperfect eyes, mainly suboptimal maculas. Hovanesian reported in a survey in Ocular Surgery News that "The subset of patients with subtly limited visual potential, usually caused by macular pathology prior to surgery, self-reported their satisfaction with surgery at a rate of about 80% at 5 years after surgery. This was compared with 90% satisfaction for patients who had perfect eyes. Patients with imperfect maculas also achieved spectacle independence for both reading and distance vision at a similar frequency to patients with healthy eyes."[2] "Grounded ethics means doing what you would for a family member. For many of us, that means that using today's tools, and some common sense, to allow spectacle independence is both possible and the right thing to do."[2]

Most patients with stable ocular comorbidities, as long as they are not ocular alignment related, with an expected potential uncorrected distance vision at the 20/30 to 20/40 level and reasonably healthy peripheral field of vision, typically do well with IOL monovision, provided that they have a desire to be less dependent on glasses in their postoperative lives. One of the reasons why monofocal pseudophakic monovision is more popular than premium IOLs is its wider suitability for patients with coexisting ocular pathology and less cost.

You may wonder, why do we have many pseudophakic monovision cases but few with MFIOL/

EDOF (extended depth of focus)/trifocal IOLs in this chapter? It was simply due to the fact that the monofocal IOL has wider suitability; MFIOL/EDOF/trifocal IOLs are not even considered when meaningful comorbidities exist in our practice. Many of these case reports had moderate or even occasionally severe ocular pathologies and we usually do not offer IOL monovision if they did not have a history of monovision created by contact lenses, or corneal refractive surgery. Typically, these patients have a strong desire to be spectacle independent. For monocular patients or amblyopic patients, we have always wanted these patients to wear safety glasses but still have excellent functional vision (at their chosen distance) when the glasses were off. We should not add additional risk for these patients. For this reason I (LBA) offered toric implants but no multifocals while fully explaining my reasoning.

It is our plan to cover the refractive cataract surgery implications of a wide spectrum of ocular pathologies in this chapter:
- Corneal astigmatism.
- RK/LASIK impact.
- Peripheral field defect due to glaucoma or PRP laser for PDR.
- Maculopathy due to ARMD, ERM, BDR, PDR, and macular hole.
- Retinal vascular occlusion.
- Retinal detachment.

15.1 Epiretinal Membrane (ERM) OU, Retinal Detachment (RD) OS, and Toric IOL

A 65-year-old male with diagnoses of visually significant cataract OU, ERM OU, and history of retinal detachment OS. Preoperative refraction OD −5.50 + 1.25 × 87 and OS −6.50 + 1.25 × 90. For preoperative topography, see ▶ Fig. 15.1. Cataract surgery OS 2/2015 with SN6A T4 at 100; OD 4/2015 with Toric SN6A T5 at 90. On his last office visit in 2018, he was happy, no glasses needed for computer and cell phone. UCDVA was 20/20−2 OD and 20/30 OS. UCNVA was J5 OD and J3 OS. CDVA OD was 20/20 with plano and 20/20 OS with −0.75 D sphere. CNVA was +2.50 J1 OD and OS. The teaching point from this case is that coexisting mild macular pathology and history of retinal detachment are not always contraindications for monofocal toric IOL use and monovision. The

history of retinal detachment did not seem to have much impact in this case (▶ Fig. 15.1).

15.2 Age-Related Macular Degeneration (ARMD) and ERM Can Affect MFIOLs

Cataract surgery was performed with a Restor SN6AD1 in each eye of a patient. The patient was happy postoperatively. She did not have to use glasses for "quite a few years" after the surgery. ▶ Fig. 15.2 and ▶ Fig. 15.3 showed no ARMD or ERM prior to cataract surgery. Her UCDVA at 1 month after her second eye surgery was 20/20 OD and 20/25 OS. UCNVA was 20/30 OD and 20/40 OS.

On a visit in August 2020, she reported, "I have to wear glasses all the time now. Even with my glasses, I still cannot see clearly, especially if I do not have strong light." CDVA was 20/30 OD and OS. (No UCDVA performed.) The reason for decreased visual function was the presence of an ERM and ARMD OU as shown in ▶ Fig. 15.4 and ▶ Fig. 15.5. Her cornea and ocular surface were unremarkable. Both IOLs were central and s/p capsulotomy. The teaching point from this case is that even mild ARMD and ERM can have significant negative impact on function with an MFIOL. This is the main reason why we typically do not consider MFIOLs if the macula has noticeable pathology prior to the surgery, given that we know this kind of pathology tends to get worse with aging. This is a strong argument for preoperative OCT in every cataract surgery patient (▶ Fig. 15.2, ▶ Fig. 15.3, ▶ Fig. 15.4, and ▶ Fig. 15.5).

15.3 ERM OS, Reading Glasses Can "Rescue" His Near Vision and He Will Still be Happy with Monofocal Toric IOL and LRI

A 73-year-old male with a history of cataract OU and ERM OS (▶ Fig. 15.6 and ▶ Fig. 15.7) was referred from his retina specialist. Preoperative distance vision was 20/40 OD with + 0.25 + 1.25 × 009 and 20/70 OS with +0.25 + 1.00 × 174. He hoped for no glasses after cataract surgery. OD was his dominant eye. Surgery OS 11/2017 aimed for −1.50 with LenSx and LRI and monofocal SN60WF; OD surgery 1/2018 used a Toric SN6AT3. Postoperative vision in 2/2018 UDVA was 20/20 OD and 20/200 OS, UNVA

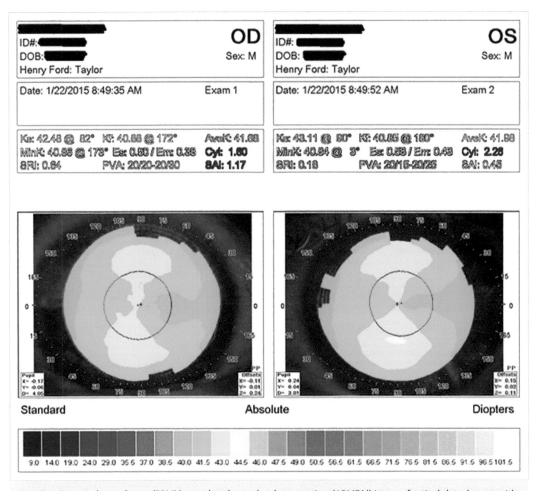

Fig. 15.1 Epiretinal membrane (ERM)/age-related macular degeneration (ARMD)/history of retinal detachment with toric. Corneal topography showed with-the-rule (WTR) astigmatism OU.

J10 OD and J5 OS; refraction was OD plano giving 20/20 and OS −2.00 + 0.50 × 173 giving 20/50. CNVA with +2.75 giving J1 in OD and +2.75 giving J3 in OS. "I see well for far and I do not need glasses for driving, day and night. I am not able to read small print without reading glasses, but I am fine to read with readers. My left eye sees much better than before although it is still not as good as my right eye." He was still happy at postoperative follow-up visits and had no need for readers for digital reading. The teaching point from this case is that IOL monovision success can be negatively affected by macular pathology, but simple backup glasses can "rescue" it. It is a good idea to give a full bilateral prescription so that such patients are capable of seeing well everywhere binocularly though many typically only use readers for fine print (▶ Fig. 15.6 and ▶ Fig. 15.7).

15.4 S/p RK OS, ERM OU, and OAG with Field Loss OD: Stable Comorbidities Can Do Well

A 66-year-old male had a history of cataract surgery OD (pseudophakic OD at presentation) and 8 cut radial keratotomy OS for monovision about 20 years ago. His main complaint was near vision

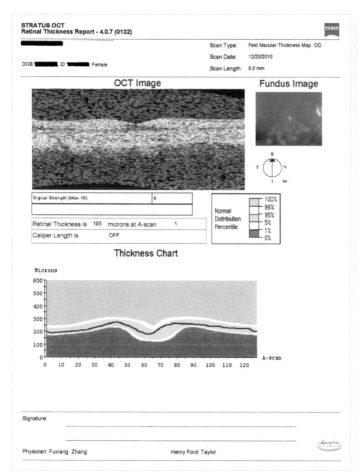

Fig. 15.2 Optical coherence tomography (OCT) in 2010 showed no ERM or AMD in OD prior to Restor IOL.

difficulty in his left eye. He strongly desired freedom from glasses and to keep his monovision. There were mild ERMs OU and open-angle glaucoma OD with moderate but very stable field loss and good IOP control OD (▶ Fig. 15.8 for HVF OD). Cup-to-disc ratios were 0.8 OD and 0.4 OS. The dominant eye was OD with the hole-in-card test. Cataract surgery on OS aimed for −1.00 D to maintain monovision. At his last office visit over 1 year later: UCDVA 20/20 OD and 20/50 OS. UCNVA J5 OD and J1 OS. Refraction: Plano OD with vision 20/20, −1.25 sphere OS with vision 20/20. He has been very happy without any glasses. The teaching point from this case report is that some field loss and ERM may still allow for monofocal IOL monovision (▶ Fig. 15.8).

15.5 Proliferative Diabetic Retinopathy (PDR) OD with PRP Laser and BDR OS, Peripheral Field Loss OD

This is a 67-year-old female patient with PDR OD with PRP laser and BDR OS. Due to PDR and PRP laser, she had some field loss in OD. See ▶ Fig. 15.9. She was also using contact lens crossed monovision for many years and doing fine; OD for near and OS for far. Her dominant eye was OD with hole-in-card and camera tests. Preoperative examination showed CDVA 20/60 OD with −7.50 + 1.50 × 175 and 20/40 OS with −5.75 + 0.75 × 180 OS. She had a strong desire to keep her monovision, although she

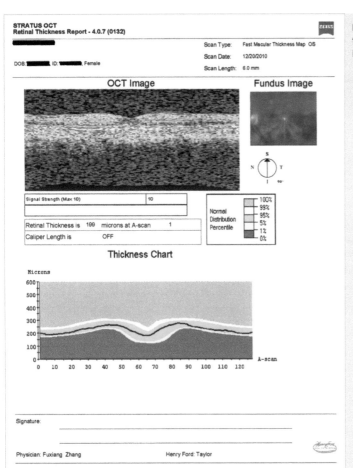

Fig. 15.3 Optical coherence tomography (OCT) in 2010 showed no ERM or AMD in OS prior to Restor IOL.

did understand that her visual function might be compromised due to her diabetic retinopathy and field loss. With the history of PDR and s/p PRP laser (▶ Fig. 15.10 and ▶ Fig. 15.11), we typically do not offer IOL monovision due to the peripheral field loss, but this patient had a strong desire to keep her monovision. An Alcon Toric SN6A T3 IOL was used for OD under ORA guidance and monofocal SN60WF for OS. Her diabetic retinopathy had been quiet with a dry macula on OCT OU for several years. At postoperative visit 2 of her second eye, she was very happy: "I see very well with no more contact lenses! I see very well for far and computer/cell phone, but I need back up readers for small print if I do not have good light." Her UCDVA was 20/100 OD and 20/20 OS. UCNVA was J1 OD and J16 OS. CDVA −1.50 sphere gave 20/20 OD and plano 20/20 OS. Customized readers with +1.00 OD and +2.50 OS were given for backup only. The teaching points from this case are that patients with stable and quiet diabetic retinopathy can still do well; limited peripheral field loss in her OD did not seem to have much effect. We chose to keep her OD for near and OS for far as crossed monovision, the same pattern as when she was using contact lens monovision; she might not have been that happy if we picked her OD for far and OS for near based on her dominance test with the hole-in-card rather than following the contact lens–induced crossed monovision pattern. MFIOLs likely would have failed in this case (▶ Fig. 15.9, ▶ Fig. 15.10, and ▶ Fig. 15.11).

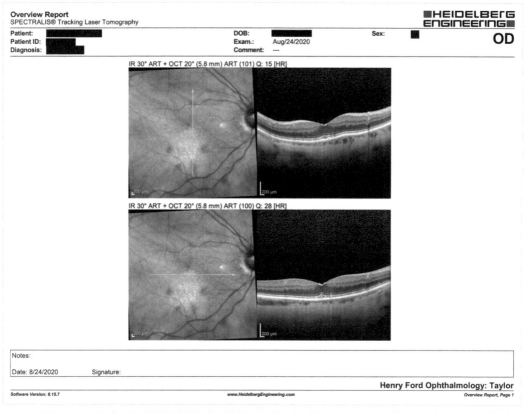

Overview Report
SPECTRALIS® Tracking Laser Tomography

■HEIDELBERG
ENGINEERING■

Patient:	DOB:	Sex:	
Patient ID:	Exam.: Aug/24/2020		**OD**
Diagnosis:	Comment: ---		

IR 30° ART + OCT 20° (5.8 mm) ART (101) Q: 15 [HR]

IR 30° ART + OCT 20° (5.8 mm) ART (100) Q: 28 [HR]

Notes:

Date: 8/24/2020   Signature:

Henry Ford Ophthalmology: Taylor

Software Version: 6.15.7   www.HeidelbergEngineering.com   Overview Report, Page 1

Fig. 15.4 OCT in 2020 showed OD ERM and dry AMD.

15.6 Monofocal IOL to Maintain LASIK-Induced Monovision; Postmacular Hole Repair OS

This 70-year-old female was s/p hyperopic LASIK OU for monovision, with OD for far and OS for near. She also had a stage 4 macular hole OS and was s/p PPV macular hole repair OS in 2015. (See ▶ Fig. 15.12 and ▶ Fig. 15.13.) She had a strong desire to have glasses independence. She was open to paying for "whatever will give me good vision without glasses." The potential impact of the macular hole OS was fully discussed before her cataract surgery. Cataract surgery was performed in OS in April and OD in June 2017 with a monofocal SN60AT (Alcon) spherical model due to increased negative corneal aberration from the hyperopic LASIK. She was very happy postoperatively with IOL monovision: UCDVA was 20/25 OD and 20/200 OS; UCNVA was J1 OD and J3 OS. (OD

had good vision both for far and for near.) Manifest refraction was –0.50 sphere giving vision of 20/20 OD and –3.00 + 0.75 × 150 giving vision 20/25 OS. "I only need glasses for nighttime driving since the cataract surgery." The teaching points from this case are the speculation that she probably would not be as happy and her visual function would not be as good if an MFIOL or EDOF IOL was used, even though she was willing and able to pay for the "best." Aberration correction should be part of the plan to improve visual quality. Patients with a history of contact lens or laser vision monovision typically do well if we can keep the same pattern (▶ Fig. 15.12 and ▶ Fig. 15.13).

15.7 Contact Lens Trial Was Needed for This Case

A 63-year-old female, practicing psychiatrist, with a history of high myopia and retinal detachment

146

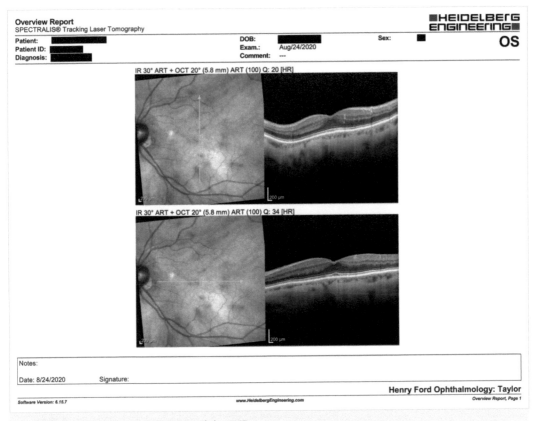

Fig. 15.5 OCT in 2020 showed OS ERM and dry AMD.

OU at age 23 had a strong desire for spectacle independence. She had a history of wearing monovision contact lenses 15 years prior to presentation as well as multifocal contact lenses for several years until a few years ago when she developed cataracts. She did not recall any issues with either type of contact lens. "Both types of contact lenses worked fine for me until I had cataract for the last few years." Preoperative refraction was OD −9.50 + 0.75 × 153 with distance vision 20/40 and OS −8.75 + 1.00 × 005 with distance vision 20/40. (Axis different from corneal topography in OD and OS, likely due to lenticular components or inaccuracy of spectacle prescription.) 2–3 + nuclear sclerotic cataracts were present in each eye with 2 + posterior subcapsular cataract OS. OD was the dominant eye. A macular ERM was present OD with mild myopic maculopathy OU. Her angle kappa was OD 0.42 mm and OS 0.38 mm. Given the history of retinal detachment

OU, ERM OD, and significant corneal astigmatism OU (▶ Fig. 15.14), IOL monovision was recommended rather than MFIOLs. Due to her history of happiness with monovision contact lenses as well as multifocal contact lenses and her personal preference, a contact lens trial was ordered. The 2-week contact lens monovision trial went well. Given that her OD was always her dominant eye and was the far vision eye when she was using contact lens monovision, the decision was to aim OD for plano and OS for near, even though her OD had a mild ERM on OCT. Surgery was performed with monofocal toric IOLs OU. Postoperative data at 2 months: UCDVA 20/20 OD and 20/40 OS; UCNVA 20/40 OD and 20/20 OS. Refractive status: Plano OD with vision 20/20 and −1.50 sphere with vision 20/20 OS. No glasses were needed after the surgery and she was very happy. She referred her husband to us to "Do the same thing what you did for me." The teaching points from this case are

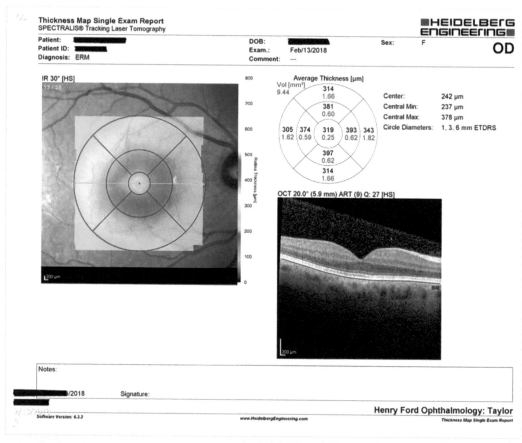

Fig. 15.6 Case report. OCT normal in OD.

that it is reasonable to give a contact lens trial in certain situations; keep the same monovision pattern as she used when she had contact lens created monovision in spite of the presence of more noticeable macular pathology in the dominant eye than the nondominant eye. As she is aging, her maculopathy may deteriorate. Correcting astigmatism is based on corneal astigmatism rather than refraction (▶ Fig. 15.14).

15.8 Crystalens Patient with Mild AMD and ERM OU Can Still Do Well

A 60-year-old gentleman with visually significant posterior subcapsular (PSC) cataract came for cataract evaluation in August 2010. He was interested in premium IOLs and decided to have

Crystalens insertion for both eyes. Surgery was done OS first a few weeks later. Crystalens AO with paired manual LRI at 155/335, 40 degrees arc 600 micros depth was done. OD surgery was done 1 month later also with a Crystalens AO. The macula was unremarkable before his cataract surgery, but in the following postoperative years, he developed mild dry ARMD as well as ERM OU (▶ Fig. 15.15 and ▶ Fig. 15.16). He has been doing well most of the time without glasses; using backup readers only "when I am tired." His last office visit in 2018 with UDVA 20/25 + 1 for OD and 20/20–1 for OS. UNVA 20/30–1 for OD and 20/40–4 for OS. CDVA was 20/20–2 with –1.00 sphere for OD and 20/20 with –0.50 for OS. CNVA was 20/20 in each eye with +2.50. The teaching point from this case is that a monofocal Crystalens can do pretty well with some mild AMD/ERM (▶ Fig. 15.15 and ▶ Fig. 15.16).

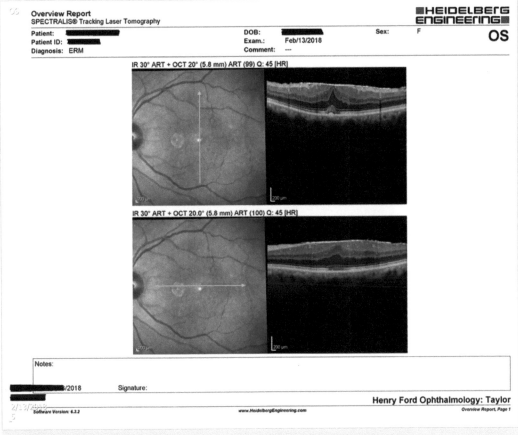

Fig. 15.7 Case Report. OCT OS ERM.

15.9 A Chronic Narrow Angle Glaucoma Patient Still Can be a Candidate for Refractive Cataract Surgery

Four things are important when a glaucoma patient wishes to have spectacle independence. Narrow angle itself is not a major concern as long as the eye is not a short amblyopic eye. The narrow angle becomes much less concerning once the cataract is removed. Sometimes, cataract surgery is one of the treatment options for narrow angle glaucoma.

The issues to be considered in this case are:

- **Ocular surface:** It can be significantly compromised due to long-term use of topical antiglaucoma medications.
- **Pupil size:** If the pupil size is too small, it can increase intraoperative difficulty if a

toric IOL is to be used, although a Malyugin Ring or other pupil expander can be used to help view the toric marks. A too small pupil can also affect MFIOL/trifocal IOL functionality.

- **Zonulopathy:** If significant zonulopathy is present, toric, MFIOL, Symfony EDOF, and trifocal IOLs should be avoided.
- **Severity:** Last but not least is the severity of the glaucoma. Significant field loss, especially central fixation involvement should be viewed as a contraindication for multifocal presbyopia-correction IOLs. According to an ASCRS survey (April 2018), EDOF was the first choice for the responders for presbyopia-correction in early/mild glaucoma patients while for mild/moderate glaucoma, IOL monovision was still the most chosen modality.[3]

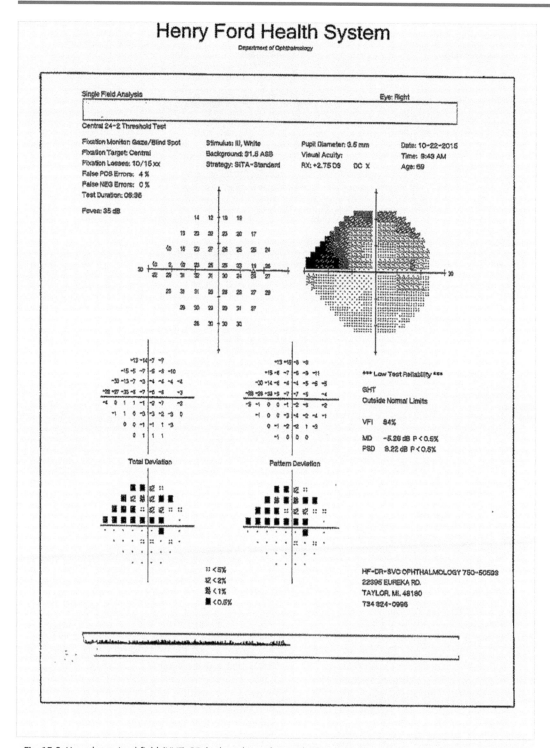

Fig. 15.8 Humphrey visual field (HVF) OD had moderate loss with MD −5.26. HVF OS unremarkable and not shown here. Source: Pseudophakic Monovision: A Clinical Guide. Zhang F, Sugar A, Barrett G, ed. 1st Edition. Thieme; 2018.

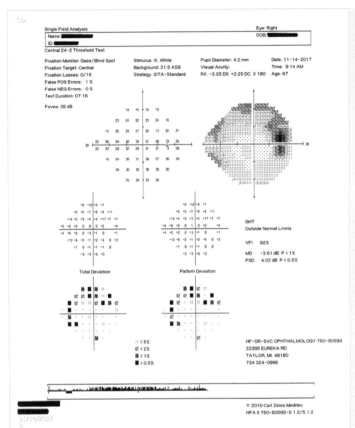

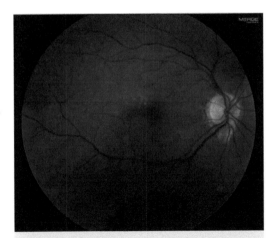

Fig. 15.10 Fundus photo showing PDR with laser panretinal photocoagulation (PRP) OD. Relatively stable with dry OCT.

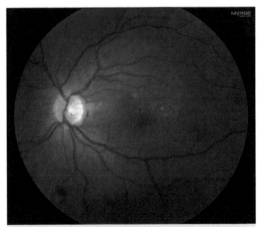

Fig. 15.9 OD had modest field loss due to PDR and PRP laser. OS field, not shown here, was within normal range.

Fig. 15.11 Fundus photo showing BDR OS. Relatively stable with dry OCT.

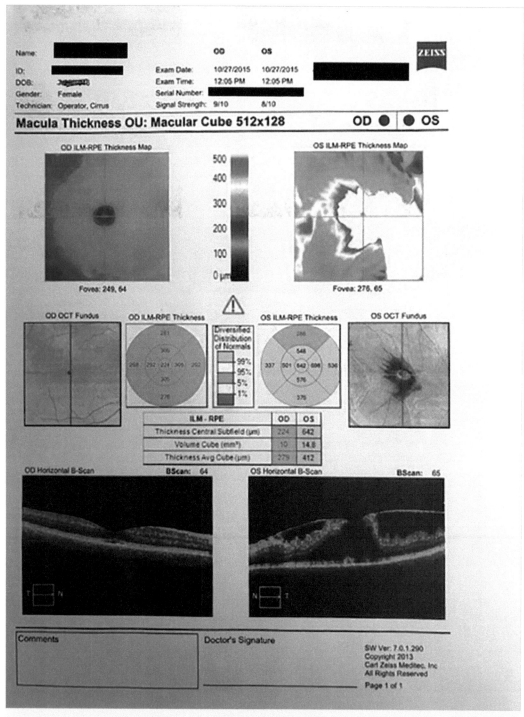

Fig. 15.12 Preoperative stage 4 full-thickness macular hole OS in 2015.

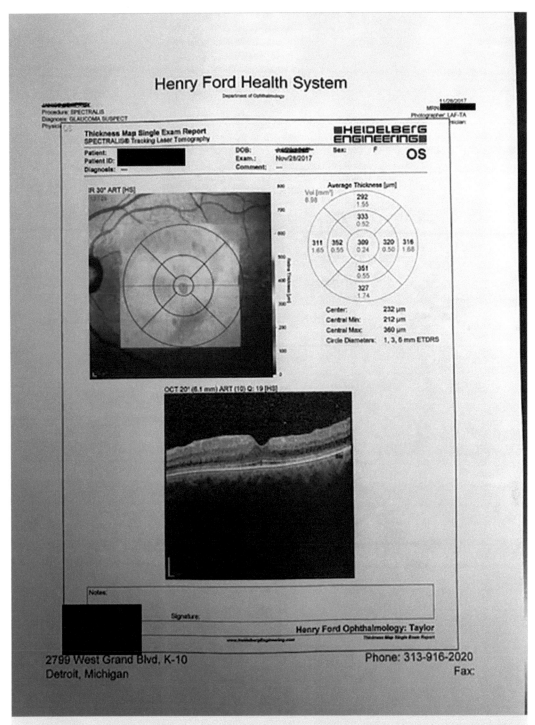

Fig. 15.13 Macular OCT OS in 2017 with some ERM, s/p pars plana vitrectomy (PPV) and macular hole repair OS. Macular hole is closed.

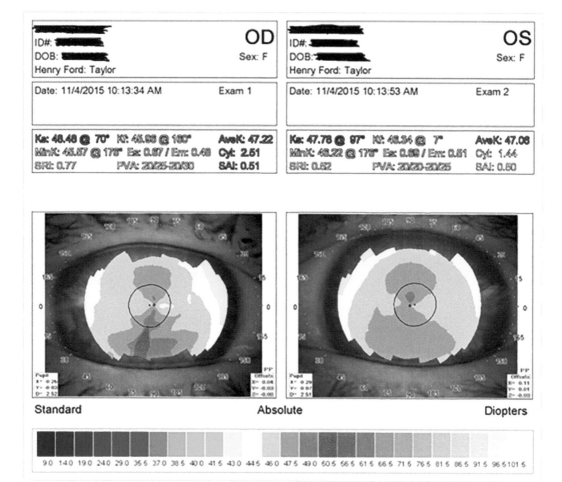

Fig. 15.14 Topography showed significant with-the-rule (WTR) astigmatism OU. Source: Pseudophakic Monovision: A
Clinical Guide. Zhang F, Sugar A, Barrett G, ed. 1st Edition. Thieme; 2018.

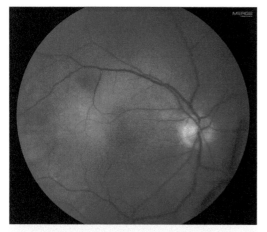

Fig. 15.15 OD fundus photo showed mild AMD/
epiretinal membrane (ERM).

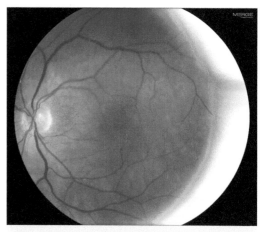

Fig. 15.16 OS fundus photo showed mild AMD/
epiretinal membrane (ERM).

References

[1] Lundström M, Barry P, Henry Y, Rosen P, Stenevi U. Evidence-based guidelines for cataract surgery: guidelines based on data in the European Registry of Quality Outcomes for Cataract and Refractive Surgery database. J Cataract Refract Surg. 2012; 38(6):1086–1093

[2] Hovanesian JA. Premium lenses in patient with maculopathy: Blasphemy? Ocular Surgery News. Published August 17, 2018. Accessed February 15, 2021. https://www.healio.com/news/ophthalmology/20200408/blog-premium-lenses-in-patients-with-maculopathy-blasphemy

[3] Intersection of refractive surgery and MIGS. EyeWorld. Published April 2018. Accessed February 15, 2021. https://www.eyeworld.org/monthly-pulse-intersection-refractive-surgery-and-migs-poll-size-102

16 Intraoperative Aberrometry

Fuxiang Zhang, Alan Sugar, and Lisa Brothers Arbisser

Abstract

New technologies usually have controversial issues and it takes time for the profession and society to test them. Intraoperative aberrometry is no exception. This chapter will focus on the basic clinical knowledge of optiwave refractive analysis (ORA). ORA does have quite a few unique benefits for optimizing refractive cataract surgery outcomes, but it also has limitations, and it may sometimes mislead the surgeon to choose incorrect intraocular lenses (IOLs). For most routine cataract surgeries, ORA does not seem to provide extra value compared with modern IOL calculation formulas. ORA has more value in astigmatism management than in spherical adjustment. It considers posterior corneal astigmatism, a deficiency of preoperative biometry measurements from some equipment, including head tilt, less-than-perfect preoperative limbal ink marking, etc. Some of these seemingly "minor errors" actually can be very significant. The role of ORA for intraoperative limbal relaxing incisions will be also discussed. The goal of this chapter is to enable beginners to feel comfortable enough to start using ORA as an adjunctive tool in their refractive cataract surgery. We will also discuss some specific questions.

Keywords: intraoperative aberrometry, Optiwave refractive analysis, ORA, refractive cataract surgery, toric IOL, limbal relaxing incision, LRL

16.1 Introduction

Technology advances: phacoemulsification replaced most extracapsular cataract extraction (ECCE); Laser-assisted in situ keratomileusis (LASIK)/photorefractive keratectomy (PRK) replaced radial keratotomy (RK) and conductive keratoplasty (CK); LenStar and IOLMaster replaced most A scans. Some older generation premium intraocular lenses (IOLs) are gradually fading away. The goal is to use the best for our patients in a professional and ethical way.

Surgeons often tend to defend the status quo. Historically, resistance to revolutions can be significant. Both Ridley and Kelman were severely criticized by their ophthalmology communities for many years until their innovations were improved and accepted. It took Edison hundreds of trial and error experiments before developing his first commercial electric light bulb. LASIK may not have become a household name if we did not previously have RK. Most new technologies take time to become optimal or near ideal situations. As physicians, we should not limit ourselves to the established successful techniques and close the door to new technology. Healthy skepticism prevents dangerous products from going too far, but resistance to changes can also harm our profession and our patients' best interests. We surgeons should be receptive to reviewing the dogma and to trying new tools if we want new technologies to be developed and optimized. On the flip side, we should not stick to new things if they are not really working as well as they are claimed to, or if they are not as good as older methods. We must follow the rules of evidence-based practice.

Wavefront aberrometry was adapted from astronomy for use in the human eye in the 1990s.[1] Intraoperative aberrometry (IA), a term describing the use of a wavefront device during cataract surgery, has been available in the United States since 2008.[1] Optiwave refractive analysis (ORA, Alcon, Ft. Worth, Texas) has been used in the United States since 2011.[1] ORA is FDA approved while another aberrometry system, HOLOS (Clarity Medical System), has not been commercialized.

16.2 What Percentage of Cataract Surgeons Use ORA?

The 2019 ASCRS clinical survey data are provided in ▶ Fig. 16.1.[2]

16.3 What Major Benefits Can a Cataract Surgeon Obtain from ORA?

The first reason we use IA is its value for those extremely short or long eyes where the prediction of effective lens position becomes difficult. As we know, most IOL formulas, including newer versions, work well for most average length eyes, but

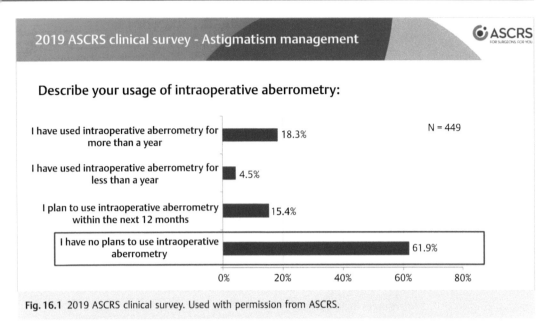

Fig. 16.1 2019 ASCRS clinical survey. Used with permission from ASCRS.

for extremes of refractive errors, even the most advanced formulas can have significant inaccuracy. In a study of 37 patients, 51 eyes, with axial length > 25.0 mm, IA was better than all formulas based on preoperative biometry in terms of predicting residual refractive error.[3] A retrospective study presented at 2019 ASCRS with 198 eyes suggested that ORA was able to provide more accurate outcomes than Barrett Universal II and Holladay 1 formulas for axial length greater than 25.0 or less than 22.0 mm.[4]

Second, the impact of the posterior corneal curvature is also measured. Corneal topography and keratometry measure only the anterior corneal surface. The contribution of posterior corneal astigmatism to total corneal astigmatism emphasized by Koch and his colleagues changed the way we manage corneal astigmatism. Even for most new formulas, we basically use a fixed theoretical ratio related to the front surface of the cornea to assume what the posterior corneal contribution would be; but there are variations and some patients can have with-the-rule astigmatism from the posterior cornea. This relationship between the front and back works for most of our patients but may not be always correct. In the visual system, astigmatism can also derive from the crystalline lens. Once the cataract is removed in an aphakic situation, ORA measures the whole optic system. This can be helpful for those who do not have the equipment to measure posterior corneal astigmatism. Based on 3159 eyes from www.astigmatismfix.com online data, a recent study revealed that use of IA resulted in significantly lower residual refractive cylinder (0.20 D, $p < .01$).[5]

Last but not least, ORA provides a new tool to measure post-keratorefractive surgery patients. Among all the merits of intraoperative wavefront mentioned here, the information ORA can provide us for post-LASIK/PRK is probably the most important. In patients with prior LASIK and PRK, these corneal curvature relationships have been altered. Numerous formulas and methods have been applied clinically, such as the clinical history method, contact lens over refraction, and the Masket, Shammas, and Haigis-L formulas, but each has its own methodology. Things became much simpler with the introduction of intraocular wavefront aberrometry, less dependent on formula-based calculations. Studies have shown that ORA is beneficial in the selection of IOL power in post-LASIK and post-PRK eyes.[6,7,8] Those studies suggest the benefit of ORA in IOL selection in post-LASIK and PRK patients when they compared the ORA with most commonly used IOL formulas. Not only are they more accurate, but direct measurement with an intraoperative aberrometer also saves the surgeon time, compared to multiple formulas preoperatively as what we used to do prior to ORA's arrival. Those of us who did cataract surgery on those patients with post-corneal refractive surgery remember how much time we spent for each case with different formulas to get the average IOL power prior to IA availability.

16.4 Modern IOL Formulas versus ORA, Which One to Follow? What If the Difference Is Very Significant?

ORA is helpful in many specific clinical situations. On the flip side, we do not believe ORA will add meaningful value in most ordinary cases. It can take care of preoperative discrepancies of biometry and photography, imperfect prediction of extreme axial lengths from most IOL formulas, imprecise ink markings, head-tilt caused inaccuracy, changed corneal curvature by laser vision correction, posterior corneal astigmatism, etc. The benefits to patients and surgeons exceed the downsides. If ORA tells us different axes for a toric IOL, which one should we trust? We would follow the ORA recommendation for toric IOL axis position because ORA also measures the posterior corneal astigmatism and the impact of incisions. Newer toric IOL calculators such as the Barrett Toric Calculator also count the posterior corneal astigmatism, but they use a theoretical model. Variation does exist between individual patients. In most situations, ORA is used to confirm preoperative calculations. For minor discrepancies, follow ORA's advice. Occasionally, you will run into a situation where the ORA's recommendation is alarmingly different from your preoperative calculation. The following list may help you out.

The first thing is to check the preoperative data entered into ORA to make sure there is no human error.

Be sure that:
- The cornea is not dried out or the corneal surface is not covered with too much BSS, such as in a very deep eye.
- The eyeball is not compressed by the lid speculum. The speculum should be away from the limbus.
- The eye is properly pressurized.
- The patient has good fixation and is not overly sedated.

- The media are clear with a clean fringe picture. (See below.)
- The implant is central without visible tilt in pseudophakic measurement.
- Significant higher order aberrations, keratoconus may also give unreliable readings, or be unable to read.

If the discrepancy remains consistent in a few consecutive measurements, we tend to use the toricity recommendation from ORA. If the ORA recommendations vary significantly between measurements, we would abandon the recommendation. In terms of the spherical recommendation, we keep the preoperatively calculated power for normal size eyes (axial length between 22 and 25 mm). Our experience tells us that the Barrett Universal II and Hill-RBF formulas are very accurate for normal range axial length eyes. In extreme eyes or eyes with a history of LASIK or PRK, we tend to take ORA's recommendation.

16.5 Do We Have Solid Literature Data to Support the Usage of Intraoperative Aberrometry?

Studies[9] in the Netherlands ($n = 41$ eyes) suggested that ORA was able to provide better predictions than the Barrett calculator in both nontoric IOLs as well as toric IOLs although the difference was not statistically significant.

Another study ($n = 123$ eyes) stated that modern IOL calculation formulas for sphere appear to produce results comparable to those achieved with IA. However, there may be some value in using IA to determine IOL cylinder power and orientation, including the Barrett Toric Calculator.[10]

A study by Cionni et al with a retrospective database analysis of more than 30,000 eyes comparing outcomes of intraoperative aberrometer (ORA) with conventional preoperative planning in eyes without previous corneal refractive surgery found that the usage of ORA significantly improved refractive outcome: use of IA could result in 82% of eyes within ±0.5 D of the intended spherical equivalent refractive error.[11]

There was a retrospective study examining 137 eyes that underwent cataract extraction and trifocal PanOptix (Alcon) implantation using the femtosecond laser, digital registration, and intraoperative aberrometer (IA).[12] Final cylinder power and axis of placement were determined by IA. Monocular uncorrected visual acuity at different distances, uncorrected distance vision (UDVA), uncorrected intermediate vision (UIVA), uncorrected near vision (UNVA), and refractive data were collected at 3 months. Postoperative residual astigmatism (PRA) determined by manifest refraction was compared to back-calculated residual astigmatism (BRA) using the cylinder power calculated preoperatively. The Barrett Universal II and Barrett Toric calculators were used. Postoperatively, mean PRA for IA was 0.07 D ± 0.19 (range 0.00–1.00 D) compared to BRA 0.31 D ± 0.33 (range 0.00–1.34 D) ($p < 0.001$). Cylinder power was changed in 50.4% of cases based on IA readings. The conclusion was that the proportion of eyes with PRA >0.50 D and mean PRA were significantly lower using IA versus the preoperative planned cylinder power.

Not all studies demonstrate superiority of ORA. A retrospective review of 132 eyes by Solomon et al noted that usage of IA for toric IOLs in normal eyes (without previous corneal refractive surgery) did not seem to add extra value in terms of improving clinical outcome.[13] When modern IOL calculators are used, such as Barrett Toric calculator, which accounts for posterior corneal astigmatism, it appears to be possible to obtain clinical results as good or better than can be achieved with IA.[13]

A recent retrospective study ($n = 949$ eyes) from Duke University suggested that in eyes without postcorneal refractive surgery, adding IA would not improve refractive outcome when Barrett Universal II or Hill-RBF formulas were used.[14] The same study also noted that the Barrett Toric Calculator outperformed ORA in the toric multifocal group. ($p = .011$)

16.6 How about Post-Keratorefractive Eyes, Barrett True-K Formula versus ORA?

There was a prospective consecutive case series of patients with cataract and prior radial keratotomy ($n = 34$ patients, 52 eyes) published in the 2019 *Journal of Refractive Surgery*. The ORA performance was similar to the Barrett True-K formula and all of the other established formulas, with no significant difference between median absolute error and mean absolute error. The Barrett True-K formula produced significantly more eyes within ±0.50 D than the SRK/T, Hoffer Q, and Holladay 1 formulas.[15] Of note, among these 52 eyes, 41 eyes (78.8%) had only four RK incisions and 11 eyes (21.2%) had eight RK incisions. Our speculation is that if most of the eyes had eight RK incisions, the outcome would be different. The reliability and validation of ORA can vary depending on the number, depth, and length of the RK incisions. See further discussion below regarding the role of ORA in eyes with a history of radial keratotomy.

A study presented at the 2019 ASCRS meeting, among those eyes with axial length greater than 25.0 mm, less than 22.0 mm, a history of LASIK/PRK, or history of RK did not find significant differences in terms of predictive accuracy between the Barrett True-K formula and IA in postcorneal refractive eyes ($p > 0.20$), although ORA did better than Barrett Universal II and Holladay formulas among those extreme eyes without history of corneal refractive surgery (all $p < 0.001$).[4]

16.7 When Can We Bill ORA?

ORA has been listed as billable for post-keratorefractive cases by AAO.[16] The other billable condition is if ORA is part of the premium IOL package.[16]

16.8 How Do You Start Learning ORA?

We recommend that beginners go through online training to get familiar with the steps. Bring an instrument specialist from the Alcon ORA team to your OR for your first few ORA cases until you feel comfortable (▶ Fig. 16.2 and ▶ Fig. 16.3).
- Focus the microscope on the apex of the cornea (a).
- Adjust alignment on the Z-axis using the focus pedal on the microscope in order to position the focus ball in the green zone (b).
- Adjust initial X and Y alignment using the microscope joystick in order to position the dot in the green circle of the wide field-of-view camera image (a).
- Fine adjustment in x and y position should be achieved by controlling the patient head position (a).

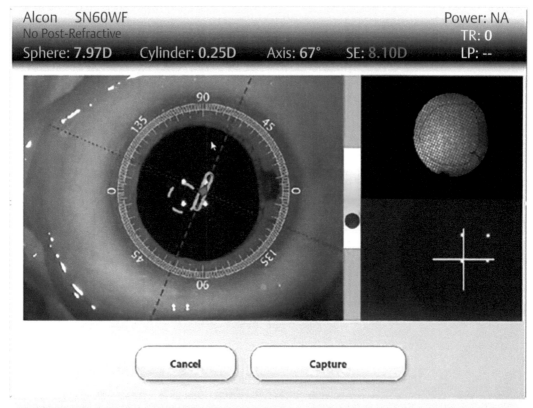

Fig. 16.2 Optiwave refractive analysis (ORA) display view for focus and alignment, not ready for capture. Used with permission from Alcon.

- If the target is red, the user must bring the target into the green circle to make it green in (a), while keeping the focus ball in the green zone in (b).
- Also pay attention to (c). That is the Fringe Pattern Screen. It is the view of the refraction camera. You want this fringe pattern to look like a "clean screen door." If there are debris, cortex, air bubbles, or large floaters in the central capture zone (center 4.5 mm), then the fringe screen will not look clean. Significant corneal scars or edema can also affect the image quality. (▶ Fig. 16.4).
- Intraocular pressure (IOP) is checked with a tonometer (the Ocular Barraquer Terry 15–21 mmHg Tonometer). The inner "smaller" ring measures 21-mmHg and the outer "larger" ring measures 15-mmHg. In between the rings would be measurements falling between 15- and 21-mg Hg.

16.9 What Kind of Special Attention Should I Pay to the Scope/Light When I Use ORA?

The scope should be perpendicular to the iris plane. We typically share OR rooms with our colleagues. If someone who did surgery the day before your OR day kept the scope tilted, then you should develop a habit to check it first thing in the morning.

We often have two rooms and two ORAs in our surgical center. It does not always mean the ORA device can be used in different scopes. The aberrometer can be "married" to the microscope. When the ORA engineer is installing, he will use the SLED for the Fringe pattern camera as a center position on a target. There is an XY adjustment on the aberrometer dovetail where it is aligned to the right ocular of the microscope. Due to the size of

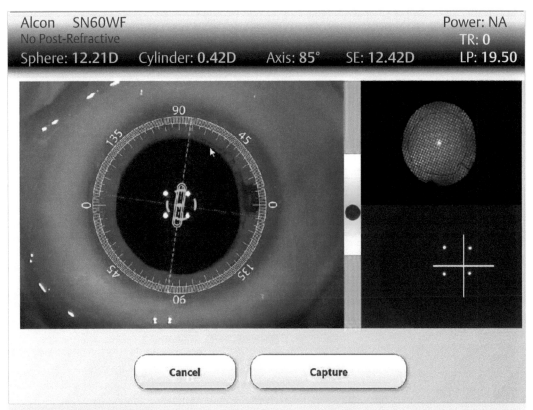

Fig. 16.3 Good alignment achieved, compared with ▶ Fig. 16.2. This is the time to capture when the target is green. Used with permission from Alcon.

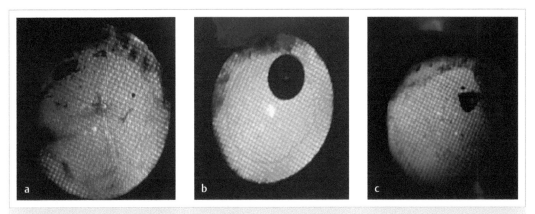

Fig. 16.4 Three samples of imperfect fringe images: **(a)** Unpolished posterior capsule. **(b)** An air bubble in the anterior chamber. **(c)** Residual cortex particle.

the mounting holes and with the +/– tolerances of the dovetails, this could lead to a significant change in alignment between microscopes, even if the microscopes are of the same make and model.

Patients can still see the small red fixation light when the main microscope light is on, but it is best to turn the scope light off to facilitate the patient's fixation. We cannot expect a reliable measurement from a patient if he/she is sedated too deeply. Before the measurement, it is also advisable to put the ORA reticles on to match the preoperative limbal reference marks (see below for further discussion).

16.10 What Attention Should I Give to the Lid Speculum?

From an ORA perspective, the eyelid speculum can have several issues if it is not managed well. First, it should be out of the limbal area so it will not directly interrupt the ORA measurements. Second, the speculum should not be extended too widely which may exert pressure on the eyeball and indirectly affect the accuracy. It is advisable to gently lift the speculum up a little bit, just away from the eyeball surface so the speculum does not touch the eyeball when the ORA captures the picture. It is important to be consistent with your ORA measurement for all your cases.

16.11 What Should I Do for the Phaco Incision So It Does Not Affect ORA Accuracy?

Too much incisional edema can negatively impact the accuracy. If your main phaco incision has a triplane structure (hinged incision or stepped incision versus one level beveled incision, as discussed by Ernest in 1995),[17] you may not need to hydrate it at all. Longer clear corneal incisions are usually more secure, with less chance of postoperative leaking,[17] but we will certainly need to avoid nearly square-shaped incisions if we are to use ORA.

16.12 Why Is It Important to Align the ORA's Reticles with the Corneal Reference Marks at the Very Beginning of the Measurement?

When we sit in the temporal position to do clear corneal incision phaco surgery, we think we are aligned well with the 180-degree meridian line. The reality is not so in most situations due to cyclorotation and due to the surgeon's position. That is why the reticles are necessary. There is a solid reason why the reticles are built in the ORA system. Once the ORA 180-degree reticle line is aligned with the eye ball's 180-degree marks, then they will be on the same page; otherwise, being 5 to 10 degrees off is very common. Some surgeons skip this reticle alignment step, thinking the no rotation recommended (NRR) will nail down the correct axis anyway, no matter if you align or not. The problem is that intraoperative information will not match preoperative or postoperative data if we skip this step. We do not have personal experience with "no marking at all." When we had the Verion device (Alcon) in the past, we still had to mark the limbal reference marks.

16.13 When Will the ORA Display NRR?

NRR will be displayed when one or both of the following conditions are met[18]:
- The measured residual astigmatism is less than 0.50 D.
- The axis of the measured residual astigmatism is within 5 degrees of the anticipated residual cylinder axis.

16.14 Should We Try to Obtain NRR Before or After Removing OVD?

Either will be fine. Trying to get NRR after you remove OVD out can be a challenge because of the difficulty rotating the IOL, especially if it is in a

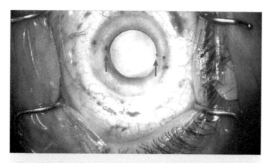

Fig. 16.5 Put these two "NRR (no rotation recommended) achieved-marks" on the cornea near the toric marks, rather than at the limbus which is far away from the toric optic marks.

counterclockwise direction. What we do is get the NRR axis before the removal of OVD. It is much easier to manipulate the toric lens when OVD is inside the bag. Once NRR is achieved, mark the axis manually or digitally, remove OVD completely, and place the implant to align the axis.

There is a trick here: where do you mark? Many people make these marks at the limbus, which is **not** the best location. It is much more accurate to make these "NRR achieved-marks" exactly on the cornea where the toric marks are aligned, rather than at the limbus which is far away from the toric optic marks. (See two *blue arrows* in ▶ Fig. 16.5.) After removing the OVD, place the IOL to realign the axis with the NRR achieved-marks *on the cornea*, rather than at limbus. If these "NRR achieved-marks" are at the limbus, you can easily place the toric 10 to 20 degrees away from the original NRR position.

16.15 What Do You Need to Look at When You Get a Red Image?

A red image suggests unacceptable quality. That typically means a large range in refractions among the 40 images from ORA so the system is unable to give you a good recommendation. Things to be ruled out include at least the following:
• Poor fixation.
• Dry corneal surface or the corneal surface is covered with too much accumulated BSS, as in a very deep eye.
• Residual OVD on corneal surface.

• Central air bubble.
• Cortex fragments in anterior chamber.
• Big posterior vitreous detachment or floaters.
• Significant retinopathy contour issues.
• Higher order aberrations, keratoconus, or any eye disease that can obstruct the normal light path to the retina.

16.16 What Do I Do If I Do Not Get NRR?

In most situations, if everything is going well, it will typically take only a few measurements to get the NRR, especially if the aphakic measurement is very close to the preoperative measurement. If you feel the axis is located at the position where you expect NRR to happen, especially after a few adjustments, but NRR still does not show, then pay attention to subtle changes: the lens centration, no tilt, no excess BSS accumulated in the conjunctival sac especially in deep set eyes (meniscus can affect the accuracy of ORA measurement), no residual OVD around the incision/paracentesis, no pressure from the lid speculum. Any of the above items can prevent ORA from displaying NRR even when the IOL power and/or toricity meet the criteria of NRR. Lens tilt and decentration, especially with MFIOL and EDOF lenses, can affect ORA measurements. The main corneal phaco incision structure and hydration can have significant impact on achieving an accurate NRR, especially if the incision is nearly square, meaning more of the central cornea is affected, or if the incision is quite edematous when the ORA measurement is taken,

If you still cannot get NRR after you checked the above items, it is better to skip NRR and leave it between the preoperative measurement and the aphakic measurement if a consecutive three aphakic measurements were consistent in a small zone. Our clinical experience suggests that this strategy usually works very well.

16.17 Is It Necessary to Obtain NRR for Every Single Case?

Some surgeons often skip the pseudophakic measurement phase; they just do the aphakic version measurement for a toric IOL without the pseudophakic version to achieve NRR. IOL centration, lens tilt, and many other factors can affect achieving NRR. A prospective randomized study

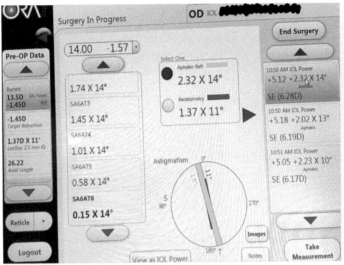

Fig. 16.6 If the preoperative measured steep axis (*blue*) and the ORA aphakic measured (*green*) axis are within five degrees in three consecutive measurements (in the figure here, *blue* was at 11 degrees and *green* was at 14 degrees), we place the toric steep axis between the *blue* and the *green*, skipping the pseudophakic measurement.

in New York[19] consisted of 40 bilateral cataract cases with toric IOLs, one eye with aphakic measurement only, and the fellow eye with both aphakic and pseudophakic measurements. No difference was noted between the two methods in terms of residual astigmatism. The average time of pseudophakic measurement was 3 minutes and 46 seconds. What we do is, if three consecutive measurements all showing the blue preoperative measurement bar and green intraoperative aphakic measurement bar by ORA are within 5 degrees, we skip the pseudophakic measurement; otherwise, we keep the pseudophakic measurement to achieve NRR (▶ Fig. 16.6).

16.18 Does NRR Always Mean the Axis Is Perfect?

NRR does not always mean the axis is at the desired location. The ORA will display NRR if the toricity magnitude is less than 0.5 D, *or* if the axis is within 5 degrees.[18] That means, when the pseudophakic refraction shows an astigmatism magnitude that's less than 0.5 D, but the axis is more than 5 degrees, the ORA will still display NRR.

The ORA will also show NRR when the measured, pseudophakic astigmatism axis is within 5 degrees of your target axis. The target axis is the axis of the aphakic refraction that *you* select on the ORA cart after aphakic refractions. For example, if you take three aphakic refractions and then select the first refraction as the basis of your pseudophakic captures, then you'll get NRR when you're within 5 degrees of 92.

$$-1.0 + 1.0 \times 92$$
$$-1.0 + 1.0 \times 94$$
$$-1.0 + 1.0 \times 90$$

It's common for wound edema to be increasing in the pseudophakic state and it will then give unreliable measurements for the magnitude of astigmatism. If there is too much edema and the magnitude of astigmatism can't be trusted, we then rely upon the axis measured pseudophakically to ensure the IOL is in the correct position.

16.19 Can ORA be Used When We Use the Malyugin Ring?

Yes, ORA can be used with the Malyugin Ring. Both 6.25-mm and 7.00-mm Malyugin rings work well for ORA (▶ Fig. 16.7). They do not seem to affect ORA function in our experience, even with toric IOLs because the central capture zoon of ORA is only 4.5 mm. The key factor is to make sure that the Malyugin ring is in the central location.

If the pupil maintains good size after the ring is taken out, the marks on the toric IOL optic are still visible. There should be no problem in this condition. If the pupil size gets smaller once the ring is taken out, you can use intracameral pupil dilation drops, such as preservative-free 1.5% Phenylephrine/1.0% Lidocaine intraoperatively. (We get this product through our Henry Ford pharmacy, for which they use a compounding pharmacy outsourced from another state.)

Alternatively, you can use an Ogawa or Kuglen hook to stretch the pupil to see the marks on the optic if indicated, but usually it is not needed.

16.20 Can We Use ORA to Guide Intraoperative LRI?

There is one study from Taiwan which demonstrated benefits of using ORA to guide manual LRI intraoperatively.[20] The proportion of patients with

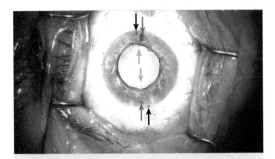

Fig. 16.7 Toric lens and optiwave refractive analysis (ORA). The toric marks (*green arrows*) are aligned between the preoperative marks (*black arrows*) and aphakic ORA measurement marks (*red arrows*) ready for pseudophakic ORA measurement.

cylinder <0.5 D 3 months postoperatively was 87% in the ORA group ($n = 60$) compared to 70% in the non-ORA group ($n = 60$, $p < 0.05$).

The guiding function of ORA for LRI is not used as often as for toric IOLs. When the fresh LRI is measured by ORA, it can be quite different from when it is healed. We still do not have solid data to demonstrate the validation of using ORA to guide intraoperative LRI, although it is a common practice to use ORA as a guide to add LRI in certain situations. For example, if the original preoperative plan is a T3 toric, but the repeated measurements by ORA suggest a T2, then we can place a manual LRI at the steep axis to decrease astigmatism since we do not have T2 in the United States. When we use spherical EDOF/MFIOL/trifocal IOLs, ORA measurement will tell us how much cylinder exists, which can be different from preoperative measurements. If the measured cylinder is significant for an LRI, but not enough to change to a more appropriate toric IOL version, and if this also matches the preoperative axis, we can add a manual LRI intraoperatively to mitigate the cylinder.

Once the LRI is done, we can still check the residual cylinder status (▶ Fig. 16.8). If the eye is still aphakic, choose LRI under aphakic. Or simply choose power calculation under aphakic to see the amount of cylinder remaining.

In pure intrastromal LRI created by femtosecond laser-assisted cataract surgery (FLACS), if the ORA shows significant undercorrection within the

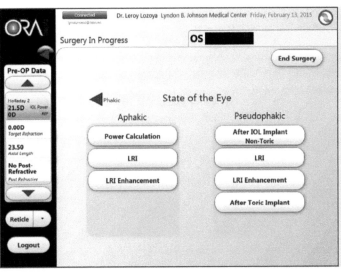

Fig. 16.8 Recheck residual astigmatism once limbal relaxing incision (LRI) is done. Used with permission from Alcon.

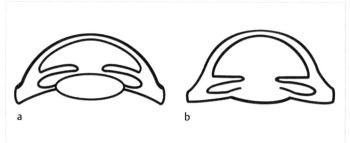

Fig. 16.9 (a) Prior to phacoemulsification. **(b)** At the end of phacoemulsification (aphakia) and at the time of optiwave refractive analysis (ORA) measurement. It is our speculation: The cornea has been stretched with swollen and weakened incisions resulting in a steeper corneal curvature, deeper anterior chamber, and longer axial length.

correct axis zone, we feel very comfortable opening it intraoperatively (▶ Video 6.1).

16.21 Is ORA Reliable for Postradial Keratotomy (RK) Eyes?

The role of IA for patients with previous radial keratotomy is still debatable. As discussed earlier, there was a study[15] from Brazil with 52 eyes of 34 patients regarding the ORA performance in RK eyes. The conclusion was that the ORA performance was similar to the Barrett True-K formula and with no significant difference between median absolute errors. In that study, however, 41 eyes had 4 cuts (78.8%) and only 8 eyes had 8 cuts (21.2%).

Our anecdotal experience tells us that accuracy and validation of IA can become an issue if the RK cuts are 8 or more, especially if the cuts are very deep or with a very small central zone. In 2018, we reported what we believe to be the first peer-reviewed case report in *American Journal of Ophthalmology* (AJO) Case Reports with a significant postoperative hyperopic surprise after cataract surgery on an eight cut radial keratotomy patient in both eyes following the ORA recommendations.[21]

16.21.1 ORA May Not Work Well in Patients with Previous History of Radial Keratotomy

The IOP during phacoemulsification can be very high, up to 80 to 90 mmHg. The high IOP can stretch the cornea and the BSS can make old RK incisions swell. In severe cases, the old RK incisions can even open up. The combination of these factors makes the cornea vulnerable to change and ORA may give misleading calculations because the depth of the anterior chamber can

vary and the corneal curvature becomes different from the situation when the cornea is back to its real condition. All these parameters are key factors for ORA calculations for IOL power recommendations (▶ Fig. 16.9).

16.22 What Are the Factors Which Can Negatively Impact the Accuracy of ORA?

- The cornea has been modified by the time we get to that point in the operation and it may not match the precision and the accuracy of the measurements that we get preoperatively.
- The impact of supine position can be different from sitting and standing, which can affect the key issue of effective lens position (ELP).
- The impact of edematous corneal incisions causes significant variation in each patient and for each surgeon.
- If we set the IOP at 21, the impact may differ from the daily baseline IOP, such as in the low teens.
- The presence of OVD versus natural aqueous humor.
- The presence of lid speculum sitting on the surface of the eye.
- The ORA will present NRR if the toricity magnitude is less than 0.5 D, *or* if the axis is within 5 degrees. The meaning of "or" is different from "and."

We hope that these issues will be addressed in the near future but not all of them can be optimized. As our preoperative biometry and topography/tomography continuously improve, as our IOL formulas get better and better, the role of intraoperative guidance from ORA may become less prominent in the future.

References

[1] Faulkner AR. Aberrometry. Cataract and Refractive Surgery Today. Published July 2011. Accessed December 28, 2020. https://crstoday.com/articles/2011-jul/aberrometry/

[2] 2019 ASCRS Clinical Survey

[3] Hill DC, Sudhakar S, Hill CS, et al. Intraoperative aberrometry versus preoperative biometry for intraocular lens power selection in axial myopia. J Cataract Refract Surg. 2017; 43 (4):505–510

[4] Passi SF, Thompson AC, Kim MJ, et al. Refractive outcomes using intraoperative aberrometry for highly myopic, highly hyperopic, and post-refractive eyes. Abstract presented at: American Society of Cataract and Refractive Surgery; May 4, 2019; San Diego CA

[5] Potvin R, Kramer BA, Hardten DR, Berdahl JP. Factors associated with residual astigmatism after toric intraocular lens implantation reported in an online toric intraocular lens back calculator. J Refract Surg. 2018; 34(6):366–371

[6] Fram NR, Masket S, Wang L. Comparison of intraoperative aberrometry, OCT-based IOL formula, Haigis-L, and Masket formulae for IOL power calculation after laser vision correction. Ophthalmology. 2015; 122(6):1096–1101

[7] Canto AP, Chhadva P, Cabot F, et al. Comparison of IOL power calculation methods and intraoperative wavefront aberrometer in eyes after refractive surgery. J Refract Surg. 2013; 29(7):484–489

[8] Yesilirmak N, Palioura S, Culbertson W, Yoo SH, Donaldson K. Intraoperative wavefront aberrometry for toric intraocular lens placement in eyes with a history of refractive surgery. J Refract Surg. 2016; 32(1):69–70

[9] Bauer NJC, Webers VSC, Nuijts RMMA. Intraoperative aberrometry versus standard preoperative biometry in non-toric and toric IOL calculations. Acta Ophthalmol. 2017; 95 Suppl. 258:34

[10] Davison JA, Makari S, Potvin R. Clinically relevant differences in the selection of toric intraocular lens power in normal eyes: preoperative measurement vs intraoperative aberrometry. Clin Ophthalmol. 2019; 13:913–920

[11] Cionni RJ, Dimalanta R, Breen M, Hamilton C. A large retrospective database analysis comparing outcomes of intraoperative aberrometry with conventional preoperative planning. J Cataract Refract Surg. 2018; 44(10):1230–1235

[12] Blaylock JF, Hall B. Astigmatic results of a diffractive trifocal toric IOL following intraoperative aberrometry guidance. Clin Ophthalmol. 2020; 14:4373–4378

[13] Solomon KD, Sandoval HP, Potvin R. Evaluating the relative value of intraoperative aberrometry versus current formulas for toric IOL sphere, cylinder, and orientation planning. J Cataract Refract Surg. 2019; 45(10):1430–1435

[14] Raufi N, James C, Kuo A, Vann R. Intraoperative aberrometry vs modern preoperative formulas in predicting intraocular lens power. J Cataract Refract Surg. 2020; 46(6):857–861

[15] Curado SX, Hida WT, Vilar CMC, Ordones VL, Chaves MAP, Tzelikis PF. Intraoperative aberrometry versus preoperative biometry for IOL power selection after radial keratotomy: a prospective study. J Refract Surg. 2019; 35(10):656–661

[16] Vicchrilli S, Glasser DB, McNett C, Burke MP, Repka MX. Premium IOLs: a legal and ethical guide to billing Medicare beneficiaries. EyeNet. 2018:79–80. https://www.aao.org/eyenet/article/premium-iols-a-legal-and-ethical-guide

[17] Ernest PH, Fenzl R, Lavery KT, Sensoli A. Relative stability of clear corneal incisions in a cadaver eye model. J Cataract Refract Surg. 1995; 21(1):39–42

[18] Scortiono G. Text For ORA SYSTEM* with VerifEye*+2.0: Operatior's Manual. Alcon; 2018. Page 132

[19] Modi SS. Clinical outcomes after aphakic versus aphakic/pseudophakic intraoperative aberrometry in cataract surgery with toric IOL implantation. Int Ophthalmol. 2020; 40 (12):3251–3257

[20] Chen M, Reinsbach M, Wilbanks ND, Chang C, Chao CC. Utilizing intraoperative aberrometry and digital eye tracking to develop a novel nomogram for manual astigmatic keratotomy to effectively decrease mild astigmatism during cataract surgery. Taiwan J Ophthalmol. 2019; 9(1):27–32

[21] Zhang F. Optiwave Refractive Analysis may not work well in patients with previous history of radial keratotomy. Am J Ophthalmol Case Rep. 2018; 10:163–164

17 Femtosecond Laser-Assisted Cataract Surgery

Fuxiang Zhang, Alan Sugar, and Lisa Brothers Arbisser

Abstract

It is not exaggerating to say that femtosecond laser-assisted cataract surgery (FLACS) is probably the most controversial procedure in modern cataract surgery. Is there a real patient-centered clinical value to using it? If most cataract surgeons prefer not to use this new technology, why do we still have a significant number of surgeons use it and why do we write this chapter to recommend FLACS be listed as part of our residency training? What are the specific advantages of FLACS over conventional cataract surgery? Who are the good candidates for FLACS? What are the indications and the contraindications? Do we have solid studies in the literature to support its validation? Based on the LenSx platform (Alcon) we will discuss these basic clinical questions as an introduction for beginners.

Keywords: femtosecond laser-assisted cataract surgery, FLACS, refractive cataract surgery, LenSx, LENSAR, docking, astigmatism correction, laser-performed arcuate keratotomy

17.1 Introduction

FLACS is an evolving technology with some existing new advances as well as real controversies. As surgeons, we must practice obeying evidence-based principles. We will also consider cost-effectiveness. It is pretty clear that for most routine cataract surgery cases, FLACS does not add much extra value. Pursuing a higher conversion rate is not professional nor ethical, because lay people do not know what exactly "laser" means. Many of them believe more expensive means a better outcome. In many situations, FLACS does have significant superiority over conventional surgery.

Femtosecond laser technology, introduced clinically for ophthalmic surgery nearly two decades ago as a new technique for creating lamellar flaps in laser in situ keratomileusis (LASIK), has been adapted as a tool for cataract surgery. Its usage in LASIK flaps has almost completely replaced manual microkeratomes, but FLACS is still debatable in our profession a decade after its FDA approval.[1] LenSx (Alcon Laboratories) was the first platform to get FDA approval in 2010 for cataract surgery. Since then, a few more platforms also got approval from the FDA, including LENSAR (LENSAR, Inc.), Victus (Bausch + Lomb), CATALYS (Johnson & Johnson), etc.

17.2 How Popular Is FLACS among Cataract Surgeons in the United States?

Based on the 2019 ASCRS clinical survey[2] ($n = 770$), 35.6% of responders were doing FLACS (US surgeons 43.3% vs. non-US surgeons 26.4%) and 50.8% said no and don't have plans to. See ▶ Fig. 17.1. The top two reasons why no FLACS were offered were "not a viable economic option for my practice" and "not enough data proving clinical benefits."[2]

17.3 Would You Choose FLACS for Your Own Eye?

Would you choose FLACS for your own eye? Which intraocular lens would ophthalmologists choose for themselves? There was a survey through the Association of University Professors of Ophthalmology (AUPO) for the surgical preferences of practicing ophthalmologists and PGY-4 ophthalmology residents with regard to cataract surgery proposed for themselves. The survey was sent to the program directors of all existing ACGME-accredited ophthalmology residency programs in 2017.[3] A total of 347 surveys were completed of which 328 were analyzed. Approximately 67% of those surveyed had been in practice for >10 years. In response to the question "If you needed cataract surgery, would you want FLACS?", 15.6% said "Yes," 31.5% "Maybe," and 52.9% "No." There were 67.7% of the responders who implanted presbyopia-correcting IOLs for their patients (diffractive, multifocal, or accommodative), but in the setting of no astigmatism, 61.3% of respondents would choose a monofocal IOL set for either distance or monovision for their own surgery.

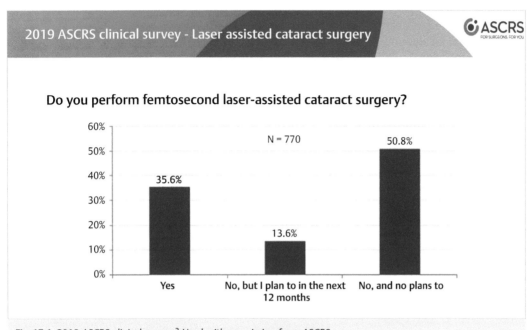

Fig. 17.1 2019 ASCRS clinical survey.[2] Used with permission from ASCRS.

17.4 What Peer-Reviewed Studies Validate the Use of FLACS?

- You reported a retrospective comparison between manual and FLACS in 2018[4] (n = 225 eyes in FLACS and 231 eyes in manual group): 94.2% of eyes in the FLACS group were within 0.5 D of the target refraction compared with 83.1% of eyes in the manual group, (p < 0.001); 53.2% of eyes in the FLACS group achieved UDVA 20/20 or better, and 28.1% of eyes in the manual group.
- A study in Germany with 100 intrapersonal cases (one eye with FLACS and one eye with conventional manual phacoemulsification) showed superior FLACS results in terms of faster visual recovery, less deviation from the target refraction, and earlier stabilization of refraction.[5]
- A prospective randomized intrapersonal study with 50 patients in Austria[6] did not show any meaningful advantage in clinically important items in the FLACS group: endothelial cell density, central corneal thickness, central

macular thickness, effective phacoemulsification time, and IOL centration.
- A large European study[7] with 2814 FLACS cases and 4987 conventional phacoemulsification cases failed to find better visual or refractive outcomes in FLACS cases. Intraocular complications were similar in both groups.
- A meta-analysis of 14,567 eyes from 15 randomized controlled trials and 22 observational cohort studies demonstrated that there were no statistically significant differences between FLACS and manual conventional cataract surgery in terms of patient-important visual and refractive outcomes and overall complications.[8] That study also found that FLACS did better with a statistically significant difference in postoperative central corneal thickness, but it was also associated with higher prostaglandin levels and a statistically higher rate of posterior capsular tear.
- A randomized trial comparing FLACS versus conventional surgery was done in the United Kingdom and published in JCRS in 2019.[9] (Total n = 400 eyes of 400 patients, n = 200 in each group.) Visual acuity, refraction, central corneal

thickness, central foveal thickness, endothelial cell loss, and rates of intraoperative and postoperative events were recorded. Quality-of-life outcomes were measured with the EuroQOL 5-dimension questionnaire (EQ-5D) and patient-reported quality of vision was assessed with a cataract surgery patient-reported outcome measures questionnaire. The study found no significant differences between the two surgery modalities, but there was a significant reduction in posterior capsule ruptures in the FLACS group with $p = .03$.

- There was a meta-analysis review[10] in JCRS (August 2020) with >25,000 eyes to compare FLACS with conventional cataract surgery (CCS). A total of 73 studies (25 randomized controlled, 48 observational) were reviewed with a total of 12,769 eyes treated with FLACS and 12,274 eyes treated with CCS. Total and effective phacoemulsification times were shorter ($p < .001$ each), cumulative dissipated energy was less ($p < .001$), circularity was more accurate ($p < .001$), central corneal thickness after 1 day and 1 to 3 months was less ($p < .001$ and $p = .004$, respectively), and endothelial cell loss after 3 to 6 weeks and 3 months was less ($p = .002$ and $p < .001$, respectively) compared with CCS. Anterior capsule ruptures occurred more often with FLACS but posterior capsule ruptures had no difference. No significant differences among groups were found in visual acuity and endothelial cell loss after 6 months.

- It is worth noting that new technologies typically take time to advance. New generation femtosecond laser machines are usually better than the older ones. Peer-reviewed studies are usually a few years behind the newest products.

17.5 Why Do We Still Do FLACS?

Based on the above literature summary and review, it is quite clear that for most routine cataract surgeries, FLACS is not superior to conventional phacoemulsification surgery and it is not cost-effective. It is basically controversial with more cost and time to use this technology, then why we are still doing this? No doubt there are industrial and financially driven reasons in this. There is also a learning curve and time frame for comparison which has been demonstrated with the change in trend. We have decreased the volume in the past few years as our enthusiasm

decreased based on clinical evidence. It is not rare to hear some patients say "I want laser and I want the best." If they do not have indications, we should honestly tell these patients not to spend extra money for something which will not add extra value. Here is the list of reasons why we like to continue doing FLACS in a professional and ethical way.

- We have witnessed many examples of technological advances over decades. Phaco in the beginning was a crude instrument. Over time, refinements were made to make it better and better. We are in favor of keeping an open mind for this technology. Newer generation lasers typically do better as the technology advances.

- There are quite a few special advantages of FLACS over conventional cataract surgery. See below for details.

- For residents and fellows, to have the basic knowledge and skill with FLACS during training time will have merit. It will be harder mentally and psychologically to learn new things years after being a busy surgeon.

- New features of femtosecond laser: Refractive Index Shaping or Refractive Indexing. No one is going to expect Refractive Indexing will use the same machine after tons of money is invested. What we hope and believe is that learning FLACS now may be also beneficial in transition to future femtosecond laser Refractive Indexing, which we believe will be the next big thing for anterior segment surgery.

As we discussed in Chapter 13, Light Adjustable Lens (LAL), there are a few concerns about the LAL: limited to silicone lens material, lock time, and unable to change once locked. Femtosecond laser was reportedly able to change IOL power by changing the refractive index without measurably changing its shape, called refractive index shaping or refractive indexing.[11] Currently two companies are evaluating the technology: Clerio Vision is working with researchers at the University of Rochester in New York and Perfect Lens is working with the University of Utah. It has the ability to change the refractive index of the existing lens implanted in the eye for most commonly used IOLs made of hydrophobic and hydrophilic acrylic materials (Alcon, Johnson and Johnson Vision, B&L. etc.) without any specific delivery devices, such as the light delivery device (LDD) used by LAL; it can be used at any time without a locking window period; and it can be done multiple times back and forth.[12,13] Each treatment is applied to only a very thin layer within the IOL, so many adjustments and retreatments are possible.[11,13] It can even change a multifocal IOL (MFIOL) back to a monofocal IOL, without compromising the original quality.[11,12,13,14] The accuracy was claimed to be 0.01 D and the changeability range can be 10 D or more. Besides lower order aberrations such as myopia, hyperopia, and astigmatism, it can also be used to treat higher order aberrations.[11] An animal study (rabbit) showed no obvious induced inflammation or toxicity up to 6 months postoperatively.

What is more exciting is the fact that not only can the femtosecond laser be used for IOL power changing, but it also can be used to change the refractive power of the human cornea and contact lens with the same mechanism of refractive index shaping.[11] It does not significantly affect corneal nerves or provoke much in the way of a wound-healing response. The laser remodels the cornea. For example, "it moves some water component out of the regional corneal stroma" and thus changes its refractive index.[15] In addition, any cornea treatments can be placed in a very thin layer so that multiple treatments could be done sequentially in future years, as the refraction changes. This is especially useful for children whose refractive status progressively changes as they grow up. At the 3-month follow-up of the first human study with 27 eyes in 2018, the data showed "an excellent safety profile."[15] All eyes were clear with no signs of inflammation, scarring, or corneal opacity. Patients exhibited a significant benefit for distance corrected near vision with no degradation of distance vision.[15] Currently, researchers are trying to shorten the treatment time, which is "the main downside."[15]

17.6 What Are the Specific Advantages of FLACS Over Conventional Cataract Surgery?

- See (▶ Fig. 17.2).
- Femtosecond laser-performed arcuate keratotomy (AK) has advantages compared to manual limbal relaxing incision (LRI) in terms of consistency in the depth, location, configuration, repeatability, and safety (less chance of perforation).

With the unopened incision model of AK with FLACS, we have one more backup if the astigmatism is undercorrected. Patients also have less pain/foreign body sensation and less risk of postoperative infection from those unopened stromal AKs. Studies have demonstrated femtosecond AK to be safe and effective,[16,17] and with better outcome than manual LRI.[16] Femtosecond laser-performed AK was reported to be effective in treating low-level astigmatism of less than 1 D. A prospective study[18] by Wortz et al ($n = 224$ patients) showed that femtolaser AK patients had significantly lower mean postoperative residual astigmatism than the conventional group (without astigmatism correction). Uncorrected distance vision (UCDVA) 20/20 was 62% in the femto AK group versus 48% in the conventional group. Preoperative astigmatism was higher in the femto AK group.

- FLACS-created stromal AK provides an opportunity for adjustment of undercorrection of astigmatism done intraoperatively (▶ Video 6.1). This can be done easily and safely in the office with a slit lamp several months postoperatively if the topography and manifest refraction match the undercorrection.
- For toric IOLs, we can use femtosecond lasers to create corneal marks at the steep axes. It eliminates the need to mark the eye intraoperatively with a second instrument. The LENSAR Laser System's proprietary Streamline software with IntelliAxis Refractive Capsulorhexis creates biomechanically stable and permanent capsular marks on the steep axis to guide toric IOL alignment, both intra- and postoperatively. Preoperative diagnostic data can be wirelessly transferred from the Pentacam or Cassini Corneal Shape Analyzer (Cassini) to the LENSAR eliminating the concerns for transcription error and cyclotorsion. The IntelliAxis Refractive Capsulorhexis iris registration-guided feature of LENSAR allows for a level of precision for toric alignment at the IOL plane that is impossible to match with manual marks or intraoperative aberrometry. (See ▶ Fig. 17.3.) The marks are on the capsule, not on or in the cornea, which will eliminate parallax errors. Toric lens misalignment and rotation happens mainly during the first hour, so the still-visible capsular marks can be of great help. Study has shown

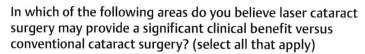

2019 ASCRS clinical survey - Laser assisted cataract surgery

In which of the following areas do you believe laser cataract surgery may provide a significant clinical benefit versus conventional cataract surgery? (select all that apply)

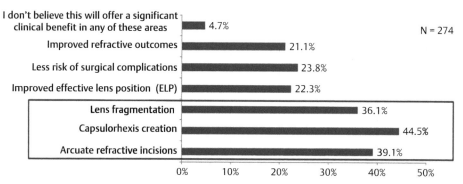

N = 274

I don't believe this will offer a significant clinical benefit in any of these areas	4.7%
Improved refractive outcomes	21.1%
Less risk of surgical complications	23.8%
Improved effective lens position (ELP)	22.3%
Lens fragmentation	36.1%
Capsulorhexis creation	44.5%
Arcuate refractive incisions	39.1%

Fig. 17.2 2019 ASCRS clinical survey. Top reasons FLACS was believed to provide benefits.[2] Used with permission from ASCRS.

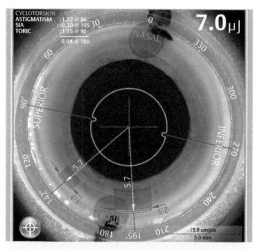

Fig. 17.3 The LENSAR Laser System's proprietary Streamline software with IntelliAxis Refractive Capsulorhexis. Used with permission from LENSAR.

that the safety and extensibility of LENSAR IntelliAxis created capsulotomy are as good as standard femtosecond laser-created capsulotomy.[19]

A prospective study with 36 patients was presented by Visco and colleagues at 2020 ASCRS to evaluate the IntelliAxis with toric IOL implantation. Astigmatism reduced significantly from mean of 2.07 ± 0.79 D to mean residual refractive astigmatism of −0.12 ±0.19 D at postoperative 6 weeks ($p < 0.001$). All eyes (100%) were within refractive astigmatism ≤0.50 D postoperatively. Assessment of toric IOL rotation from its intended axis of implantation with reference to capsular marks showed no IOL misalignment in any of the eyes. No adverse events were reported.[20]

- FLACS can provide a near-perfect capsulotomy. If the rhexis is too small, it can increase surgical difficulty intraoperatively and increase risk of future phimosis; if it is too big, not covering 100% of the optic, it can cause astigmatism, especially when pressure from the vitreous is high by the end of cataract surgery, pushing the IOL forward and resulting in a tilted optic; it can affect effective lens position (ELP). Too big a rhexis is also associated with a higher rate of posterior capsular opacification.[21] There is controversy regarding centration which is typically based on the dilated pupil. While FLACS does have the control of continuous curvilinear capsulorrhexis (CCC) size/shape/location, it may not have perfect centration for visual access. If the laser machine can image the location and size of the lens, based on which, the CCC is placed, it will have a better centration. Centration with a dilated pupil is not equal to centration on the visual axis. Zepto precision pulse capsulotomy (Centricity Vision) may provide a better centration in this perspective.[22] The center of the Zepto device can be aligned with the Purkinje light reflex, and suction is then applied and activated.

- Femtosecond laser can create a new rhexis in cases of old phimosis.

A demonstration on the use of the femto laser to assist IOL exchange with a phimotic anterior capsule can be seen in the following video: https://youtu.be/35ZilIBE8CQ. The patient was 2.5 years after an MFIOL. She had dry age-related macular degeneration (ARMD) and epithelial basement membrane dystrophy (EBMD), a poor MFIOL candidate. It's almost impossible to enlarge or make a new rhexis mechanically unless you strip all of the fibrotic tissue from the bag, but the laser did it nicely. She had a BCVA of 20/40, but improved to 20/25 with a standard IOL.

- Shallow anterior chamber (AC). FLACS can be an advantage in shallow ACs, especially with dense cataract, where maneuvering space is less and there are higher chances of rhexis tear and endothelial damage from phacoemulsification.
- Endothelial dystrophy and dense cataract. Reduced effective phaco time and cumulative dissipated energy may make this safer for patients with Fuchs corneal dystrophy and dense cataracts.
- White cataracts are a special group which can benefit from FLACS.

17.7 Are All White Cataracts Good Candidates for FLACS?

White cataracts, especially those intumescent cataracts with anterior capsule bulging anteriorly, can be good candidates for FLACS with safer capsulorhexis creation. When it is done manually, the intralenticular pressure is higher than the pressure inside the AC. Once the capsulorhexis is initiated, this forward push can cause the capsulorhexis to run out and result in what was called the Argentinian flag sign due to trypan blue staining. The opaque liquefied cortex may rush into the AC and block the surgeon's view. We certainly can keep the pressure in the AC higher than the intralenticular pressure by inflating it with ophthalmic viscosurgical device (OVD), but the balance is dynamic and can change quickly, especially if the incision is not small enough or if the main incision is unintentionally lifted up as happens often with inexperienced surgeons.

Although occasionally capsulorhexis in hypermature cataracts can still be incomplete because of release of milky fluid interfering with the laser, the fast speed of capsulotomy makes a difference. Increased laser energy will also help. An interesting study was presented at 2020 ASCRS by Chao and Page.[23] The authors used slow motion videography to analyze the timing of anterior capsule tear out in intumescent cataracts from the point of contact with a capsulotomy instrument to when the capsulorhexis extends beyond the pupillary margin and compared it to femtosecond capsulotomy speeds. The average tear-out time for the 11 cases was 12.95 +/− 10.05 seconds. The fastest recorded tear out occurred within 1.53 seconds, whereas femtosecond laser capsulotomy can be performed in 1.1 seconds (Catalys, Johnson & Johnson, Personal communication with Tim Page, MD). The capsular tear out was not instantaneous and even the fastest observed tear out was slower than the time that it takes to perform a femtosecond laser capsulotomy in this study.

There was a prospective consecutive case series of white cataracts that underwent FLACS with Victus (Bausch + Lomb, Munich, Germany) at the Singapore National Eye Centre ($n = 58$ eyes of 54 patients).[24] White cataract types included dry white (24 eyes), intumescent (28 eyes), and Morgagnian (6 eyes). Incomplete capsulotomies occurred in 10 eyes (17.2%). Lens fragmentation was attempted in 38 eyes and it was effective or partially effective in 31 (81.6%). With white intumescent cataracts, the high water component can make efficient lens fragmentation difficult. No anterior or posterior capsule tears occurred. LogMAR BCVA at 1 month was 0.073 (SD 0.09). Risk factors for incomplete capsulotomy were Morgagnian cataract (5 out of 6) and lens thickness. The authors recommend that Morgagnian cataract is not a good candidate for FLACS. The anatomic shape as well as intracapsular milky fluid in Morgagnian cataract does not suit laser treatment. Lens thickness was identified as a significant risk factor for incomplete capsulotomy. The amount of fluid in a swollen lens is one factor that can be altered. In systemically fit patients, the authors recommend the routine administration of intravenous 20% mannitol, 30 min to 1 hour prior to the laser procedure, to reduce the lens thickness and intralenticular pressure. This may help to retard the rate of expulsion of liquefied lens material into the AC and thus reduce the risk of an incomplete capsulotomy.[24]

There was a prospective consecutive non-randomized comparative cohort study about white cataract in China published in 2019 JCRS ($n = 132$ eyes, 66 in each group).[25] Anterior capsule tears were significantly more common in the conventional manual group than the FLACS group (12.1% vs. 0%). Six FLACS cases developed incomplete capsulotomies. The incidences of posterior capsular rupture and vitreous loss were also higher in the manual group, although it was not statistically significant. Other studies[1,26] also suggested that femtosecond lasers can be used successfully in cases of white cataracts, dense brunescent lenses, and cataracts in which zonulopathy is encountered.

17.8 What Can Happen if I Have a Tilted Docking?

- Suction can be lost if the docking is too tilted although mild tilt usually will not lose suction.
- Tilted docking can affect AK symmetry.
  - ► Fig. 17.4 could be due to a tilted docking and the consequences will be increased irregular astigmatism and higher order aberration.
- Decentration of docking will affect capsulotomy centration. Uneven capsulorhexis with a postage stamp edge can be the result of tilted docking. Postage stamp edge can also be due to corneal folds. Liquid interface FLACS has less chance of causing corneal folds than curved contact lens interface FLACS.[1]
- Tilted docking can also have the risk of lasering the posterior capsule.
- It is very important to avoid lens tilt when docking for an intumescent white cataract in order to avoid incomplete or oval shaped capsulotomy and even capsular tear.

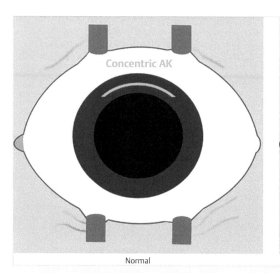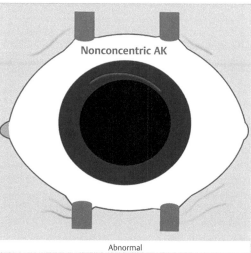

Fig. 17.4 Concentric arcuate keratotomy (AK) versus nonconcentric AK. Tilted docking can result in nonconcentric AK.

17.9 What Are Contraindications/Relative Contraindications for FLACS?

- Significant corneal pathology, such as scar, corneal blood vessels, pterygium.
- Different from traditional cataract surgery, soft cushions cannot be used in FLACS because of accurate and stable fixed distance required by the laser. Patients with severe neck problems or severe kyphosis should be considered relative contraindications. Being able to lie flat and keep still for a few minutes is also necessary.
- Very narrow palpebral apertures cause docking difficulty.
- Docking can be a challenge for a very nervous patient. If a patient is asking for general anesthesia and refuses to have topical cataract surgery, then that patient should not be a candidate for FLACS no matter what.
- The increased intraocular pressure due to FLACS is not as high as in LASIK,[27] but the safety of FLACS for glaucoma patients still needs to be studied. Liquid interface docking has advantages of causing less increase in intraocular pressure as opposed to the curved contact lens interface docking group.[1]
- Small pupils are not suitable for capsulotomy and lens fragmentation with FLACS, although these patients can still have arcuate keratotomy (AK) and corneal incisions.

17.10 What Should I Do if the Patient Has a Prominent Nose and I Cannot Dock on the Cornea?

For a patient with a prominent nose, you may need to turn the face a little bit to the side so the operated eye can be docked. Of note, when you turn the face a little bit, you must ask the patient to look at the fixation light to secure a straight, central, and untilted docking.

17.11 What Should I Do if the Suction Is Lost When the Laser is Firing?

Fortunately this rarely happens. The footswitch should be turned off immediately if suction loss happens. If suction is lost during capsulotomy, then the capsulotomy should be completed manually. If the patient moves his/her eye during the procedure, suction loss also can happen even with good docking. A small air bubble between the eye and the contact lens typically is ok for docking with the LenSx platform, but the presence of a large air bubble requires redocking. Redundant conjunctiva can be a risk factor for possible suction loss.

17.12 What Are the Pros and Cons of Laser-Created Main Phaco and Paracentesis Incisions?

A sophisticated triplane incision can be created nicely with the laser. The main incision is designed to be incomplete, so there is no concern for conventional sterilization processes. At this point, we still recommend manual incision and paracentesis for beginners.

Many surgeons still prefer manual incision rather than a laser created one. As of this writing, we definitely preferred a manual incision. The annual survey by *Review of Ophthalmology* in March 2019 showed that only 41% of responders use the femtosecond laser to make the main entry wound and only 33% for the paracentesis.[28] Manual incision has more control in the accuracy of incision location in relation to the limbal vascular arcade. Laser-created incision locations can be expected to get better as imaging technology improves in the future, but an ideal location is not always easy to obtain at this time; often you find it is either too central or too peripheral. Too central can cause intraoperative difficulty with more postoperative aberration while if too peripheral, the laser cannot cut accurately and may cause bleeding and intraoperative conjunctival edema. A prominent senile arcus may interfere with recognition of the limbus while positioning the clear corneal incisions and may result in too anteriorly placed incisions and difficult cataract extraction.[1] A suboptimal tilted position as well as docking may also affect precision of the incision location. A recent prospective randomized study has statistically shown significantly more incision edema at postoperative 1 day and 1 week in laser-created than in manually created incisions.[29] The same study also statistically revealed significantly more surgically induced astigmatism (SIA) at postoperative 1 day, 1 week, 1 month, and 3 months in the laser group than in the manual group. The reason for the increased SIA in the laser group was believed to be more incision location variation, a closer distance from the incision to the central corneal apex even though the incision was intentionally placed as far peripherally as possible per study protocol.

The best location of the paracentesis should be determined under the microscope after the laser procedure, based on patient head position/orbit anatomy and if there is presence of arcuate keratotomy. This is likely to provide a safer approach for the eye and a more comfortable postural position for the surgeon.

17.13 What Can We Do for Laser-Induced Miosis?

FLACS-induced pupillary miosis is well known. It is believed to be due to increased release of prostaglandins.[1,26,30] All steps can contribute to the miosis but the capsulotomy is believed to be the main reason.[30] The following steps can be used to decrease the severity of miosis.

- Topical NSAID drops a couple of days preoperatively.
- 10% topical phenylephrine drops immediately after the laser procedure as long as the patient does not have cardiovascular contraindications, such as increased blood pressure and/or tachycardia.
- Intracameral 1.5% preservative-free phenylephrine/1% lidocaine (JCB Laboratories, Wichita, Kansas).
- Omidria (0.3% ketorolac and 1% phenylephrine) in balanced salt solution (BSS) irrigating bottles. Omidria is the only FDA-approved medication for use during cataract surgery in preventing pupillary miosis.[31]
- The timing of the interval between laser and cataract removal should be as short as possible.

17.14 Is There Any Special Technique I Can Use if I See an Incomplete CCC with Postage Stamp Tags?

In the presence of capsular tags, shallowing of the AC can result in a radial tear. For this reason, the first step is to fill the AC with an OVD through the paracentesis with a blunt cannula to maintain

the AC, then advance the cannula to the middle of the lens capsule, and press downward with the tip of the cannula at the center of the capsule. This central dimple-down maneuver[32] indents the capsule disc, pulls it gently centrally, separates the free edge from the surrounding peripheral capsule, and confirms that there is a continuous 360-degree cut with a free flap. If a tag is present, this maneuver will identify its location and usually "pop" it free without causing a radial tear. An alternative is to fill the AC with OVD once the main incision is made and then use an Utrata forceps to perform this central dimple-down maneuver.

17.15 What Special Attention Should I Pay to Hydrodissection for FLACS Cases?

The femtosecond laser generates intracapsular gas resulting in a high intracapsular pressure. Manual hydrodissection will further add extra liquid volume worsening the intracapsular pressure and thereby may increase the risk of capsular block syndrome (CBS). CBS is believed to occur because of a rapid increase in intracapsular pressure during hydrodissection if fluid egress from the capsular space is impeded from occlusion of the capsulorhexis by the lens nucleus and cortex, resulting in posterior capsular rupture. In the presence of a gas bubble inside the capsular bag from femtosecond laser application, CBS with nucleus drop may have a higher chance to occur. The nucleus may be gently rocked to allow this gas to be burped out. CBS is prone to happen if you do not modify hydrodissection to make it slower and gentler. In patients with shallow AC, it is critical not to overdo hydrodissection, otherwise the AC will be shallower. Some FLACS surgeons rely on the intracapsular gas to create a pneumodissection, obviating the need for hydrodissection; this may potentially weaken the zonules if there is a lack of full separation.

17.16 Why Is It More Difficult to Aspirate Cortex in FLACS and What Should I Do Differently for Cortex Aspiration?

Cortex aspiration can be more difficult than conventional cataract surgery due to the fact that the subcapsular cortex is also cut in line with the capsulorhexis. This layer of cortex is fused together with the rhexis edge. Increased aspiration power may help to clean this fused cortex. Try to be very gentle not to exert pulling pressure on the zonules because of the increased aspiration power. There is a technique reported in JCRS as "second-wave hydrodissection" to facilitate the clearance of cortex material.[33] Under high magnification, search for an opening between the cortex and the capsule and then do the second-wave hydrodissection. In most situations, this second-wave hydrodissection technique does not seem to be necessary. Bimanual irrigation and aspiration can be very helpful in FLACS cases.

References

[1] Agarwal A, Jacob S. Current and effective advantages of femto phacoemulsification. Curr Opin Ophthalmol. 2017; 28(1):49–57

[2] 2019 ASCRS Clinical Survey. ASCRS Database

[3] Logothetis HD, Feder RS. Which intraocular lens would ophthalmologists choose for themselves? Eye (Lond). 2019; 33(10):1635–1641

[4] Yeu E. Surgeons hold strong opinions for and against FLACS vs. manual cataract surgery. Ocular Surgery News. Published July 3, 2018. Accessed January 28, 2021. https://www.healio.com/news/ophthalmology/20180629/surgeons-hold-strong-opinions-for-and-against-flacs-vs-manual-cataract-surgery

[5] Conrad-Hengerer I, Al Sheikh M, Hengerer FH, Schultz T, Dick HB. Comparison of visual recovery and refractive stability between femtosecond laser-assisted cataract surgery and standard phacoemulsification: six-month follow-up. J Cataract Refract Surg. 2015; 41(7):1356–1364

[6] Mursch-Edlmayr AS, Bolz M, Luft N, et al. Intraindividual comparison between femtosecond laser-assisted and conventional cataract surgery. J Cataract Refract Surg. 2017; 43(2):215–222

[7] Manning S, Barry P, Henry Y, et al. Femtosecond laser-assisted cataract surgery versus standard phacoemulsification cataract surgery: study from the European Registry of Quality Outcomes for Cataract and Refractive Surgery. J Cataract Refract Surg. 2016; 42(12):1779–1790

[8] Popovic M, Campos-Möller X, Schlenker MB, Ahmed II. Efficacy and safety of femtosecond laser-assisted cataract surgery compared with manual cataract surgery: a meta-analysis of 14,567 eyes. Ophthalmology. 2016; 123(10): 2113–2126

[9] Roberts HW, Wagh VK, Sullivan DL, et al. A randomized controlled trial comparing femtosecond laser-assisted cataract surgery versus conventional phacoemulsification surgery. J Cataract Refract Surg. 2019; 45(1):11–20

[10] Kolb CM, Shajari M, Mathys L, et al. Comparison of femtosecond laser-assisted cataract surgery and conventional cataract surgery: a meta-analysis and systematic review. J Cataract Refract Surg. 2020; 46(8):1075–1085

[11] Stuart A. Cataract innovations. EyeNet. American Academy of Ophthalmology. 2018:43–47

[12] Kent C. New high-tech IOL options in the pipeline. Rev Ophthalmol. 2018; 25:12–16

[13] Mamalis N, Lindstrom R, Chang D, et al. Refractive Index Shaping of IOLs with Femtosecond Laser. Presented at American Society of Cataract & Refractive Surgery Master Class in Refractive Cataract Surgery 20/Happy in 2020. December 5, 2020. https://ascrs.org/20happy

[14] Waring GO, Gouvea L. Modifiable intraocular lens technology with light adjustment and refractive index shape changing. Cataract & Refractive 360. 2018; 3(2):1–5

[15] MacRae SM. Femtosecond laser-induced refractive index change may lead to paradigm shift in refractive correction. Ocular Surgery News. 2019: 9. https://www.healio.com/news/ophthalmology/20190702/femtosecond-laserinduced-refractive-index-change-may-lead-to-paradigm-shift-in-refractive-correction

[16] Roberts HW, Wagh VK, Sullivan DL, Archer TJ, O'Brart DPS. Refractive outcomes after limbal relaxing incisions or femtosecond laser arcuate keratotomy to manage corneal astigmatism at the time of cataract surgery. J Cataract Refract Surg. 2018; 44(8):955–963

[17] Visco DM, Bedi R, Packer M. Femtosecond laser-assisted arcuate keratotomy at the time of cataract surgery for the management of preexisting astigmatism. J Cataract Refract Surg. 2019; 45(12):1762–1769

[18] Wortz G, Gupta PK, Goernert P, et al. Outcomes of femtosecond laser arcuate incisions in the treatment of low corneal astigmatism. Clin Ophthalmol. 2020; 14:2229–2236

[19] Teuma EV, Gray G, Bedi R, Packer M. Femtosecond laser-assisted capsulotomy with capsular marks for toric IOL alignment: Comparison of tensile strength with standard femtosecond laser capsulotomy. J Cataract Refract Surg. 2019; 45(8):1177–1182

[20] Visco DM, Hill WE, McKee Y. Prospective Evaluation of Iris Registration-Guided Femtosecond Laser-Assisted Capsular Marks for Toric IOL Alignment during Cataract Surgery. Paper presented at Annual Meeting of the American Society of Cataract & Refractive Surgery; May 16–17, 2020. https://ascrs.confex.com/ascrs/20am/meetingapp.cgi/Paper/64629

[21] Kovács I, Kránitz K, Sándor GL, et al. The effect of femtosecond laser capsulotomy on the development of posterior capsule opacification. J Refract Surg. 2014; 30(3):154–158

[22] Devgan U. Centration of capsulorhexis an important part of cataract surgery. Ocular Surgery News. Published August 19, 2019. Accessed April 24, 2021. https://www.healio.com/news/ophthalmology/20190814/centration-of-capsulorrhexis-an-important-part-of-cataract-surgery

[23] Chao JT, Page TP. Slow Motion Videography and Timing of Manual Anterior Capsular Tear Outs in Intumescent Cataracts Compared to Femtosecond Capsulotomy Speed. Paper presented at Annual Meeting of the American Society of Cataract and Refractive Surgery; May 16, 2020

[24] Chee SP, Chan NSW, Yang Y, Ti SE. Femtosecond laser-assisted cataract surgery for the white cataract. Br J Ophthalmol. 2019; 103(4):544–550

[25] Zhu Y, Chen X, Chen P, et al. Lens capsule-related complications of femtosecond laser-assisted capsulotomy versus manual capsulorhexis for white cataracts. J Cataract Refract Surg. 2019; 45(3):337–342

[26] Taravella MJ, Meghpara B, Frank G, Gensheimer W, Davidson R. Femtosecond laser-assisted cataract surgery in complex cases. J Cataract Refract Surg. 2016; 42(6):813–816

[27] Trikha S, Turnbull AMJ, Morris RJ, Anderson DF, Hossain P. The journey to femtosecond laser-assisted cataract surgery:

new beginnings or a false dawn? Eye (Lond). 2013; 27(4): 461–473

[28] Bethke W. Cataract surgeons eye new techniques. Rev Ophthalmol. 2019; 26:46–49

[29] Zhu S, Qu N, Wang W, et al. Morphologic features and surgically induced astigmatism of femtosecond laser versus manual clear corneal incisions. J Cataract Refract Surg. 2017; 43(11):1430–1435

[30] Schultz T, Joachim SC, Stellbogen M, Dick HB. Prostaglandin release during femtosecond laser-assisted cataract surgery: main inducer. J Refract Surg. 2015; 31(2): 78–81

[31] Osher RH, Ahmed IK, Demopulos GA. OMS302 (phenylephrine and ketorolac injection) 1%/0.3% to maintain intraoperative pupil size and to prevent postoperative ocular pain in cataract surgery with intraocular lens replacement. Expert Rev Ophthalmol. 2015; 10(2):91–103

[32] Arbisser LB, Schultz T, Dick HB. Central dimple-down maneuver for consistent continuous femtosecond laser capsulotomy. J Cataract Refract Surg. 2013; 39(12):1796–1797

[33] Lake JC, Boianovsky C, de Faria Pacini T, Crema A. Second-wave hydrodissection for aspiration of cortical remains after femtosecond laser-assisted cataract surgery. J Cataract Refract Surg. 2018; 44(6):677–679

18 Intraocular Lens Formulas

Fuxiang Zhang, Alan Sugar, and Lisa Brothers Arbisser

Abstract

If the goal of refractive cataract surgery is to hit the refractive target, it will be very important to be familiar with IOL power formulas. From a clinical practice point of view, this chapter aims at helping the beginner sort out the current, most commonly used formulas. Based on published peer-reviewed studies in the literature, this chapter lists and discusses three categories of formulas: nontoric IOL, toric IOLs, and formulas for eyes with history of corneal refractive surgery. Based on parameters, such as the axial length (long or short), the curvature of the cornea (steep or flat), and the depth of anterior chamber (deep or shallow), we summarize the winning formulas for each subgroup so our readers can adapt them accordingly in their practices. Besides recommendations of which formulas are likely to provide the best possible outcome in each clinical subcategory, we also introduce a quick and easy mental calculation formula for every single IOL chosen in daily routine cataract surgery to avoid refractive surprises.

Keywords: IOL formulas, toric IOL formulas, IOL formulas for s/p LASIK/PRK/RK, Barrett Universal II formula, Hill-RBF formula, Barrett Toric formula, Barrett True-K formula, refractive cataract surgery

18.1 Introduction

Numerous intraocular lens (IOL) power calculation formulas have been developed and used since the publication of Fyodorov's paper describing the first theoretical IOL calculation formula in 1967.[1] The selection of an IOL calculation formula is considered one of the four potential sources of inaccurate IOL power calculations.[2] The remaining three are corneal curvature measurement, axial length measurement, and effective lens position (ELP) prediction, the one over which we still have inadequate control.

Like our equipment, the new generation of formulas is usually, but not always, better than old ones. With numerous options, which formulas should we use for our daily practice? Many factors influence this decision, including peer review studies demonstrating superiority, the length of a particular eye, the curvature of the cornea, the depth of anterior chamber, specific available biometry equipment containing built-in formulas, convenience of access, personal experience, etc.

Many young surgeons use what they were taught during their residency or use whatever their colleagues have been using after they joined a group. It is not rare to find that some surgeons are using some very old generation formulas, and this is, at this stage of our knowledge, nearly unforgivable. Better to bring a practice you join up to date for the betterment of all. For those who have to make a decision to choose which formula(s) to use for your new practice, we think this chapter is particularly valuable. Knowing the strength and weakness of commonly used IOL formulas will also benefit every cataract surgeon, because one can intentionally run a specific formula for some certain conditions to optimize the outcome. For example, if one has SRK-T as the default formula in their IOLMaster machine, and the patient's keratometry reading was >46.00 D, the surgeon can use the measurement data to run the Hill-RBF (radial-basis function) formula if he knows the fact that SRK-T was noted, in a peer reviewed study, to be the least accurate and Hill-RBF was the most accurate one in eyes with very steep K readings.

Of note, no formula can work without accurate measurements and appropriate input of data; this is one of the reasons to use the right biometer with the formula indwelling to prevent transcription errors. Another thing to keep in mind is that "those who don't count, don't count," meaning that it is important to look at one's own data and outcomes to be sure that we are on track. The concept of refractive outcomes is like sailing to a particular destination. To stay on course, one sometimes has to "tack" this way or that. Similarly, the concept of a personal A constant that is periodically tweaked keeps us getting great results.

18.2 Nontoric IOL Calculation Formulas

For the past few years, we have seen how artificial intelligence (AI) has changed our lives. The big data approach has proved to be more and more powerful in many fields. Hill-RBF and Kane formulas are examples of AI application in this regard.[3,4] The downside of relying solely on AI-generated formulas is the risk of ending up out-of-bounds in certain rare types of eyes. Moving forward, we expect AI-based IOL formulas to have great potential to optimize, because big data will get bigger as time goes on and therein lies its unique beauty. With the use of a sophisticated optical biometer and careful scrutiny of raw data, the Hill-RBF formula was reported to have a prospective predicted accuracy in 91% of eyes within ±0.50 D of the target in eyes with axial lengths of 21.0 to 29.0 mm, most between 22.50 and 24.5 mm.[5] The Hill-RBF formula is an algorithm to select IOL power independent of a distinct ELP; therein lies its advantage, since ELP is unknowable with precision.[6,7] Hill-RBF was reported to be one of the best formulas for short eyes,[8,9] and for steep K, >46.00 D.[10] The first test case for the Hill-RBF formula was our patient (LBA, personal communication). "It just happened that when the RBF was ready to be tested clinically, I had a challenging case to decide which IOL power to use. I consulted Warren. He used the formula for the first time and it came out within .25 D of aim."

A large retrospective study[11] published in the *Journal of Cataract & Refractive Surgery* (JCRS) in 2016 with 3241 patients compared accuracy of IOL power predictions among the most commonly used formulas: Barrett Universal II, Haigis, Hoffer Q, Holladay 1, Holladay 2, SRK/T and T2. The Barrett Universal II formula had the lowest mean absolute prediction error over the entire axial length (AL) range ($p < .001$, all formulas). Overall, the Barrett Universal II formula resulted in the highest percentage of eyes with prediction errors between ±0.25 D, ±0.50 D, and ±1.00 D. The superiority of Barrett Universal II has also been reported by other peer-reviewed studies.[9,12,13,14,15] In the past few years, there have been studies which suggest that the Kane formula, which combines theoretical optics with regression and AI components,[4] was not inferior to or even better than the Barrett Universal II.[4,16]

A study published in *Ophthalmology* in February 2018 with an analysis of 18,501 eyes[17] compared accuracy among seven commonly used formulas: Barrett Universal II, SRK/T, Hoffer Q, Haigis, Holladay 1 and Holladay 2, Olsen when SN60WF and SA60AT IOLs were used (13,301 with SN60WF and 5200 with SA60AT). Lenstar 900 (Haag-Streit) was used for preoperative biometry. One eye from each study subject was used and best-corrected vision worse than 20/40 eyes was excluded. About 15% of study patients would have to be excluded if the Hill-RBF formula were included for comparison, so the Hill-RBF formula was not compared. The study concluded: Overall, the Barrett Universal II appears to be the most accurate in postoperative refraction prediction ($p < 0.001$) for both SN60WF and SA60AT IOLs.

- For short eyes (<22.50 mm), the Barrett had the lowest mean absolute prediction error. Contrary to expectation, the study also suggested that the Hoffer Q (traditionally chosen for short eyes in the past) had the greatest mean absolute prediction error for short eyes for both IOLs. That suggestion seems to be consistent with studies by Kane,[11] Cooke and Cooke,[13] and Gökce.[6]
- For long eyes (>25.50 mm), the Olsen had the lowest mean absolute prediction error and the Holladay 1 and the Hoffer Q had the greatest.
- For flat or steep keratometry, SRK-T was particularly adversely affected with worse outcomes.

In short eyes it is usually more difficult to achieve accurate refractive target predictions than in normal length and long eyes. Prediction of ELP is more challenging in short eyes; high IOL powers and the relatively short distance between the IOL and the retina also play important roles in generation of errors. A study has shown that a 0.25-mm error in measurement of postoperative ACD corresponds to a 0.1-D error in an eye with an axial length of 30.0 mm and a 0.5-D error in an eye with an AL of 20.0 mm.[18] With extremely high-power IOLs, 0.1-mm forward placement in the capsular bag can cause a 1.0-D refractive error.[19] Short eyes tend to have postoperative myopic errors. Some early studies suggested that the Hoffer Q formula provided the most reliable results in short eyes.[20,21] A recent retrospective case series[6] consisting of 86 eyes of 67 patients with axial lengths of 22.0 mm or shorter compared seven commonly used formulas (Barrett Universal II, Haigis, Hill-RBF, Hoffer Q, Holladay 1, Holladay 2 and Olsen). That study has shown that when the mean numerical refractive prediction error for each formula was adjusted to zero, no significant differences in median absolute error were found between these seven formulas, but without adjusting the mean refractive prediction error to zero, as what we use clinically, no significant differences were found between the seven formulas except that the Hill-RBF formula had a significantly smaller median absolute error than the Hoffer Q formula. Another study[9] in Australia of 400 consecutive patients undergoing implantation of an SN60WF suggested that the Hill-RBF and Barrett Universal II formulas provide the lowest mean numerical errors compared with existing formulas in short and long eyes, respectively. The Barrett Universal II formula had the lowest percentage of refractive surprises (>1 D from predicted error) across all axial lengths.[9] A recent study suggests that the Kane formula provides the most accurate outcome in short eyes when the IOL power is 30 D or higher.[22]

Very steep (>46.00 D) and very flat (<42.00 D) keratometry readings have always been a challenge for accurate power predictability. A recent retrospective study in Israel comparing commonly used third- and fourth-generation IOL calculation formulas with 171 eyes (79 eyes with average K reading >46.00 D and 92 eyes with average K reading <42.00) revealed that the Barrett Universal II had the highest predictability with 96.7% within ±0.50 D in those patients with average K reading <42.00, and Hill-RBF method had the highest predictability within ±0.50 D from target refraction for K reading >46.00 D.[10] It is not surprising to associate the good prediction for Hill-RBF in short eyes and steep K reading, because short eyes often also have steep K readings.

Let us look at the differences from the anterior chamber depth (ACD) perspective. A recent study[14] consisting of 270 eyes with normal axial length 22.0 to 25 mm, preoperative measurement with Lenstar LS-900 (Haag-Streit), IOLs with ZCBOO or ZCT IOL (both from Johnson & Johnson Vision) noted no significant differences among all eight commonly used IOL formulas (Barrett Universal II, Haigis, Hoffer Q, Holladay 1 and 2, Olsen PV, Olsen OLCR, and Hill-RBF) if the ACD is in a normal range, between 3.01 and 3.49 mm, but for the subgroup where the ACD was 3.0 or less

(shallow ACD group), as well as the subgroup of ACD 3.50 or more (deep ACD group) eyes, the Barrett Universal II formula produced significantly lower median absolute error (MAE) and a higher percentage of eyes within ±0.25 D of error than the Haigis and Holladay 2. It also produced a greater percentage of eyes within ±0.50 D of error compared with the Hoffer Q, Holladay 1, and Olsen OLCR formulas and a smaller MAE than the Hoffer Q, Hill-RBF, and Olsen OLCR formulas in shallow ACD patients. In addition, the Barrett Universal II had a smaller MAE than the Hoffer Q in deep ACD patients. The best results with the Hill-RBF formula were encountered in the normal ACD group in this study.[14]

Refractive outcomes after cataract extraction in vitrectomized eyes are more variable than in virgin eyes regardless of the calculation method.[23] A retrospective study reviewed 61 eyes of 57 patients from 2013 to 2017 and noted more variable and hyperopic than the predicted outcomes. One of the possible explanations why these vitrectomized eyes tend to have a hyperopic refractive outcome is due to the lack of anterior hyaloid and vitreous body, resulting in more posterior positioned IOL. The ELP of the IOL will likely be more posterior and therefore a slightly higher IOL power should be chosen to achieve the desired refraction.[24] The formula with the highest percentage of predictions within ±0.50 D of the postoperative outcome in these vitrectomized eyes was Holladay 2 (60.4%). Significant differences ($p < 0.05$) between the predicted and actual refractive outcomes were found with all methods (including Barrett and Hill-RBF) except the Wang/Koch adjusted Holladay 1 and Wang/Koch adjusted SRK/T.[23] Zonular integrity could also be another potential cause to affect the ELP. Significant macular pathology like macular holes and membranes can change the outcome as it subtly affects axial length, especially when the cataract surgery is done before the retinal surgery. Sometimes it doesn't matter that much when there is poor central vision but for those with great visual results it can be frustrating.

18.3 Toric IOL Calculation Formulas

Nearly a decade ago, based on their initial work on 715 corneas of 435 consecutive patients with ray tracing techniques, Koch and colleagues demonstrated that when corneal astigmatism was calculated based only on anterior surface curvature, the with-the-rule (WTR) group are usually overcorrected and against-the-rule (ATR) undercorrected.[25] Further, the same team at Baylor College of Medicine measured corneal astigmatism with five devices (IOLMaster, LenStar, Atlas, manual keratometer, and Galilei combined Placido-dual Scheimpflug analyzer). The conclusion from these multiple device measurements was that in eyes with toric IOL implantation, in the WTR eyes, there were significant WTR prediction errors (0.5–0.6 D) with all devices. In ATR eyes, WTR prediction errors were 0.2 to 0.3 D by all devices except the Placido-dual Scheimpflug analyzer.[26] They also noted that the steep meridian of the anterior corneal surface gradually changes from a vertical orientation to a horizontal orientation, that is from WTR to ATR, as we age. The steep meridian of the posterior surface of the cornea, however, does not have that change trend in most people, regardless of age, remaining vertically oriented.[25] This steep vertical orientation on the posterior surface of the cornea adds more ATR because the posterior surface provides negative power while the anterior surface provides positive power. When corneal astigmatism was calculated based only on the anterior surface, on average the WTR group frequently was overcorrected by 0.5 D and the ATR group was often undercorrected by 0.3 D.[26]

The power of the status quo can be strong. About 30% of cataract surgeons queried in the 2018 ASCRS survey still did not integrate the impact of posterior corneal astigmatism into their plan when they corrected astigmatism,[27] and this was about 35% in the 2018 ESCRS survey.[28] Educational programs help; the percentage decreased to 21.4% based on 2019 ASCRS Clinical survey.[29]

A study[30] of 86 eyes comparing 11 toric calculators/methods published in JCRS in 2017 demonstrated that the Barrett toric calculator and the new Alcon calculator which both have a fudge factor for posterior corneal astigmatism yielded lower astigmatic prediction errors overall and in subgroups with WTR astigmatism or ATR astigmatism.

Adjusted to include the Baylor nomogram for posterior corneal astigmatism, both the Alcon toric calculator and Holladay toric calculator did significantly better than the standard Alcon and Holladay

toric calculators (both $p < .001$), but the results were still not as good as the Barrett toric calculator.[31] The Barrett toric calculator does not need further adjustment with the Baylor nomogram, so it is easier to use and less time-consuming. Studies have shown significantly improved clinical outcomes, resulting in significantly lower levels of residual refractive cylinder than might be expected with standard calculators.[32,33,34]

With the advent of the Barrett toric calculator, the necessity for instruments such as the Pentacam to directly measure the astigmatism of the posterior cornea has become less important.[33,34,35,36] Posterior corneal astigmatism is hard to measure. The main challenge is believed to be the small difference of refractive index between the cornea and the aqueous humor and the lack of a gold standard to validate the measurement.[37] That was probably the reason why the refractive outcome of actual direct measurement of the posterior corneal astigmatism was not superior to the outcome of the Barrett toric calculator.[33,34,35,36] According to a recent study in Germany, there is still considerable variability of total corneal power measurement between the IOLMaster 700 (Zeiss) and Pentacam (Oculus).[38] That suggests the difficulty of accurately measuring posterior corneal astigmatism. This is an advantage to those who may not have the capital required to keep up with all the new expensive tools for routine refractive cataract surgery, especially for those of you who recently completed your residency training. The trend, however, appears to favor direct measurement as technology advances.

Based on the 2019 ASCRS survey, the Barrett toric calculator was the most frequently used (▶ Fig. 18.1).

18.4 Formulas for Patients with Previous History of Refractive Surgery

Laser in situ keratomileusis (LASIK), photorefractive keratectomy (PRK), and radial keratotomy (RK) have been the main corneal-based refractive surgery for decades (excluding arcuate incisions for astigmatism). RK played an important role in the history of refractive surgery and was the primary procedure for treating myopic patients until the 1990s. The excimer laser was originally

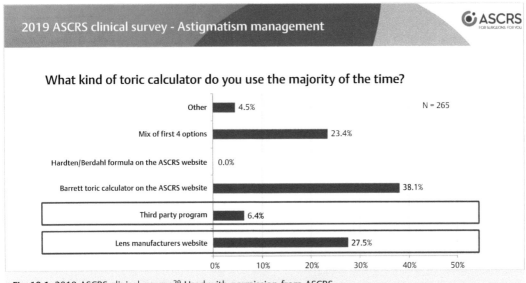

Fig. 18.1 2019 ASCRS clinical survey.[29] Used with permission from ASCRS.

applied to the cornea to produce more accurate RK incisions, not for surface ablation or laser in situ keratomileusis (LASIK), for which the excimer laser is now used.[39] Millions of patients around the world underwent RK in the 1980s and 1990s. Over two million procedures were done in the United States and Canada alone.[40] There were about 1.2 million to 1.4 million refractive surgery cases per year from 2001 to 2007 in the United States.[41] By 2009, more than 16 million LASIK procedures had been performed worldwide, and annual LASIK cases were up to a million in the United States alone.[42] The accumulated cases are huge and they now gradually are becoming our cataract patients. This group of patients are always challenging for cataract surgeons.

There was a study of 21 eyes to compare the most commonly used seven formulas (Atlas 0–3, Barrett True-K, Barrett True-K No-history, Haigis-L, Masket, Modified Masket, and the Shammas P-L); investigators considered the percentages of eyes within 0.5 D of predicted refraction as well as variations in the median absolute refractive prediction error in those patients who had history of LASIK or PRK for the treatment of hyperopia. There was no significant difference in accuracy in

these patients among those seven formulas in terms of refractive prediction.[43] Our concern for that study is the small sample size.

There was another retrospective consecutive series[44] (n = 25 eyes) in patients with a history of myopic LASIK. Mean prediction error, mean absolute error (MAE), and the number of eyes within ±0.5 D, ±1.0 D, ±1.5 D, and ±2.0 D were calculated with the following formulas from the ASCRS calculator: Shammas, Haigis-L, Barrett True-K, Barrett No History, Masket, modified Masket. In this study, the Shammas and Haigis-L formulas performed best regarding MAE and percentage of eyes within ±0.5 D. Again, our concern is the sample size.

Haigis-L, Shammas, and Barrett True-K (no history) are reliable formulas for IOL power calculation in patients who received RK or LASIK.[45] A study published in *Ophthalmology* in 2020, compared seven methods of IOL power calculation in cataract surgery after RK (52 eyes of 34 patients) and demonstrated that the Barrett True-K (history) formula delivers the greatest accuracy.[46] A recent study published in March issue of 2021 JCRS with 107 eyes of 107 patients of myopic LASIK noted that the predictive accuracy of no-history IOL formulas depends on the AL. The

Barrett True-K had the highest accuracy when AL was <28.0 mm and the Triple-S when it ranged from 28.0 to 30.0 mm, whereas the Shammas-PL was more accurate when AL was ≥30.0 mm.[47]

With a total of 104 eyes with a previous history of myopic LASIK/PRK and subsequent cataract surgery, comparison among OCT-based formulas, Barrett True-K, Wang-Koch-Maloney, Shammas, Haigis-L, concluded that "The OCT-based and the Barrett True-K formulas are promising formulas."[48]

A retrospective study[49] by Serels et al was presented at the 2020 ASCRS meeting looking into whether the Barrett True-K formula with anterior keratometry is as good as the total corneal power (TK) measurement, and if intraoperative aberrometry provides better outcomes in postmyopic LASIK patients. One-hundred and nine post-myopic LASIK eyes, 46 of which had TK available were analyzed. Using TK, the Wang-Koch formula had the highest percentages of eyes with expected spherical equivalent refractive errors within 0.50 and 1.00 D of plano (57% and 87%, respectively). With anterior Ks the Barrett True-K formula had the highest percentages within 0.50 and 1.00 D of plano (64% and 92%, respectively), but was not significantly better than Wang-Koch with TK (McNemar test, $p > 0.2$). Expected mean spherical equivalent results based on ORA were not significantly different than the Barrett True-K for outcomes within 0.50 D or within 1.00 D (McNemar test, $p > 0.2$). The authors conclude that using measured total corneal (TK) power in existing post-LASIK formulas did not appear beneficial. The formulas themselves may have to be adjusted to account for TK. The best results were obtained with the Barrett True-K formula with anterior keratometry. ORA did not appear to materially improve sphere power determination.

There was another retrospective study presented at ASCRS 2020[50] to compare the accuracy of intraoperative wavefront aberrometry (IWA) and modern intraocular lens (IOL) formulas including Hill-RBF Version 2.0, Barrett True-K, Holladay 1 ± Wang-Koch adjustment, SRK/T, Haigis, (total n = 34 eyes: 25 myopic LASIK, 7 hyperopic LASIK, and 2 RK). A capsular tension ring was placed in all eyes. The study suggests that in postmyopic and posthyperopic LVC eyes undergoing cataract surgery, the accuracy of IWA

and Barrett True K are comparable, but Barrett True K yielded fewer hyperopic surprises than ORA in post-myopic LASIK eyes.

18.5 Conclusions from Peer-Reviewed Studies in the Past Few Years

- Overall Barrett Universal II has been suggested by most recently published peer-reviewed studies to be the most accurate IOL power predictor.[11,12,13,14,15,17]

- For short eyes, although Hoffer Q was once widely believed to be the most accurate formula,[20,21] many recent peer-reviewed studies suggested otherwise.[6,11,13,17,22] Hill-RBF is probably the best formula for short eyes,[8,9] especially when seen together with steep Ks >46.00 D.[10] Barrett Universal II is probably the best for short eyes when the K reading is <42.00D.[10] A recent study suggests that the Kane formula provides the most accurate outcome in short eyes when the IOL power is 30 D or higher.[22]

- From the keratometry curvature perspective, SRK-T did not perform well in very flat or very steep K reading eyes.[17] Barrett Universal II had the highest predictability for K reading <42.00 D, and Hill-RBF method had the highest predictability for K reading >46.00 D.[10]

- The Barrett toric calculator, which takes into account the posterior corneal astigmatism and the impact of the phacoemulsification incision with the concept of the centroid, has been the winner[29,30,31,51] among toric IOL formulas, but a recent study based on 823 eyes in 2020 noted the Kane toric formula had a slight edge.[52]

- For postmyopic LASIK[47,48,49,53] as well as hyperopic LASIK[43,50] and RK,[46,54,55] the Barrett True-K formula proved to provide best results. In post-RK patients, Barrett True-K with history provides a more accurate outcome if RK data are available, especially the post-RK refraction and the pre-RK refraction.[46] When no refractive history is available, the True-K (No History) and Haigis formulas both perform well, with the added advantage of not requiring data from separate biometric devices.[46]

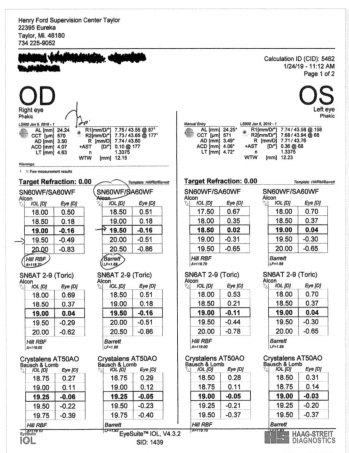

Fig. 18.2 Copy of dual formula format for every patient intraocular lens (IOL) selection.

18.6 Recommendation for a Dual Format for Each IOL Selection

- It may be beneficial to list two evidence supported formulas for each eye as a dual format, as in ▶ Fig. 18.2. Either Barrett Universal II plus Hill-RBF or Barrett Universal II plus Olsen will be good options. The Olsen formula tends to do very well for long eyes.
- If you prefer not to have this default setting, then run another one for comparison. See below a case report discussion.
- If you do not have convenient access from a biometry machine, go to ASCRS or APACRS online. The downside is the possibility of

human error due to data transcription (▶ Fig. 18.2).

18.7 A Quick and Easy Mental Calculation to Estimate IOL Power

Once we identify the IOL power for a given eye, there is still a quick and easy way to roughly estimate if the picked power is within the "correct range." This mental math has likely been used by others, but our search failed to find any published study in literature.

The major parameters are axial length, in which 1 mm equals 3 D, and the keratometry reading which yields a 1:1 D ratio. Assuming an average eye pattern: AL = 23.50 mm, K = 43.50 D. Then the

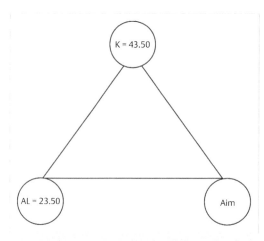

Fig. 18.3 Three major elements of this quick mental calculation about the intraocular lens (IOL) power.

Final End Point (FEP) of the IOL power will be somewhere between 21.00 and 22.00 D when we use SN60WF/SA60WF, ZCB00/DCB00, and most commonly used PCIOLs. If the FEP is less than 21.00 or more than 22.00, then either IOL power is wrong, or it is an extreme eyeball (▶ Fig. 18.3).

18.7.1 Case 1

Average K reading 46.95 D.
AL 22.35 mm.
The differences (d) of case 1 and the pattern are the following:
K (d) = 46.95 − 43.50 = 3.45 D, meaning the K is steeper than average, so we need to take 3.45 D out from the IOL power.
AL (d) = 23.50 − 22.35 = 1.15 mm, which is about (1.15) × 3 = 3.45 D; meaning the AL is shorter than average 23.50, so we need to give extra 3.45 D to the IOL power.
Barrett Universal II recommends +22.00 SN60WF when refractive target aims −0.50 D, which will give the eye another +0.50 D because it is aiming for −0.50 D.
So the balance equation will be:
+3.45 − 3.45 + 0.50 = +0.50 D
The IOL power suggested by Barrett II, which is 22.00. Take the extra +0.50 D out, then FEP is +21.50 D.

18.7.2 Case 2

K 44.19 D.
AL 23.09 mm.
The differences (d) of case 2 and the pattern are the following:
K (d) = 44.19 − 43.50 = 0.69 D, meaning the cornea is steeper than average 43.50, so we need to take 0.69 D out of the IOL.
AL (d) = 23.50 − 23.09 = 0.41 mm, which yields 0.41 × 3 = 1.23 D, meaning the eye is shorter than the average 23.50 mm, and we need to give extra 1.23 D to the IOL.
Aiming for −0.50 D, Barrett II recommends 22.50 D SN60WF. Since we are aiming −0.50, it will give the eye another 0.50 D.
So the balance equation will be:
−0.69 D + 1.23 D + 0.50 D = 1.04 D
The IOL power suggested by Barrett II is 22.50. Take the extra 1.04 D out, then FEP is 22.50 − 1.04 = 21.46 D.

18.7.3 Case 3

K 44.43 D.
AL 27.29 mm.
K (d) = 44.43 − 43.50 = 0.93 D. K is steeper than the average 43.50 D, so we need to take away 0.93 D.
AL (d) = 27.29 − 23.50 = 3.79 mm; 3.79 × 3 = 11.37 D.
AL is longer than the average 23.50 mm, so we need to take away 11.37 D.
Barrett Universal II recommends 9.50 D ZXR00, aiming for −0.50 D, so we need to add 0.50 D.
The balance equation is −0.93 − 11.37 + 0.50 = −11.8 D.
The FEP is 9.50 + 11.8 = 21.3 D.

18.7.4 Summary

- If the FEP is between 21.00 and 22.00 D, refractive surprises should be very rare. It works very well in the overwhelming majority of virgin eyes. Patients with corneal refractive surgery will need integration of the amount of correction by the corneal refractive surgery.
- Extreme eyes, the FEP may be out of 21 to 22 D.

- This is a very simple and easy estimate. It will only take about one minute or less when you become familiar with it.
- This off-the-cuff calculation will give you peace of mind. It is useful for every single case, especially in situations where:
  - The cataract is very dense and regular biometry (IOLMaster/LenStar) is not able to provide a reliable measurement or immersion ultrasound shows irregular spike patterns when you are not sure of the accuracy.
  - In eyes that are status post scleral buckles, corneal transplant, and other unusual conditions.
  - It will help to detect data transfer errors as well.

18.8 Questions from Our Residents and Colleagues

I have a patient with a history of retinal detachment with a scleral buckle. When I make decisions regarding IOL power, do I need to make any adjustments because the eye is much longer than the fellow eye?

No, you do not need to make adjustments because of the scleral buckle. In a given IOL calculation formula, it automatically gives you the suggested IOL power based on the axial length, the corneal curvature, the depth of anterior chamber, white to white distance, and other parameters. Our experience echoes a study that there is no need to adjust IOL power because of the presence of scleral buckle.[56]

I am consulting you about this patient. I did her OS cataract last year aiming at plano with the implant SN60WF+16.50 D, but I got an almost −2.0 refractive surprise. SRK-T formula was used. Retrospectively, no human error was identified. Would you be able to tell me the possible reason for this near −2.0 surprise?

The preoperative data are (▶ Table 18.1): Postoperative refractive surprises can have many potential causes. Most of them are due to preoperative measurements, human errors, or are formula related. IOL mislabeling can also occur, but they are very rare.[57,58] If you cannot find any errors from remeasurement, then attention should be paid to formulas. Among all the measurement parameters, the corneal curvature seemed to be the only one belonging to the extreme category. Very steep (>46.00 D) and very

Table 18.1 Preoperative data

	OD	OS
Axial length	24.07	24.12
K readings	46.69/ 47.03@64	46.62/ 46.86@116
AC depth	3.26	3.23
White to white	11.55	11.57

Abbreviations: AC, anterior chamber; OD; OS.

flat (<42.00 D) keratometry readings can be a challenge for accurate predictability when we choose IOL power. The study discussed earlier found that the Barrett Universal II had the highest predictability, with 96.7 within ±0.50 D in those patients with an average K reading <42.00, and Hill-RBF method had the highest predictability percentage within ±0.50 D from target refraction for K reading >46.00 D.[10] I also ran an IOL calculation based on your measurement: Aiming for plano, both Barrett Universal II and Hill-RBF would choose 15.00 D rather than +16.50 D. So, I believe the SRK-T formula was at least part of the reason for her myopic surprise. In a study published in *Ophthalmology* with over 18,000 eyes with SN60WF and SA60AT IOLs to compare seven commonly used IOL calculation formulas, SRK-T was noted to be in particular adversely affected by eyes that have flat or steep keratometry,[17] although the 2017 ESCRS survey still showed that SRK-T was still the most popularly used IOL formula, about four times more than Barrett's for the survey question "What is your preferred lens formula for the majority of your cataract surgeries?"[59] In the 2019 ESCRS survey, SRK-T was still the most preferred formula, with 64%, while Barrett was the second with 42%.[60]

When we measure the total corneal power with the IOLMaster 700, can we still use the current Barrett toric calculator?

The current Barrett toric calculator uses a unique eye model to predict the posterior corneal surface. Using total keratometry (TK) with the Barrett toric calculator would thus lead to overcompensation for posterior corneal astigmatism. Because of this, Graham Barrett, MD, has developed two new IOL power calculation formulas: the Barrett TK Universal II for nontoric IOLs, and the Barrett TK Toric for toric IOLs.[61] Both new formulas use posterior corneal surface measurements. So if you use the current Barrett toric calculator, you should not use the TK measurement.

What happens when you get a refractive surprise in one eye, can't pin down the etiology, and have to choose a lens for the fellow eye?

It has been a very common strategy to use the first eye predictive error to tailor the IOL power for the second eye for a better refractive outcome.[62,63,64] This clinical modality usually works and it is probably the reason why many cataract surgeons arrange the more important eye to be operated as the second eye (such as in pseudophakic monovision, operate the nondominant eye first) so they can fine-tune the second eye IOL power. A common method is to make 50% adjustment of what was missed from the first eye prediction error.[63] It works better when symmetric biometric findings are present.[62] The correlation is weaker when interocular corneal power differences are >0.60 D.[63] With modern IOL calculation formulas, the need for adjustment for the second eye has become less significant and it does not always seem to be beneficial.[65,66]

References

[1] Koch DD, Hill W, Abulafia A, Wang L. Pursuing perfection in intraocular lens calculations: I. Logical approach for classifying IOL calculation formulas. J Cataract Refract Surg. 2017; 43(6):717–718

[2] Wang L, Shirayama M, Ma XJ, Kohnen T, Koch DD. Optimizing intraocular lens power calculations in eyes with axial lengths above 25.0 mm. J Cataract Refract Surg. 2011; 37 (11):2018–2027

[3] Kieval JZ, Al-Hashimi S, Davidson RS, et al. ASCRS Refractive Cataract Surgery Subcommittee. Prevention and management of refractive prediction errors following cataract surgery. J Cataract Refract Surg. 2020; 46(8):1189–1197

[4] Reitblat O, Gali HE, Chou L, et al. Intraocular lens power calculation in the elderly population using the Kane formula in comparison with existing methods. J Cataract Refract Surg. 2020; 46(11):1501–1507

[5] Hill WE. IOL power selection: Think Different. Presented at: The 11th annual Charles D Kelman Lecture for American Academy of Ophthalmology Annual Meeting; November 2015; Las Vegas, NV

[6] Gökce SE, Zeiter JH, Weikert MP, Koch DD, Hill W, Wang L. Intraocular lens power calculations in short eyes using 7 formulas. J Cataract Refract Surg. 2017; 43(7):892–897

[7] Hill WE. Something Borrowed, Something New: Improved Accuracy of IOL Power Selection. Presented at Charles D. Kelman Innovator's Lecture for the ASCRS Symposium on Cataract, IOL and Refractive Surgery; April 2014; Boston, MA

[8] Lopes D. Calculation comparison. EuroTimes. 2018; 23(6): 19

[9] Roberts TV, Hodge C, Sutton G, Lawless M, contributors to the Vision Eye Institute IOL outcomes registry. Comparison of Hill-radial basis function, Barrett Universal and current third generation formulas for the calculation of intraocular lens power during cataract surgery. Clin Exp Ophthalmol. 2018; 46(3):240–246

[10] Reitblat O, Levy A, Kleinmann G, Lerman TT, Assia EI. Intraocular lens power calculation for eyes with high and low average keratometry readings: comparison between various formulas. J Cataract Refract Surg. 2017; 43(9):1149–1156

[11] Kane JX, Van Heerden A, Atik A, Petsoglou C. Intraocular lens power formula accuracy: comparison of 7 formulas. J Cataract Refract Surg. 2016; 42(10):1490–1500

[12] Kane JX, Van Heerden A, Atik A, Petsoglou C. Accuracy of 3 new methods for intraocular lens power selection. J Cataract Refract Surg. 2017; 43(3):333–339

[13] Cooke DL, Cooke TL. Comparison of 9 intraocular lens power calculation formulas. J Cataract Refract Surg. 2016; 42(8):1157–1164

[14] Gökce SE, Montes De Oca I, Cooke DL, Wang L, Koch DD, Al-Mohtaseb Z. Accuracy of 8 intraocular lens calculation formulas in relation to anterior chamber depth in patients with normal axial lengths. J Cataract Refract Surg. 2018; 44 (3):362–368

[15] Shajari M, Kolb CM, Petermann K, et al. Comparison of 9 modern intraocular lens power calculation formulas for a quadrifocal intraocular lens. J Cataract Refract Surg. 2018; 44(8):942–948

[16] Darcy K, Gunn D, Tavassoli S, Sparrow J, Kane JX. Assessment of the accuracy of new and updated intraocular lens power calculation formulas in 10 930 eyes from the UK National Health Service. J Cataract Refract Surg. 2020; 46(1): 2–7

[17] Melles RB, Holladay JT, Chang WJ. Accuracy of intraocular lens calculation formulas. Ophthalmology. 2018; 125(2): 169–178

[18] Olsen T. Calculation of intraocular lens power: a review. Acta Ophthalmol Scand. 2007; 85(5):472–485

[19] Morselli S. Precise preoperative planning optimizes premium IOL outcomes. Strategies for success with toric & presbyopia correcting IOLs. EuroTimes. April 2019

[20] Hoffer KJ. The Hoffer Q formula: a comparison of theoretic and regression formulas. J Cataract Refract Surg. 1993; 19 (6):700–712

[21] Hoffer KJ. Clinical results using the Holladay 2 intraocular lens power formula. J Cataract Refract Surg. 2000; 26(8): 1233–1237

[22] Kane JX, Melles RB. Intraocular lens formula comparison in axial hyperopia with a high-power intraocular lens of 30 or more diopters. J Cataract Refract Surg. 2020; 46(9):1236–1239

[23] Lamson TL, Song J, Abazari A, Weissbart SB. Refractive outcomes of phacoemulsification after pars plana vitrectomy using traditional and new intraocular lens calculation formulas. J Cataract Refract Surg. 2019; 45(3):293–297

[24] Devgan U. Cataract surgery after prior vitrectomy. Cataract Coach. Published August 27, 2018. Accessed March 13, 2021. https://cataractcoach.com/2018/08/27/cataract-surgery-after-prior-vitrectomy/

[25] Koch DD, Ali SF, Weikert MP, Shirayama M, Jenkins R, Wang L. Contribution of posterior corneal astigmatism to total corneal astigmatism. J Cataract Refract Surg. 2012; 38(12): 2080–2087

[26] Koch DD, Jenkins RB, Weikert MP, Yeu E, Wang L. Correcting astigmatism with toric intraocular lenses: effect of posterior corneal astigmatism. J Cataract Refract Surg. 2013; 39 (12):1803–1809

[27] ASCRS Clinical Survey 2018. EyeWorld. Published November 10, 2018. Accessed March 26, 2021. https://supplements.eyeworld.org/eyeworld-supplements/december-2018-clinical-survey

[28] ESCRS Clinical trends survey 2018 Results. EuroTimes. Accessed April 9, 2020. https://www.eurotimes.org/wp-content/uploads/2019/11/Clinical-Survey-Results-2018-12pp-Supplement-press.pdf

[29] ASCRS Database

[30] Ferreira TB, Ribeiro P, Ribeiro FJ, O'Neill JG. Comparison of astigmatic prediction errors associated with new calculation methods for toric intraocular lenses. J Cataract Refract Surg. 2017; 43(3):340–347

[31] Abulafia A, Barrett GD, Kleinmann G, et al. Prediction of refractive outcomes with toric intraocular lens implantation. J Cataract Refract Surg. 2015; 41(5):936–944

[32] Gundersen KG, Potvin R. Clinical outcomes with toric intraocular lenses planned using an optical low coherence reflectometry ocular biometer with a new toric calculator. Clin Ophthalmol. 2016; 10:2141–2147

[33] Abulafia A, Koch DD, Wang L, et al. New regression formula for toric intraocular lens calculations. J Cataract Refract Surg. 2016; 42(5):663–671

[34] Abulafia A, Hill WE, Franchina M, Barrett GD. Comparison of methods to predict residual astigmatism after intraocular lens implantation. J Refract Surg. 2015; 31(10):699–707

[35] Koch DD. The enigmatic cornea and intraocular lens calculations: The LXXIII Edward Jackson Memorial Lecture. Am J Ophthalmol. 2016; 171:xv–xxx

[36] Abulafia A, Koch DD, Wang L, et al. A novel regression formula for toric IOL calculations. Paper presented at: European Society of Cataract and Refractive Surgeons Congress; September 5–9, 2015; Barcelona, Spain

[37] Koch D. Inaugural Steinert Refractive Lecture: Posterior cornea is missing key in refractive outcomes. ASCRS EyeWorld. Published June 2017. Accessed March 26, 2021. https://www.eyeworld.org/inaugural-steinert-refractive-lecture-posterior-cornea-missing-key-refractive-outcomes

[38] Shajari M, Sonntag R, Ramsauer M, et al. Evaluation of total corneal power measurements with a new optical biometer. J Cataract Refract Surg. 2020; 46(5):675–681

[39] Waring GO, III, Lynn MJ, McDonnell PJ. Results of the prospective evaluation of radial keratotomy (PERK) study 10 years after surgery. Arch Ophthalmol. 1994; 112(10):1298–1308

[40] GVR scleral lens and RK. All radial keratotomy posts. Published September 22, 2014. Accessed on September 7, 2020. https://sclerallens.com/all-radial-keratotomy-posts

[41] Helzner J. Can you revive your refractive surgery practice? Ophthalmology Management. Published September 1, 2010. Accessed March 26, 2021. https://www.ophthalmologymanagement.com/issues/2010/september-2010/can-you-revive-your-refractive-surgery-practice

[42] Khor WB, Afshari NA. The role of presbyopia-correcting intraocular lenses after laser in situ keratomileusis. Curr Opin Ophthalmol. 2013; 24(1):35–40

[43] Hamill EB, Wang L, Chopra HK, Hill W, Koch DD. Intraocular lens power calculations in eyes with previous hyperopic laser in situ keratomileusis or photorefractive keratectomy. J Cataract Refract Surg. 2017; 43(2):189–194

[44] Lwowski C, Pawlowicz K, Hinzelmann L, Adas M, Kohnen T. Prediction accuracy of IOL calculation formulas using the ASCRS online calculator for a diffractive extended depth-of-focus IOL after myopic laser in situ keratomileusis. J Cataract Refract Surg. 2020; 46(9):1240–1246

[45] Liu CF, Sun CC, Lin YH, Peng SY, Yeung L. Intraocular lens power calculation after radial keratotomy and LASIK: a case report. Am J Ophthalmol Case Rep. 2019; 15:100495

[46] Turnbull AMJ, Crawford GJ, Barrett GD. Methods for intraocular lens power calculation in cataract surgery after radial keratotomy. Ophthalmology. 2020; 127(1):45–51

[47] Whang WJ, Hoffer KJ, Kim SJ, Chung SH, Savini G. Comparison of intraocular lens power formulas according to axial length after myopic corneal laser refractive surgery. J Cataract Refract Surg. 2021; 47(3):297–303

[48] Wang L, Tang M, Huang D, Weikert MP, Koch DD. Comparison of newer intraocular lens power calculation methods for eyes after corneal refractive surgery. Ophthalmology. 2015; 122(12):2443–2449

[49] Serels CM, Sandoval HP, Potvin R, Solomon KD. Evaluation of IOL power calculation formulas using different keratometries in post-refractive surgery cases. Presented at 2020 Virtual Annual Meeting for American Society of Cataract and Refractive Surgery; May 16, 2020

[50] Chen AL, Long CP, Lu T, Heichel C. Accuracy of intraoperative aberrometry and modern preoperative biometry for IOL power selection in post-refractive surgery patients. Presented at 2020 Virtual Annual Meeting for American Society of Cataract and Refractive Surgery; May 16, 2020

[51] Holladay JT. Achieving optimal outcomes with toric IOLs. Ocular Surgery News. Published April 15, 2016. Accessed March 30, 2021. https://www.healio.com/news/ophthalmology/20160415/achieving-optimal-outcomes-with-toric-iols

[52] Kane JX, Connell B. A comparison of the accuracy of 6 modern Toric intraocular lens formulas. Ophthalmology. 2020; 127(11):1472–1486

[53] Abulafia A, Hill WE, Koch DD, Wang L, Barrett GD. Accuracy of the Barrett True-K formula for intraocular lens power prediction after laser in situ keratomileusis or photorefractive keratectomy for myopia. J Cataract Refract Surg. 2016; 42(3):363–369

[54] Ma JX, Tang M, Wang L, Weikert MP, Huang D, Koch DD. Comparison of newer IOL power calculation methods for eyes with previous radial keratotomy. Invest Ophthalmol Vis Sci. 2016; 57(9):OCT162–OCT168

[55] Curado SX, Hida WT, Vilar CMC, Ordones VL, Chaves MAP, Tzelikis PF. Intraoperative aberrometry versus preoperative biometry for IOL power selection after radial keratotomy: a prospective study. J Refract Surg. 2019; 35(10):656–661

[56] Eshete A, Bergwerk KL, Masket S, Miller KM. Phacoemulsification and lens implantation after scleral buckling surgery. Am J Ophthalmol. 2000; 129(3):286–290

[57] Kohnen S. Postoperative refractive error resulting from incorrectly labeled intraocular lens power. J Cataract Refract Surg. 2000; 26(5):777–778

[58] Solebo LA, Eades Walker RJ, Dabbagh A. Intraocular lens exchange for pseudophakic refractive surprise due to incorrectly labeled intraocular lens. J Cataract Refract Surg. 2012; 38(12):2197–2198

[59] ESCRS 2017 Clinical Trends Survey. EuroTimes. Accessed March 30, 2021. https://www.eurotimes.org/wp-content/uploads/2018/11/Clinical_Survey_Supplement-2017Results-12pp-final.pdf

189

[60] ESCRS Clinical Trends Survey 2019 Results. EuroTimes. Accessed March 30, 2021. https://www.eurotimes.org/wp-content/uploads/2020/11/Clinical-Survey-Results-2019-Supplement_PQ.pdf

[61] Total Keratometry. Zeiss. Accessed September 12, 2020. https://www.zeiss.com/meditec/int/c/iolmaster-700/total-keratometry.html#:~:text=The%20IOLMaster%C2%AE700%20from,Total%20Keratometry%20(TK%C2%AE)

[62] De Bernardo M, Zeppa L, Forte R, et al. Can we use the fellow eye biometric data to predict IOL power? Semin Ophthalmol. 2017; 32(3):363–370

[63] Aristodemou P, Knox Cartwright NE, Sparrow JM, Johnston RL. First eye prediction error improves second eye refractive outcome results in 2129 patients after bilateral sequential cataract surgery. Ophthalmology. 2011; 118(9): 1701–1709

[64] Henderson BA, Schneider J. Same-day cataract surgery should not be the standard of care for patients with bilateral visually significant cataract. Surv Ophthalmol. 2012; 57(6):580–583

[65] Landers J, Goggin M. An inter-eye comparison of refractive outcomes following cataract surgery. J Refract Surg. 2010; 26(3):197–200

[66] Jabbour J, Irwig L, Macaskill P, Hennessy MP. Intraocular lens power in bilateral cataract surgery: whether adjusting for error of predicted refraction in the first eye improves prediction in the second eye. J Cataract Refract Surg. 2006; 32(12):2091–2097

19 Refractive Cataract Surgery for Post-Keratorefractive Surgery Patients

Fuxiang Zhang, Alan Sugar, and Lisa Brothers Arbisser

Abstract

Patients with a history of corneal refractive surgery are often difficult candidates for refractive cataract surgery (RCS). This chapter will review the ophthalmic literature to show which post-refractive surgery patients have been good candidates for premium intraocular lenses (IOL). We will focus on preoperative consultation, biometry, and topography and characteristics of wavefront profile to analyze who can be reasonable candidates. The principles of how to decide which IOL for what patients will be reviewed. The role of Optiwave refractive analysis (ORA) is different when it is used in patients with a history of laser-assisted in situ keratomileusis (LASIK) and photorefractive keratectomy (PRK) versus radial keratotomy (RK). The light adjustable lens and small aperture IC-8 extended depth of focus (EDOF) lens have a role in this special group of patients when they require spectacle independence. The impact of history of conductive keratoplasty, phakic IOL/implantable contact lens to RCS will also be briefly discussed.

Keywords: refractive cataract surgery, s/p LASIK/PRK, s/p RK, Optiwave refractive analysis, ORA, spectacle independence, IC-8 lens

19.1 Background of Post-Keratorefractive Patients

Millions of nearsighted patients chose to get out of their glasses by having radial keratotomy (RK) in the 1980s and 1990s. Over two million RK procedures were done in the United States and Canada alone.[1] Due to delayed hyperopic regression, secondary to the loss of structural integrity of the cornea from the incisions, RK was gradually phased out and replaced by more predictable and safer laser vision correction—laser-assisted in situ keratomileusis (LASIK) and photorefractive keratectomy (PRK). By 2009, more than 16 million LASIK procedures had been performed worldwide, and it is estimated that up to a million are performed each year in the United States alone.[2]

According to statistics from the Refractive Surgery Council, the volume of laser vision correction procedures in the United States grew for the third consecutive year in 2018. The overall number of LASIK, PRK, and SMILE procedures performed was more than 843,000 in 2018, a 6.2% increase over 2017.[3] When these patients later present with cataracts, most are still very motivated to minimize spectacle dependence after cataract surgery. They still do not like glasses or contact lenses and we face more difficulties when they are in our offices and operating rooms. They have preconceived expectations for their perfect youthful vision and spectacle freedom. The challenges are focused mainly on the cornea, but we should also make sure that other parts of the eye have the potential to meet spectacle independence as these eyes may not be as healthy as when they had corneal refractive surgery performed. Frequently, they are not good candidates for premium IOLs.

19.2 What Important Things Should I Cover during Preoperative Consultation?

Patients should have realistic expectations. They need to know that the outcome may not be as great as the initial "WOW" vision they experienced after their corneal refractive surgery. Literature indicates that after laser vision correction, >90% of eyes were within ±0.50 D of the intended optical target[4] while with respect to cataract surgery, the "benchmark" established by the National Health Service of the United Kingdom indicate that only about 60% of eyes were within ±0.50 D of the intended refractive target.[5] Only 1% of cataract surgeons can achieve 90% of eyes within ±0.50 D of the intended refractive target.[6] It is even tougher to achieve this goal when there is a history of previous corneal refractive surgery. Compared to virgin eyes, patients with a history of corneal refractive surgery have a higher chance of requiring laser enhancement to correct residual refractive error after they receive premium IOLs. One study reported the need in 42.9% of 49 eyes

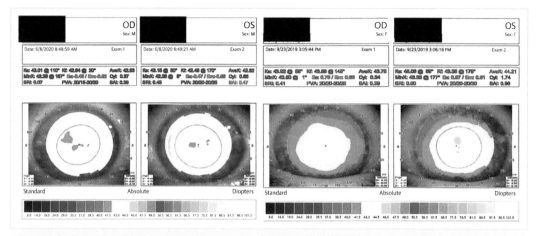

Fig. 19.1 On the left, postmyopic laser-assisted in situ keratomileusis (LASIK) with central cornea flatter than peripheral cornea OD and OS. On the right, Posthyperopic LASIK OD and OS. Central cornea is steeper than the peripheral cornea OD and OS.

(38 patients) with history of myopic LASIK after AcrySof ReSTOR (Alcon) implantation.[7]

All of these patients should have a good understanding and consent for the possibility of needing glasses, touch-up, or even IOL exchange after the cataract surgery. While it is necessary to discuss all the major concerns and difficulties, we do not want to scare these patients away from refractive cataract surgery since this group of patients is typically well motivated to seek spectacle independence. Many post-LASIK/PRK patients can do well with premium IOLs or pseudophakic monovision. Do not hesitate to tell them your statistics, which pushes surgeons to be more perfect and makes patients more comfortable. With the art of preoperative consultation honed, most patients will have realistic expectations and end up happy.

19.3 What Pertinent History and Tests Do We Need for These Patients If They Desire Spectacle Independence?

We first need to know what corneal refractive surgery was done. Some patients do not really know if they were myopic or hyperopic. Original documents or old spectacle prescriptions are helpful, but often they are not available. A simple corneal topography can typically tell the difference. See

▶ Fig. 19.1 for postmyopic LASIK and posthyperopic LASIK. In postmyopic LASIK, the central cornea will be flatter than peripheral cornea (oblate) while in posthyperopic LASIK, the central cornea will be steeper than peripheral cornea (prolate). Corneal topography will also provide information about whether the ablation is central or decentered. In cases of significantly decentered ablation, IOLs with zero spherical aberration (SA) are preferred, such as SN60AT or SA60AT (Alcon), enVista (Bausch & Lomb), or SofPort AO (Bausch & Lomb).[8] Because these IOLs are do-no-harm lenses suitable in situations involving decentration. If the ablation is decentered, an SA-correcting IOL that is centered will cause coma and nighttime glare. AcrySof IQ SN60WF/SA60WF (Alcon) and ZCB00 (Johnson & Johnson) are among the most commonly used SA-correcting IOLs on the market.

In most situations, the postoperative ablative pattern is easily identifiable, but rarely it can be a challenge. A recent study demonstrated that tangential curvature maps could more accurately demonstrate postoperative curvature patterns than those with axial curvature maps and facilitate identification of myopic and hyperopic ablations for novice ophthalmologists.[9] We can also look at wavefront measurement. Myopic LASIK typically has increased positive higher order aberration (HOA) while hyperopic LASIK typically has increased negative HOA, although variations do occur. For example, hyperopic LASIK eyes can still have positive HOA if the LASIK correction is small because the human cornea typically has positive SA.[8,10] With aging, total SA increases, mainly from the aging lens,[8,10] while it is not conclusive if corneal positive SA also increases with aging. In rare cases where it is not possible to accurately determine the pattern (myopic vs. hyperopic), especially if the keratorefractive surgery correction was mild, intraoperative aberrometry will be helpful.

We need to ask the patient if he/she achieved great quality of vision after refractive surgery. This question is very important and should never be missed. If he/she was never happy with the corneal refractive surgery, this should be a red flag initiating careful evaluation with topography/ tomography and slit lamp examination and assessment for a demanding personality.

Dry eyes are very common among these patients and they sometimes need pre-biometry treatment with lubricants and punctal plugs. (See detailed discussion in Chapter 3.) They may have had a large angle kappa to start with when they had previous corneal surgery. High myopia patients may have myopic maculopathy or lattice with holes or tears.

Compared with virgin corneas, those patients with a history of corneal refractive surgery may have increased corneal irregular astigmatism, multifocal corneal changes, significant SA, coma, and even ectasia. These patients should have an aberration profile test preoperatively, even if they do not plan to pursue premium IOLs. ▶ Fig. 19.2 is from a patient who had RK surgery, OD 16 incisions, and OS 8. She wanted "the best implant available, cost is not an issue." She wished to need

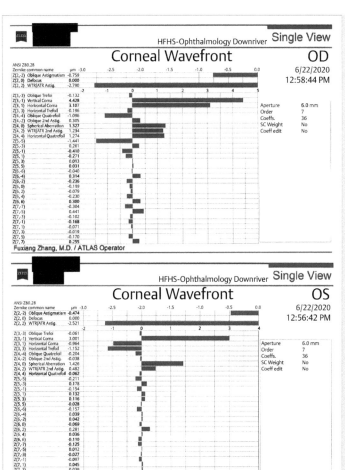

Fig. 19.2 OD had 16 cuts radial keratotomy (RK) and OS 8 cuts. Both eyes had significant higher order aberration (HOA) and coma, OD worse than OS.

no spectacles for far or near after cataract surgery. Corneal wavefront with Atlas (Zeiss) showed severe HOA and coma, OD worse than OS. The coma in her OD was about 15 times and OS 10 times more than our cutoff of 0.3 μm. SA was also significant. That patient was not a good candidate for multifocal IOL (MFIOL), extended depth of focus (EDOF), or trifocal IOLs. She might be a good candidate for IC-8 (Chapter 14) or XtraFocus (Chapter 20) pinhole IOLs.

19.4 Do We Have Evidence to Support the Suitability of Premium IOLs for Patients with History of Corneal Refractive Surgery?

Studies have demonstrated the suitability with encouraging outcomes of MFIOLs in postmyopic LASIK[2,11,12,13,14] and posthyperopic LASIK patients.[2,11,15] Some studies have shown that best corrected visual acuity can be compromised in postmyopic LASIK and posthyperopic LASIK patients when they receive MFIOLs.[16,17,18] A study[19] in the Netherlands summarized visual outcomes of MFIOL (ReSTOR SN6AD1, Alcon) implantation in 40 eyes of 40 patients with a history of hyperopic LASIK: 62.5% were within ±0.50 D and 87.5% within ±1.00 D of refractive target at the 3-month postoperative visits. Nine eyes (22.5%) had a laser enhancement after IOL implantation in that study. A study in Portugal[20] consisting of 22 patients and 44 eyes in each group demonstrated the suitability and success of the Symfony lens (Johnson & Johnson) in postmyopic LASIK patients with comparable uncorrected distance vision (UDVA) but statistically significantly better binocular uncorrected intermediate as well as binocular uncorrected near vision; and similar contrast in any special frequency when compared with the same company's monofocal ZCB00 IOL patients. Subjective complaints of mild halo were equal (13.6%) but mild glare was more frequent in the Symfony IOL group (22.7%) than the ZCB00 group (9.1%). A study at Baylor showed that toric IOLs effectively corrected preexisting corneal astigmatism in eyes with previous excimer laser corneal refractive surgery, with postoperative astigmatism of ≤0.50 D in 80% of eyes with previous myopic and 84% hyperopic LASIK/PRK.[21]

To our knowledge, there is a lack of large studies to suggest the suitability of MFIOL for post-RK patients, although some case reports are available.[22,23,24] It is a known phenomenon that radial keratotomy can induce significant HOAs.[25,26] The increased HOA is negatively correlated with the central clear zone diameter,[26] and positively associated with the magnitude of radial keratotomy refractive correction.[27] Post-RK patients were reported to do well with the Symfony EDOF.[28,29] The small aperture IC-8 IOL also showed promising outcomes for RK patients.[28,30]

In our limited experience, with good corneal conditions on topography as well as good aberration profiles, Symfony EDOF lenses can do well. (Vivity EDOF lenses are being evaluated as of this writing.) In terms of monofocal toric IOLs, we have found great success for these patients. We agree with the three preoperative selection criteria by Koch[31]:
- Good or near good bow tie pattern.
- Magnitude of cylinder <0.75 with two trusted devices.
- Axis difference <15 degree with two trusted devices.

19.5 Do I Need to Consider Spherical versus Aspherical Lenses for These Patients?

Young human crystalline lenses have negative SA which is about the same level as the positive SA in the cornea.[10] As aging progresses, total SA increases, mainly from lens aging. As corneal astigmatism increases, SA also increases.[32] Corneal refractive surgery will change the corneal profile. Hyperopic LASIK increases negative aberration while myopic LASIK increases positive corneal SA.[15,33,34] SA in hyperopic PRK also changed from positive before surgery to negative after surgery.[35] Hyperopic LASIK induced more third- and fifth-order coma-like aberration than myopic LASIK.[33] AcrySof ReSTOR MFIOL/PanOptix trifocal (Alcon), Tecnis MFIOL/Symfony EDOF (Johnson & Johnson), and others are designed to compensate for positive SA, which is typical for virgin eyes. So, theoretically, post-hyperopic corneal refractive surgery patients may not be the best candidates for these lenses which have built-in negative SA.

Quantitative measurement of corneal aberration profile is necessary among post-keratorefractive patients before they have cataract surgery. Even if they do not want to have a premium IOL for RCS, the information about HOAs is still helpful in terms of consultation and IOL selection. For example, hyperopic LASIK typically induces negative SA and if we use some of the most commonly used posterior chamber intraocular lens, PCIOL, such as SN60WF/SA60WF (Alcon) and ZCBOO (Johnson & Johnson), the built-in negative SA in these lenses will worsen the outcome, especially if the LASIK ablation zone is decentered. In this scenario, neutral SA lenses, such as SofPort or enVista (both from Bausch & Lomb), SN60AT/SA60AT (Alcon) and AABOO (Johnson & Johnson) would be preferred. Posthyperopic LASIK patients can often still have positive SA if the correction of corneal refractive surgery was small (▶ Fig. 19.3). Karakelle cited studies suggesting that a young adult at peak visual performance typically has very small positive SA and that was the reason why Alcon IOLs had only −0.2 μm built in spherical correction.[8] Studies in the literature suggest that some positive SA can be preserved or added in the nondominant eye by selecting a traditional nonspherical-correcting IOL that could increase near vision and extend depth of focus.[36,37]

One study has shown that *spherical* MFIOLs have done well for posthyperopic LASIK patients.[15] For postmyopic LASIK/PRK patients, who have increased positive SA, *aspherical* MFIOLs could provide better visual quality and optical quality than spherical IOLs under mesopic

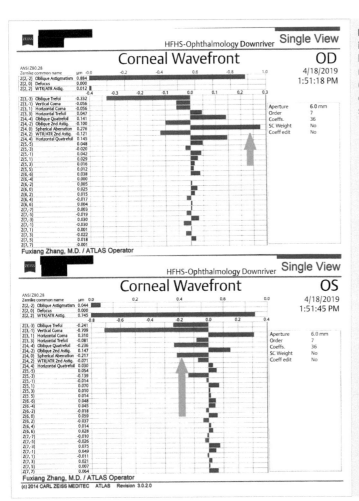

Fig. 19.3 S/p Hyperopic laser-assisted in situ keratomileusis (LASIK) OU. OD had small LASIK correction and it remained positive spherical aberration (*short blue arrow*). OS had large LASIK correction which resulted in negative spherical aberration (*long blue arrow*).

conditions.[18] AcrySof PanOptix and ReSTOR +3.0 D add have −0.10-μm SA[38] and ReSTOR +2.5 D add has −0.2-μm SA. Symfony EDOF and Tecnis MFIOLs both have −0.27-μm SA correction built-in to compensate for the positive SA of the cornea. Johnson & Johnson Tecnis IOLs may be better options for postmyopic LASIK/PRK than Alcon's IOL because the former have more SA correction. Even for conventional monofocal IOLs, we still recommend the same principle. For example, as in ▶ Fig. 19.3, posthyperopic LASIK OS with increased negative SA, a SN60AT was used while in OD, SA was still positive, a SN60WF was used. AcrySof IQ SN60WF/SA60WF lenses (Alcon) have −0.2-μm SA correction[8] while SN60AT/SA60AT do not have either positive or negative built-in SA correction. Post-RK patients typically have increased positive SA, so aspherical lenses with built-in negative SA correction are preferred.

19.6 How Do I Decide Which IOL for What Patients?

There are many factors to consider for this question. Many patients believe a myth: the more expensive the IOL, the better quality and better visual outcomes. It is a good thing that most patients make decisions mainly based on their doctors' recommendations and very few based on their knowledge or research results.

- Patient's desire:
  - Some want to have as much spectacle independence as possible. In our practice, traditional monofocal monovision has been the most commonly used option. It can be easily achieved now with the light adjustable lens (LAL).
  - Some want to have best quality far and intermediate vision, but do not mind needing readers. Aspheric monofocal IOLs with mini-monovision or modified monovision can be chosen for this group of patients. In modified monovision, the dominant eye receives an aspheric monofocal IOL aiming for emmetropia while the nondominant eye receives an EDOF Vivity (Alcon) or an EDOF Symfony (Johnson & Johnson) aiming for −0.50.
  - Some like to need no glasses at home, but do not mind using glasses for driving. If they do not like to deal with any dysphotopsia or to pay the extra money, choose a monofocal IOL aiming the first eye at −1.50 D. Adjust the second eye refractive target based on the

outcome of the first eye. If the patient does well with the first operated eye for home-based activities and wishes the second eye to have better distance vision, then set the target at −1.0 D. Or set it at −2.0 D if the patient wishes to have a bit better reading.
  - Often, there is a quick and easy way to ask about the patient's desires. Which one would you like to have? (A) To have the best quality of vision for far, but you will need to wear readers for small print or even the computer. (B) To have the most convenience, no need for spectacles for far or near, but there is a compromised quality of vision in contrast and nighttime halo/glare. The answer to this question will lead to the next discussion.
- Ocular examination conditions:
  - Ocular surface should be pretty much perfect if EDOF/MFIOL/trifocal IOL are to be used. Intensive treatment can make ocular surfaces temporarily look good with improved and acceptable corneal topography, but this may not realistically be maintainable in real life postoperatively; it is better to avoid premium IOLs.
  - Other significant comorbidities, especially potentially progressive macular pathologies and glaucoma, avoid premium IOLs except toric IOLs to correct significant astigmatism.
- Preoperative tests conditions:
  - Corneal topography is the most important test. If there is significant irregular astigmatism from previous corneal refractive surgery, diffractive premium IOLs are best avoided. Sometimes, it is worthwhile to have an in-office trial of rigid contact lenses to see whether the actual visual disturbance is from the aberrated cornea or the cataract. This can be very enlightening and help the patient to understand what the best outcome can be after the cataract surgery; helps create realistic expectations and, occasionally, the cataract is a small part of the visual disturbance and contact lens fitting is more appropriate than cataract surgery.
  - Corneal aberration profile and angle kappa also need to meet the recommendations if MFIOL/trifocal IOLs are to be considered.
  - OCT of macula should be performed for every single RCS patient.
- Corneal refractive surgery type:
  - In our limited experience, most post-RK patients are not good candidates for premium

IOLs due to the presence of irregular astigmatism, increased HOA, and diurnal variation, especially if there are eight or more corneal incisions.

- If the corneal refractive surgery created monovision and the patient was doing well and happy for many years until the cataract developed, keeping the same pattern with monofocal IOL or LAL will offer the most likelihood of a happy patient.
- Patients with a history of enhancement with more than one laser treatment are tougher to hit spherical targets, and potentially to enhance postoperatively.

19.7 What Is the Role of Symfony EDOF IOLs in Post-Keratorefractive Surgery Patients?

Given that we do not have IC-8 EDOF lenses in the United States yet, Symfony EDOF IOLs (Johnson & Johnson) are frequently used for refractive cataract surgery in patients who have a history of corneal refractive surgery. The following are favorable factors: First, photic phenomena are typically less than those with MFIOLs.[39,40] Second, due to the elongated optical focus, there is less chance of missing the refractive target. Third, recent studies have shown that the higher tolerability of postoperative residual astigmatism is favorable for this lens in post-LASIK patients.[41,42] Our limited experience also suggests that Vivity (Alcon) EDOF IOLs are also promising with similar outcomes as Symfony EDOF IOLs, although we have not used Vivity lenses for a long time yet.

19.8 What Are the Advantages of Using ORA for Post-Keratorefractive Surgery Patients?

Among all the merits of intraoperative aberrometry, the information Optiwave refractive analysis (ORA, Alcon) provides for post-LASIK/PRK probably has the most value. There are many studies that have shown that ORA is beneficial in the selection of IOL power in post-LASIK and post-PRK eyes.[43,44,45] Those studies suggest the benefit of ORA in IOL selection in post-LASIK and PRK

patients when they compared the ORA with other IOL formulas, but most studies in the literature as of today did not compare ORA with the Barrett True-K formula which has been widely considered as the most accurate formula in choosing IOL power among cataract patients with a history of LASIK/PRK/RK. In the 2019 ESCRS survey, SRK-T was still the most preferred formula, with 64%, while Barrett was the second with 42%.[46]

We have found a few studies comparing the Barrett True-K formula and intraoperative aberrometry/ORA for cataract patients with a history of corneal refractive surgery.

- In eyes with prior RK surgery, the ORA's performance was similar to the Barrett True-K formula and all of the other established formulas, with no significant difference between median absolute error and mean absolute error. The Barrett True-K formula produced significantly more eyes within ±0.50 D than the SRK/T, Hoffer Q, and Holladay 1 formulas.[47] In that study, however, 41 eyes had 4 cuts (78.8%) and only 8 eyes had 8 cuts (21.2%).
- A study presented at 2019 ASCRS did not find significant differences in terms of predictive accuracy between Barrett True-K formula and intraoperative aberrometry in postcorneal refractive eyes.[48]
- In a retrospective chart review study with 44 post-LASIK cataract surgery eyes, Fisher et al did not find significant differences in prediction error between ORA and the Barrett True-K formula.[11]

Our limited experience suggests that the Barrett True-K formula alone is as good as ORA in terms of previous LASIK/PRK, both myopic and hyperopic. We recommend that ORA be a backup to confirm IOL power. The Barrett True-K formula alone is probably better than ORA in post-RK patients, but there is a lack of peer-reviewed studies in the literature. Limitations of intraoperative aberrometry for post-RK patients will be discussed later in this chapter.

19.9 What If I Do Not Have an Intraoperative Aberrometer?

Not all cataract surgeons have an ORA (Alcon) and not all believe the necessity to have an ORA. As discussed in Chapter 18, IOL Formulas, for postmyopic as well as hyperopic LASIK/PRK and RK, the Barrett True-K formulas do better than other formulas. In post-RK patients, Barrett True-K with history provides a more accurate outcome if RK data are available, especially the post-RK refraction and pre-RK refractions.[49] When no refractive history is available, the Barrett True-K (No History) and Haigis formulas both perform well.[49] Thanks to Drs. Hill, Wang and Koch, the ASCRS Postrefractive IOL Calculators are also excellent and popular tools for this special group of patients.

19.10 What Impact Does Postconductive Keratoplasty Have and Do I Need to Change the IOL Formula?

Conductive keratoplasty (CK) was an in-office procedure for the correction of hyperopia, hyperopic astigmatism, and presbyopia. One of the most common approaches using CK was to make the nondominant eye myopic for near vision and reading. The US Food and Drugs Administration approved CK in 2002.[50] Due to the procedure's regression trend, CK was not widely used after its FDA approval. The negative impact of CK on refractive cataract surgery is not as significant as LASIK/PRK/RK. The CK treatment spots are farther away from the central cornea. Thermal waves were believed to steepen the cornea at almost full corneal thickness and CK does not disrupt the relationship between the anterior and posterior curvatures,[51] although CK may induce negative SA,[52] so special attention is needed for corneal astigmatism and aberration profiles. No special formulas or further adjustments have to be used.[51]

19.11 Can I Use Standard Biometry and IOL Calculation Formulas for Patients Whose Cataracts Are due to Phakic IOLs/ Implantable Contact Lenses? Are There Any Special Intraoperative Considerations?

Generally speaking, we do not have to change our biometry technique, such as with the IOLMaster (Zeiss Meditec AG) or Lenstar (Haag Streit) for most commercially available posterior chamber phakic IOL (pIOL) or implantable contact lens (ICL) in situ with coexisting cataracts because the measured axial lengths (AL) with the pIOL/ICL in situ are usually very close to the measurements prior to the pIOL/ICL implantation.[53,54,55,56] Refractive surgeons typically do measurements prior to pIOL/ICL and this reference data does have utility, but it may not always be accurate for IOL calculation because the AL may increase progressively in some highly myopic patients; therefore, AL measurements taken before pIOL implantation are not always accurate for IOL power calculation.[57] In terms of IOL calculation formulas, we do not have to have any specific modification either.[53,54,56] Most of these lenses are very thin, sitting on top of the crystalline lens/cataract. The long AL for most axial myopic eyes is another factor making the impact of ICL in situ on the IOL power minimal. The SRK-T formula with the Wang/Koch adjustment had good results and the Barrett Universal II has become more popular lately.[53] Intraoperative aberrometry can also be used after the bi-lensectomy and the cataract extraction in an aphakic state. Accurate predictability can be a challenge in these eyes, usually because of their extreme length, effective lens position, and macular anatomy. Having a pIOL/ICL in situ does not have a significant negative effect on IOL calculation.[53,54,56]

Most foldable pIOLs/ICLs are very soft and thin implants, so bi-lensectomy itself is not technically challenging, although attention is needed to avoid tearing during explantation; the grasping forceps should grab the optic portion of the implant. Make sure that an ample amount of dispersive OVD is used to protect the corneal endothelium. High axial myopia eyes typically have a deep anterior chamber which is prone to reverse pupillary block. These patients also often have weaker zonules due to excessive stretching of the zonular fibers.[58] If reverse pupillary block does occur, a second instrument should be used to lift the iris off the capsule to allow fluid to circulate back to the posterior chamber and return the iris/lens diaphragm to its normal position.

Benjamin Franklin once said that "an ounce of prevention is worth a pound of cure." It is best to prevent this from happening with a low bottle height and slow motion technique.

It is better to prevent retropulsion of the Iris in all high myopes by placing a jot of OVD between the iris and anterior capsule rhexis edge nasally near the paracentesis when filling the anterior chamber. We then enter on foot position zero in an OVD filled anterior chamber in a controlled manner while lifting the iris off the capsule with the chopper. Once this is done, irrigation can commence without allowing deepening of the chamber as this guarantees distribution of BSS between anterior and posterior chambers. Care must be taken, of course, to establish flow prior to beginning phaco to prevent wound burn. This small maneuver eliminates the pain and zonular stretching associated with reverse pupillary block which is predictable and nearly ubiquitous in high myopes.

These eyes also tend to have large anterior segments and bags, so extra effort to measure the appropriate size continuous curvilinear capsulorhexis (CCC) just before execution with a caliper can prevent a too large rhexis. Lastly, very large bags may permit standard one-piece IOL decentration. Consideration can be given to using a three-piece lens for standard optic capture or posterior optic capture through a primary hyaloid sparing posterior capsulorhexis into Berger's space with the advantage of eliminating secondary cataract in these retinal detachment prone eyes.

19.12 What Are the Two Postoperative Hyperopic Changes after Cataract Surgery in Post Radial Keratotomy Patients?

Most of us realize the benefit of knowing the first eye refractive outcome in terms of making some adjustment for the second eye IOL power decision. There is certainly merit to allowing enough time between surgeries on the two eyes until the first eye has achieved a relatively stable refraction. This becomes more important for post-RK than post-LASIK patients because the LASIK corneal flap incision typically does not change radically after cataract surgery. In contrast, with RK, swelling of the cornea incisions, immediately after cataract surgery, can result in significant hyperopia. The greatest hyperopia often happens in the first week after cataract surgery.[59] After the first one month or so the immediate postoperative hyperopic shift

tends to disappear. One of the ways to objectively check this is to do a corneal topography and then compare it with the preoperative baseline. The secondary slow and long duration hyperopic drift after the cataract surgery might be the same as we observed in almost all RK patients regardless of cataract surgery. The phase two hyperopic drift is the reason why we add extra myopic power, not phase one. The 10-year prospective evaluation of radial keratotomy (PERK) study data showed that an eight-incision RK shifts hyperopically about 1 D per decade.[60]

19.13 Why Do You Say Most RK Patients Are Not Good Candidates for Most Premium IOLs?

The impact from previous RK surgery on the outcomes of cataract surgery is more complicated than from LASIK/PRK and CK. It depends on multiple factors: the number of radial cuts, the presence of arcuate keratotomy cuts, the size of the central cut-free optical zone, the length of the cuts toward the limbus, wound scar, and new blood vessels, etc. Post-RK patients are typically not good candidates for MFIOL/EDOF/trifocal due to increased irregular astigmatism, increased SA/coma (▶ Fig. 19.2) and diurnal variation. It is common for post-RK patients to have more than 1-µm HOA and often in excess of 1.5 µm. Occasionally, in significant diurnal variation patients, different spectacles are used for morning and for afternoon/evening. As we have discussed in other chapters, a Placido ring image (▶ Fig. 19.4) can be helpful for our surgeon's decision as well as education for our patients.

19.14 Monofocal Toric IOLs Can Do Well for Some Post-RK Patients

Many post-RK patients do well with pseudophakic monovision. Monofocal toric IOLs can work well if the astigmatism is fairly regular and stable, typically with lower number of RK cuts patients. In most situations, we use a monofocal IOL for these patients for IOL monovision if the patient requires spectacle independence. The Symfony EDOF lens

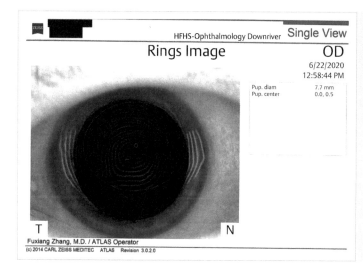

Fig. 19.4 Irregular Placido rings in a patient with a history of radial keratotomy (RK).

(Johnson & Johnson) has been reported to be successful in post-RK patients.[28,61]

A patient with 4-cut RK OD and 8-cut RK with 2 AK cuts OS did well with a monofocal toric IOL in OD. His OD Lenstar measurement was *39.40/42.03@48* and his preop spectacle OD was −0.75 + 3.25 × 62. Manual keratometry OD read as 39.62/41.00 × 48. Atlas topography (▶ Fig. 19.5) showed *39.49/41.53@51* with a fairly regular astigmatism pattern and reasonable wavefront profile of SA, 0.113 μm, vertical coma 0.646 μm, and horizontal coma 0.061 μm. OD's Placido rings (▶ Fig. 19.6) showed fairly regular astigmatism with an oval shape matching the rest of the preop tests. All these preop tests seemed to agree well and indicated this to be a reasonable candidate for a monofocal toric IOL. OS did not need a toric IOL. That gentleman was happy at 1-month follow-up of his second eye surgery. UDVA 20/30 OD and 20/80 OS. UNVA 20/30 OD and 20/25 OS. Manifest −1.00 + 0.50 × 30 OD 20/25 and −2.00 + 0.50 × 160 OS 20/25. Of note, it is advisable to leave some mild myopia for post-RK patients preparing for future hyperopic shifts.

19.15 Are There Other Options for s/p RK Refractive Cataract Surgery Patients?

Before the availability of Refractive Index Shaping (See Chapter 17, FLACS), the LAL (RxSight, Aliso Viejo, California) and IC-8 small aperture IOL (AcuFocus, Irvine, California) may be the two most suitable lenses for s/p RK patients. The unique benefit of the LAL is the ability to adjust the lens power, both sphere and cylinder, after the cataract surgery. Even in the situation of RK, the LAL has been shown to do well, although postoperative UV-blocking glasses will be needed for a couple of months until the cornea becomes stable, compared to only a few weeks required in non-RK cases. See Chapter 13, Light Adjustable Lenses. The small-aperture design (IC-8 AcuFocus, Irvine, California) blocks *unfocused* peripheral light rays via its 3.23-mm-wide opaque mask while allowing central and paracentral light rays through its 1.36-mm central aperture.[62] This unique design theoretically should work well for those patients whose cornea has significant irregular astigmatism such as s/p RK, corneal transplant, keratoconus, trauma, etc. One study has shown that overall quality of life improved significantly with the IC-8 IOL.[63] A study by Dick et al found that the small-aperture IOL, when combined with a −0.75 D myopic defocus, could extend the range of functional near vision by 1.0 D without any loss to distance vision.[64] It can tolerate up to 1.5 D of residual astigmatism. When asked if they were willing to consider the same implant, 95.9% of these patients reported yes.[64] The fellow eyes were implanted with monofocal IOLs aimed at plano. For more details refer to Chapter 14, IC-8 Lens.

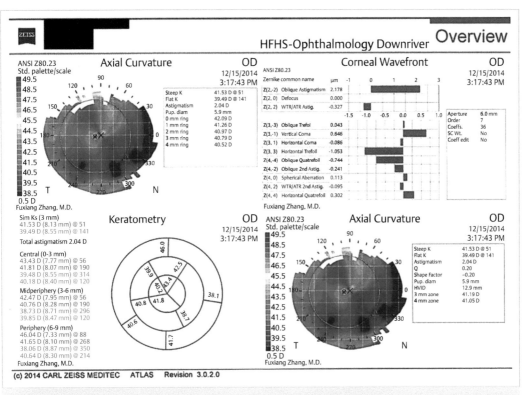

Fig. 19.5 Corneal topography (Atlas, Zeiss). S/p four radial keratotomy (RK) cuts in OD.

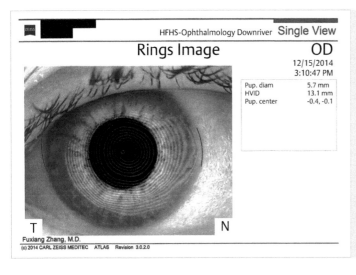

Fig. 19.6 Placido ring of four radial keratotomy (RK) cuts OD with pretty regular astigmatism.

19.16 If I Consider a Post-RK Patient for IOL Monovision, What Requires Special Attention?

- Not all RK patients are good candidates for IOL monovision. We do not recommend IOL monovision for post-RK patients who have significant irregular astigmatism (especially in the dominant eye) or significant diurnal vision change.
- The dominant eye should have reasonable UDVA potential of around 20/30 or better with a lower number of RK cuts, typically less than 8.
- Some monocular RK patients have RK-induced monovision. These patients can be expected to do well maintaining monovision with the IOL.
- Use multiple formulas to calculate the IOL power. Pick the highest IOL power. Barrett True-K is the one we have used exclusively in the past few years.
- Do biometry measurement in the morning when the corneas are flat. A higher power IOL will then be chosen. In this way, the patient may have some myopic shift in the afternoon or evening, it will be better than if they cannot see well in the early morning when the eyes are more hyperopic.
- If the cut number is 8 or fewer, the main incision is probably best at the limbus-cornea junction with incision size 2.4 mm or less; but if there are 12 or more cuts, it is better to use a scleral tunnel. The length of the tunnel incision may need to be a bit shorter than one's routine incisional length to avoid touching or stretching the RK cuts.
- Lower flow and lower bottle height to lower intraoperative IOP is recommended for every RK patient. If you notice any leaking, be cautious, since that will compromise AC stability with higher chance of PC tears. You may need to suture the leak immediately, when it is still near the limbus, before the leaking extends to the central cornea. Make it routine to paint the whole cornea at the end of the surgery with a sterile fluorescein strip to make sure no leaking wound needs suturing.

19.17 Is Intraoperative Aberrometry Reliable in Post-RK Patients?

ORA will not give a reliable recommendation in certain conditions. Unlike post-LASIK or post-PRK, the validation of ORA in patients with a history of RK has not been well studied in the peer-reviewed literature.[44] ORA has been, however, widely used among cataract surgeons on post-RK patients. The structural changes after LASIK/PRK versus RK are quite different. As we know, IOP can be very high, up to 80 to 90 mmHg, during phacoemulsification, which may weaken the cornea and make RK cuts gape or even open in severe cases. The corneal shape and curvature at a pressure of 21 mmHg prior to the ORA reading may be quite different from the preoperative measurements or a few months after the surgery. Because of this acute change, it is also possible to have subsequent changes in anterior chamber depth (deeper) and axial length (longer). These artificial changes will affect the accuracy of ORA's recommendations for the IOL power.

A retrospective chart review[65] at 2013 ARVO consisted of 30 eyes with 12 postradial keratotomy eyes and 18 post-LASIK/PRK eyes. ORA was used for all eyes in that study. That paper demonstrated that the ORA's ability to predict IOL power was significantly better in LASIK/PRK patients than in RK patients ($p = 0.0064$). To our knowledge, the first peer-reviewed case report of a significant refractive surprise was by us in the *American Journal of Ophthalmology* case reports where a significant hyperopic refractive surprise happened in both eyes of a post-RK patient using the ORA recommendation (https://www.sciencedirect.com/science/article/pii/S2451993617301810).[66]

We recommend that surgeons be cautious when using ORA on RK patients, especially for those who have more than six cuts.

References

[1] All Radial Keratotomy Posts. ScleralLens.com. Published September 22, 2014. Accessed September 7, 2020. https://sclerallens.com/all-radial-keratotomy-posts

[2] Khor WB, Afshari NA. The role of presbyopia-correcting intraocular lenses after laser in situ keratomileusis. Curr Opin Ophthalmol. 2013; 24(1):35–40

[3] Baartman B. Laser refractive surgery gradually regains ground since peaking in early 2000s. Ocular Surgery News. Published April 10, 2019. Accessed March 3, 2021. https://www.healio.com/news/ophthalmology/20190329/laser-refractive-surgery-gradually-regains-ground-since-peaking-in-early-2000s#:~:text=According%20to%20statistics%20released%20by,a%206.2%25%20increase%20over%202017

[4] Schallhorn SC, Venter JA. One-month outcomes of wavefront-guided LASIK for low to moderate myopia with the VISX STAR S4 laser in 32,569 eyes. J Refract Surg. 2009; 25 (7) Suppl:S634–S641

[5] Gale RP, Saldana M, Johnston RL, Zuberbuhler B, McKibbin M. Benchmark standards for refractive outcomes after NHS cataract surgery. Eye (Lond). 2009; 23(1):149–152

[6] Hill WE. IOL power selection by pattern recognition. CRSTEurope. Accessed June 4, 2021. https://crstodayeurope.com/articles/new-frontiers-in-iol-prediction-for-improved-refractive-outcomes/iol-power-selection-by-pattern-recognition/

[7] Muftuoglu O, Dao L, Mootha VV, et al. Apodized diffractive intraocular lens implantation after laser in situ keratomileusis with or without subsequent excimer laser enhancement. J Cataract Refract Surg. 2010; 36(11):1815–1821

[8] Karakelle M. The science behind the AcrySof IQ. Cataract & Refractive Surgery Today. 2018:4

[9] Shah RS, Khandelwal SS, Goshe JM, Haberman ID, Randleman JB. Comparative postoperative topography pattern recognition analysis using axial vs tangential curvature maps. J Cataract Refract Surg. 2020; 46(10):1368–1373

[10] Smith G, Cox MJ, Calver R, Garner LF. The spherical aberration of the crystalline lens of the human eye. Vision Res. 2001; 41(2):235–243

[11] Fisher B, Potvin R. Clinical outcomes with distance-dominant multifocal and monofocal intraocular lenses in post-LASIK cataract surgery planned using an intraoperative aberrometer. Clin Exp Ophthalmol. 2018; 46(6):630–636

[12] Chow SSW, Chan TCY, Ng ALK, Kwok AKH. Outcomes of presbyopia-correcting intraocular lenses after laser in situ keratomileusis. Int Ophthalmol. 2019; 39(5):1199–1204

[13] Chang JSM, Ng JCM, Chan VKC, Law AKP. Visual outcomes, quality of vision, and quality of life of diffractive multifocal intraocular lens implantation after myopic laser in situ keratomileusis: a prospective, observational case series. J Ophthalmol. 2017; 2017:6459504

[14] Vrijman V, van der Linden JW, van der Meulen IJE, Mourits MP, Lapid-Gortzak R. Multifocal intraocular lens implantation after previous corneal refractive laser surgery for myopia. J Cataract Refract Surg. 2017; 43(7):909–914

[15] Alfonso JF, Fernández-Vega L, Baamonde B, Madrid-Costa D, Montés-Micó R. Refractive lens exchange with spherical diffractive intraocular lens implantation after hyperopic laser in situ keratomileusis. J Cataract Refract Surg. 2009; 35 (10):1744–1750

[16] Alfonso JF, Fernández-Vega L, Baamonde B, Madrid-Costa D, Montés-Micó R. Visual quality after diffractive intraocular lens implantation in eyes with previous hyperopic laser in situ keratomileusis. J Cataract Refract Surg. 2011; 37(6):1090–1096

[17] Alfonso JF, Madrid-Costa D, Poo-López A, Montés-Micó R. Visual quality after diffractive intraocular lens implantation in eyes with previous myopic laser in situ keratomileusis. J Cataract Refract Surg. 2008; 34(11):1848–1854

[18] Fernández-Vega L, Madrid-Costa D, Alfonso JF, Montés-Micó R, Poo-López A. Optical and visual performance of diffractive intraocular lens implantation after myopic laser in situ keratomileusis. J Cataract Refract Surg. 2009; 35(5):825–832

[19] Vrijman V, van der Linden JW, van der Meulen IJE, Mourits MP, Lapid-Gortzak R. Multifocal intraocular lens implantation after previous hyperopic corneal refractive laser surgery. J Cataract Refract Surg. 2018; 44(4):466–470

[20] Ferreira TB, Pinheiro J, Zabala L, Ribeiro FJ. Comparative analysis of clinical outcomes of a monofocal and an extended-range-of-vision intraocular lens in eyes with previous myopic laser in situ keratomileusis. J Cataract Refract Surg. 2018; 44(2):149–155

[21] Cao D, Wang L, Koch DD. Outcome of toric intraocular lenses implanted in eyes with previous corneal refractive surgery. J Cataract Refract Surg. 2020; 46(4):534–539

[22] Kim KH, Seok KW, Kim WS. Multifocal intraocular lens results in correcting presbyopia in eyes after radial keratotomy. Eye Contact Lens. 2017; 43(6):e22–e25

[23] Gupta I, Oakey Z, Ahmed F, Ambati BK. Spectacle independence after cataract extraction in post-radial keratotomy patients using hybrid monovision with ReSTOR(®) multifocal and TECNIS(®) monofocal intraocular lenses. Case Rep Ophthalmol. 2014; 5(2):157–161

[24] Nuzzi R, Monteu F, Tridico F. Implantation of a multifocal toric intraocular lens after radial keratotomy and crosslinking with hyperopia and astigmatism residues: a case report. Case Rep Ophthalmol. 2017; 8(2):440–445

[25] Hjortdal JØ, Olsen H, Ehlers N. Prospective randomized study of corneal aberrations 1 year after radial keratotomy or photorefractive keratectomy. J Refract Surg. 2002; 18(1):23–29

[26] Applegate RA, Howland HC, Sharp RP, Cottingham AJ, Yee RW. Corneal aberrations and visual performance after radial keratotomy. J Refract Surg. 1998; 14(4):397–407

[27] Applegate RA, Hilmantel G, Howland HC. Corneal aberrations increase with the magnitude of radial keratotomy refractive correction. Optom Vis Sci. 1996; 73(9):585–589

[28] Waring GO IV. EDOF lenses in post-refractive eyes. Ocular Surgery News. 2018:19

[29] Mah F. "Blended" monofocal monovision. Our refractive IOL armamentarium, more choices than ever. The ASCRS Master Class in Refractive Cataract Surgery, 20/Happy in 20 webinar. August 29, 2020. https://ascrs.org/20happy/agenda/our-refractive-iol-armamentarium

[30] Agarwal S, Thornell E. Spectacle independence in patients with prior radial keratotomy following cataract surgery: A case series. Int Med Case Rep J. 2020; 13:53–60

[31] Koch DD. Post-refractive eyes. Hitting the refractive target. The ASCRS Master class in Refractive Cataract Surgery, 20/Happy in 20 webinar. August 15, 2020. https://ascrs.org/20happy/agenda/hitting-the-refractive-target

[32] Labuz G, Khoramnia R, Auffarth GU. Corneal Spherical Aberration in an Elderly Population with High Astigmatism. Paper presented at 2020 ASCRS virtual annual meeting. May 16–17, 2020

[33] Kohnen T, Mahmoud K, Bühren J. Comparison of corneal higher-order aberrations induced by myopic and hyperopic LASIK. Ophthalmology. 2005; 112(10):1692–1698

[34] Wang L, Koch DD. Anterior corneal optical aberrations induced by laser in situ keratomileusis for hyperopia. J Cataract Refract Surg. 2003; 29(9):1702–1708

[35] Oliver KM, O'Brart DP, Stephenson CG, et al. Anterior corneal optical aberrations induced by photorefractive keratectomy for hyperopia. J Refract Surg. 2001; 17(4):406–413

[36] Zheleznyak L, Sabesan R, Oh JS, MacRae S, Yoon G. Modified monovision with spherical aberration to improve presbyopic through-focus visual performance. Invest Ophthalmol Vis Sci. 2013; 54(5):3157–3165

[37] Worrall EB, Jung HC. Blended vision with multifocal intraocular lenses. EyeNet. 2019:31–32

[38] Sudhir RR, Dey A, Bhattacharrya S, Bahulayan A. AcrySof IQ PanOptix intraocular lens versus extended depth of focus intraocular lens and trifocal intraocular lens: a clinical overview. Asia Pac J Ophthalmol (Phila). 2019; 8(4):335–349

[39] Gundersen KG. Rotational stability and visual performance 3 months after bilateral implantation of a new toric extended range of vision intraocular lens. Clin Ophthalmol. 2018; 12:1269–1278

[40] Coassin M, Di Zazzo A, Antonini M, Gaudenzi D, Gallo Afflitto G, Kohnen T. Extended depth-of-focus intraocular lenses: power calculation and outcomes. J Cataract Refract Surg. 2020; 46(11):1554–1560

[41] Carones F. Residual astigmatism threshold and patient satisfaction with bifocal, trifocal and extended range of vision intraocular lenses (IOLs). Open J Ophthalmol. 2017; 7(1):1–7

[42] Cochener B. Tecnis Symfony intraocular lens with a "sweet spot" for tolerance to postoperative residual refractive errors. Open J Ophthalmol. 2017; 7(1):14–20

[43] Fram NR, Masket S, Wang L. Comparison of intraoperative aberrometry, OCT-based IOL formula, Haigis-L, and Masket formulae for IOL power calculation after laser vision correction. Ophthalmology. 2015; 122(6):1096–1101

[44] Canto AP, Chhadva P, Cabot F, et al. Comparison of IOL power calculation methods and intraoperative wavefront aberrometer in eyes after refractive surgery. J Refract Surg. 2013; 29(7):484–489

[45] Yesilirmak N, Palioura S, Culbertson W, Yoo SH, Donaldson K. Intraoperative wavefront aberrometry for toric intraocular lens placement in eyes with a history of refractive surgery. J Refract Surg. 2016; 32(1):69–70

[46] ESCRS Clinical Trends Survey 2019 Results. EuroTimes. Accessed March 30, 2021. https://www.eurotimes.org/wp-content/uploads/2020/11/Clinical-Survey-Results-2019-Supplement_PQ.pdf

[47] Curado SX, Hida WT, Vilar CMC, Ordones VL, Chaves MAP, Tzelikis PF. Intraoperative aberrometry versus preoperative biometry for IOL power selection after radial keratotomy: a prospective study. J Refract Surg. 2019; 35(10):656–661

[48] Passi SF, Thompson AC, Kim MJ, et al. Refractive outcomes using intraoperative aberrometry for highly myopic, highly hyperopic, and post-refractive eyes. Paper presented at: American Society of Cataract and Refractive Surgery Annual Meeting; San Diego, CA. May 4, 2019

[49] Turnbull AMJ, Crawford GJ, Barrett GD. Methods for intraocular lens power calculation in cataract surgery after radial keratotomy. Ophthalmology. 2020; 127(1):45–51

[50] Azar DT. In: Azar D, Gatinel D, Hoang-Xuan T, eds. Refractive Surgery. 2nd ed. Mosby; 2006:475–482

[51] Brinton JP, Durrie DS, Khodabakhsh J, Wiley WF, Raviv T. Cataracts after conductive keratoplasty. Cataract & Refractive Surgery Today. 2012:31–35. https://crstoday.com/articles/2012-sep/cataracts-after-conductive-keratoplasty/

[52] Pascucci S. Negative spherical aberration after CK is desirable: greater degree of negative spherical aberration seen with great number of spots applied. Ophthalmology Times 2004:73

[53] Vargas V, Alió JL, Barraquer RI, et al. Safety and visual outcomes following posterior chamber phakic intraocular lens bilensectomy. Eye Vis (Lond). 2020; 7:34

[54] Meier PG, Majo F, Othenin-Girard P, Bergin C, Guber I. Refractive outcomes and complications after combined copolymer phakic intraocular lens explantation and phacoemulsification with intraocular lens implantation. J Cataract Refract Surg. 2017; 43(6):748–753

[55] Pitault G, Leboeuf C, Leroux les Jardins S, Auclin F, Chong-Sit D, Baudouin C. Optical biometry of eyes corrected by phakic intraocular lenses. J Fr Ophtalmol. 2005; 28(10):1052–1057

[56] Yu A, Wang Q, Zhu S, Xue A, Su Y, Pan R. Effects of posterior chamber phakic intraocular lens on axial length measurements. Zhonghua Yan Ke Za Zhi. 2015; 51(3):206–209

[57] Saka N, Ohno-Matsui K, Shimada N, et al. Long-term changes in axial length in adult eyes with pathologic myopia. Am J Ophthalmol. 2010; 150(4):562–568.e1

[58] Eleftheriadis H, Amoros S, Bilbao R, Teijeiro MA. Spontaneous dislocation of a phakic refractive lens into the vitreous cavity. J Cataract Refract Surg. 2004; 30(9):2013–2016

[59] Stakheev AA. Intraocular lens calculation for cataract after previous radial keratotomy. Ophthalmic Physiol Opt. 2002; 22(4):289–295

[60] Lindstrom RL. Many points need to be considered in cataract patients with prior corneal refractive surgery. Ocular Surgery News 2019:3–5

[61] Baartman BJ, Karpuk K, Eichhorn B, et al. Extended depth of focus lens implantation after radial keratotomy. Clin Ophthalmol. 2019; 13:1401–1408

[62] Kohnen T, Suryakumar R. Extended depth-of-focus technology in intraocular lenses. J Cataract Refract Surg. 2020; 46(2):298–304

[63] Shajari M, Mackert MJ, Langer J, et al. Safety and efficacy of a small-aperture capsular bag-fixated intraocular lens in eyes with severe corneal irregularities. J Cataract Refract Surg. 2020; 46(2):188–192

[64] Dick HB, Piovella M, Vukich J, Vilupuru S, Lin L, Clinical Investigators. Prospective multicenter trial of a small-aperture intraocular lens in cataract surgery. J Cataract Refract Surg. 2017; 43(7):956–968

[65] Tannan A, Epstein R, Virasch V, Majmudar P, Faron C, Rubenstein J. Utility of intraoperative wavefront aberrometry in post-refractive cataract patients. Invest Ophthalmol Vis Sci. 2013; 54(15):3004

[66] Zhang F. Optiwave Refractive Analysis may not work well in patients with previous history of radial keratotomy. Am J Ophthalmol Case Rep. 2018; 10:163–164

20 Piggyback Intraocular Lenses

Fuxiang Zhang, Alan Sugar, and Lisa Brothers Arbisser

Abstract

This chapter focuses on three basic issues for piggyback intraocular lenses (IOLs): indications, lens selection, and power calculation. The advantages and disadvantages of current commonly used piggyback IOLs are reviewed. The commonly used calculation methods are discussed in detail. This chapter also briefly discusses topics such as the alternative options for piggyback IOLs, relative contraindications, and enhancement principles when a refractive surprise occurs. There is also a brief discussion to introduce a logical way to consider polypseudophakia in a situation when the single IOL power is not enough in situations like high hyperopia. There is a brand new proposal for design of a 360-degree sulcus piggyback IOL.

Keywords: piggyback lenses, piggyback IOL calculation, interlenticular film, IOL exchange, new design for sulcus IOLs

20.1 Introduction

Three major factors are important for piggyback intraocular lenses (IOLs): indications, lens selection, and power calculation. Surgical skill is usually not challenged to place a piggyback IOL because there is already a posterior intraocular lens (PCIOL) in place, although space is limited compared to primary IOL insertion. We use the term "primary piggyback IOL" to mean having both lenses placed at the same procedure (▶ Fig. 20.1) while "secondary piggyback IOL"

means having the piggyback lens placed from a later secondary procedure (▶ Fig. 20.2).

20.2 What Are the Alternatives and Relative Contraindications for Piggyback IOLs?

A post–cataract surgery refractive surprise is a leading indication for piggyback IOLs. Another usage of piggyback IOLs is for the management of negative dysphotopsia,[1] although reverse optic capture may be an easier method for management.[2] If one uses the latest generation IOL calculations formulas, the need for a piggyback IOL should be rare. With the increased popularity of intraoperative aberrometry and light adjustable lenses, piggybacking for this indication will become even rarer.

Not all refractive surprise cases need a piggyback IOL. If a patient can and is willing to use glasses or contact lenses, it is not necessary to consider surgery. Laser vision correction is another option, especially if the eye also has significant residual astigmatism to correct. If the surgery is recent and there is an intact posterior capsule, it is usually better to consider IOL exchange, especially if there is a significant spherical power discrepancy.

Be careful if a patient has a history of glaucoma or has a short eye or shallow anterior chamber depth due to the risk of pigmentary dispersion syndrome and UGH (uveitis glaucoma hyphema)

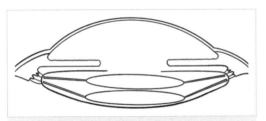

Fig. 20.1 Primary piggyback with both lenses placed at the same procedure. Here, both IOLs are in the bag. We should try to avoid both lenses in the bag due to increased risk of interlenticular fibrosis.

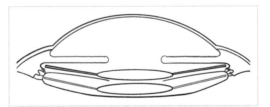

Fig. 20.2 Secondary piggyback intraocular lens (IOL) with the first lens in the bag from the initial surgery and the second lens in the sulcus from a later secondary surgery. This pattern can also be used for primary piggyback lens insertion, meaning the two IOLs are placed within a single surgery.

syndrome. We also avoid those patients who have a history of uveitis for two reasons: one is the tendency for recurrence and one is the increased likelihood of deposits on the lens surface as well as interlenticular film formation. A good slit lamp examination with gonioscopy is recommended, although we know the extra lens is not going to be placed as an anterior chamber lens. It is not advisable to consider a piggyback lens if there is already significant preexisting anterior chamber angle pathology, such as peripheral anterior synechiae, angle neovascularity, etc., because we may not be able to predict if the piggyback lens will negatively impact these angle comorbidities.

There is no FDA approved sulcus IOL in the United States, so whenever we place a lens in the sulcus it is "off-label." This should be mentioned to our patients and documented in the medical notes.

20.3 What Are the IOL Selection Options?

Most commonly used routine PCIOLs are made from acrylic materials. There is a unique issue of interlenticular opacification with piggyback IOLs. The literature has shown this problem when both lenses are made of the same materials, especially when both lenses are hydrophobic acrylic implanted in the capsular bag.[3] The adhesive semitacky texture of the hydrophobic acrylic material may have contributed to this complication due to retained or regenerative cortex and pearls. For that reason, we typically try to use a silicone optic IOL as the sulcus-placement secondary IOL. The interlenticular opaque membranes are usually not removable mechanically or manageable with an Nd:YAG laser; the IOLs usually need to be removed. It is still relatively rare, however, to have interlenticular opaque membranes with secondary piggyback lenses because the second lens is not in the bag, even when the two lenses are both hydrophobic acrylic. A single-piece acrylic IOL (such as commonly used SN60WF/SA60WF from Alcon, ZCBOO from J&J and enVista from B&L) is contraindicated as a sulcus-placed piggyback IOL.

- STAAR AQ 2010V and AQ 5010V were the go-to piggyback lenses for many cataract surgeons due to their large optic diameters (6.3 mm), silicone material, round edge design, 13.5 mm length for AQ 2010V and 14 mm length for AQ

5010V, and negative power availability for AQ 5010 (−4 to +4 D), but they are no longer available. This was a huge loss to the refractive cataract surgical armamentarium. Do manufacturers have any responsibility to have devices available for rare but essential use? Then who will compensate them financially? Should the AAO, ASCRS, industry, or government explore a potential solution for this kind of problem?

- Sensar three-piece AR40E (+2.00 to + 5.50 D) and AR40 M (−10.00 to +1.50 D) (Johnson & Johnson Vision). Both E and M lenses have 6.00-mm optics, 13.5-mm haptics, and OptiEdge (rounded front).[4] They are hydrophobic acrylic. The AR40 M lens has a meniscus optic. The AR40E and AR40e are biconvex. AcrySof Alcon lenses are probably the most commonly used primary PCIOL in the world. Since the introduction of the AcrySof IQ IOL, over 100 million of these lenses had been implanted worldwide by 2018.[5] Sensar lenses (J&J) and AcrySof are both hydrophobic acrylic materials, but they have different molecular structures.[6] Interlenticular opacification is still a potential risk; however, this typically happens when both lenses are in the bag. If the piggyback lens is placed in the sulcus, the interlenticular opacification rate can be decreased.[7] These are probably the reasons why Sensar lenses are commonly used as the piggyback lens of choice since the Starr AQ lenses were no longer available. We also like the Sensar AR40 lenses as our backup choice three-piece IOL when we are not able to use a single-piece IOL because of its rounded anterior edge.

- Z9002 (Johnson & Johnson Vision) has the advantage of being a silicone lens, 6-mm optic and 13-mm haptic length, and the OptiEdge design as a rounded front.[4] The diameter of 13 mm is a concern for risk of tilt and unstable status in the sulcus if it is placed asymmetrically. Pseudophakodonesis can cause mild chronic iritis or even UGH. It is not made in a low power low power (availability is +6.00 to +30.00 D) or negative power.

- LI 61AO SofPort (Bausch & Lomb) is a silicone lens with 6-mm optic and 13-mm overall diameter. It does have lower powers starting from 0.0 D, but it does not have negative powers. It is designed with both anterior and posterior square edges, a feature that can reduce posterior capsular opacification (PCO) compared to round-edged IOLs, but a concern as a piggyback IOL leading to chafing and chronic inflammation.[7,8,9]

- For surgeons outside the United States, the Sulcoflex IOL (Rayner) is an option. It is designed just for sulcus usage.[10] Interestingly, it is single piece and it is hydrophilic acrylic, but a cadaver eye experiment[10] suggested its suitability as a sulcus piggyback IOL. The optic diameter is 6.5 mm with an overall diameter of 14.0 mm with a round edge and 10-degree posterior angulation. The Sulcoflex family of supplementary IOLs has included monofocal, toric, multifocal, and multifocal toric versions.[11] Because the supplementary IOL is reversible and exchangeable, it is also an adaptive option. Should a patient develop some pathology in the future, such as diabetic retinopathy or macular degeneration, a multifocal Sulcoflex IOL can be easily removed, returning the patient to monofocal vision with better contrast.

- The pinhole intraocular lenses (XtraFocus, Morcher GmbH, Germany) have two versions, the old tripod Model 93E and the newer open-loop Model 93 L.[12] They have no power (plano) for sulcus use.[13] Both lenses were made of a black hydrophobic acrylic material, had a concave-convex design, as well as a posterior optic-haptic angulation. The newer model (93L) has an open-loop design, an overall diameter of 14.0 mm, a 6.0-mm occlusive portion with a 1.3-mm central opening, an optic-haptic angulation of 14 degrees, and a thinner occlusive portion.[13] Small aperture piggyback lenses can be especially good for those who have had corneal refractive surgeries, significant corneal astigmatism, keratoconus, s/p corneal transplant, etc. There are some concerns about their centration and tilt based on a human pseudophakic cadaver study where it was placed in the ciliary sulcus.[13] It is not available in the United States. One study noted that there was about a 9% rate of need to recenter the decentered sulcus-placed XtraFocus lenses with a mean postoperative follow-up 2.3 months.[14]

The XtraFocus was designed for ciliary sulcus use, but a recent study in Brazil ($n = 60$ eyes: keratoconus 38, s/p post-PKP 12, s/p RK 8 and others 2) with a mean follow-up of 16 months demonstrated the following encouraging facts[14]:

- All 60 Xtrafocus intraocular pinhole (IOPH) lenses were implanted as primary piggyback IOLs, meaning the IOPH was implanted in the bag at the same surgery following the main IOL. (IC-8 pinhole lens could be a better option in this regard. See Chapter 14.)

- All the primary IOLs had the same hydrophobic acrylic material although from different companies, such as Alcon, Johnson & Johnson, Bausch & Lomb, etc. The XtraFocus IOPH is also hydrophobic acrylic.

- During this mean 16-month postoperative period, there was no case with noticeable interlenticular fibrosis. The authors hypothesized that the lack of interlenticular opacification was due to the concave-convex design to avoid direct contact with the primary in-the-bag IOL. Also, the pinhole could let aqueous flow through the pinhole and between the space of the two lenses, which could further inhibit lens epithelial cell proliferation.

- As expected for a primary in the bag piggyback, much better centration was observed, compared to decentration, a common concern for sulcus-placed piggyback IOLs. Decentration for the pinhole piggyback can result in significant vision issues due to the nature of the small aperture.

- Both uncorrected distance vision and corrected distance vision were dramatically improved compared to preoperative vision: improved from logMAR 1.34 ± 0.338 and 0.57 ± 0.145 preoperatively to 0.14 ± 0.012 ($p < .001$) and 0.12 ± 0.008 ($p = .001$) at 1 year postoperatively, respectively.

- It can also be used as a secondary piggyback IOL in the ciliary sulcus.

- The nature of the XtraFocus IOPH can allow transmittance of infrared light through it, so future ND:YAG laser for posterior capsular opacification can be performed and posterior segment pathologies can be examined.

- It can also be used as the sole implant in the bag.

- The major downside of this lens is that Argon laser light cannot penetrate it and if there is a need for retinal surgery, the IOPH must be explanted first. Another downside of this lens is the frequent complaint of "darkness" from bilateral XtraFocus patients[15] (▶ Fig. 20.3).

20.4 A Proposal for Design of a 360-degree Sulcus Piggyback IOL

A cataract surgeon typically needs to suture a PCIOL onto the iris or in the sclera or choose an anterior chamber intraocular lens (ACIOL) when there is no capsular bag support. When suturing of a PCIOL is necessary, it is time-consuming, with challenging techniques and other risks, such as intraoperative bleeding. Many surgeons are reluctant to use these suturing techniques. An ACIOL is widely believed to have potential long-term risk to the cornea and is not the first choice in many situations. We are considering a new design of a 360-degree Sulcus PCIOL (▸ Fig. 20.4, ▸ Fig. 20.5, ▸ Fig. 20.6, and ▸ Fig. 20.7). It can be used as a PCIOL placed in the sulcus with 360-degree ciliary sulcus support. We also consider the optic shape design, biconvex versus biconcave front or back so

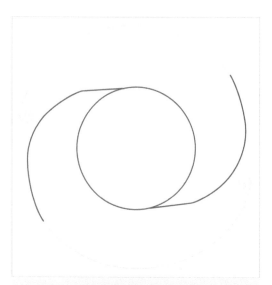

Fig. 20.3 XtraFocus pinhole piggyback intraocular lens. Used with permission from Morcher.

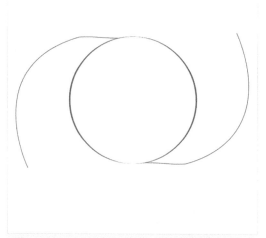

Fig. 20.4 Three-piece 360 sulcus PCIOL piggyback intraocular lens (IOL).

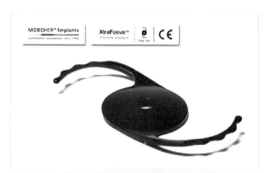

Fig. 20.5 Three-piece 360 sulcus PCIOL piggyback intraocular lens (IOL) with an option of eyelet for scleral fixation when needed.

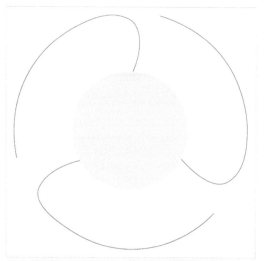

Fig. 20.6 Four-piece 360 sulcus PCIOL piggyback intraocular lens (IOL) with advantage of better stability and disadvantage of insertion.

that the two lens optics do not "kiss." The size of the lens can be customized to fit **any** given eye. Accurate measurement of ciliary sulcus diameter by optical coherence tomography (OCT) imaging technology should not be a remote practice. Those of us who have done femtosecond laser-assisted cataract surgery know how clearly we can see intraocular structures with the OCT technique. To precisely place this 360-degree lens in the sulcus is possible. That should be easier than suturing a PCIOL onto the iris or in the sclera. Industrial companies are welcome to discuss details by email fzhang1@hfhs.org (▶ Fig. 20.4, ▶ Fig. 20.5, ▶ Fig. 20.6, ▶ Fig. 20.7, ▶ Fig. 20.8, and ▶ Fig. 20.9).

20.5 How Do We Determine Piggyback IOL Power?

The calculation for a piggyback IOL is relatively simple and straightforward in most situations. Usually, we only need to know the refractive surprise at the spectacle plane and the required refractive target. Usually, we do not need to know the power of the primary IOL. The following are some commonly used methods.

- An easy but only approximate method: Every 0.5 D change in IOL power will give 0.35 D at the spectacle plane.

- Holladay/Nichamin Nomogram (Personal communication with and courtesy of Dr. Nichamin):
  - Overpowered pseudophake (Myope) 1:1 ratio. If Rx is −2.0D SE, then give −2.0 D IOL if the target is plano.
  - Underpowered pseudophake (Hyperope) 1:1.5 ratio. If Rx is +2.0 D, then give 2 × 1.5 = 3.0 D IOL to aim for plano.
- Gills Nomogram is based on axial length, more detailed than the above two methods.[17]
  - Residual hyperopia. Short eye (<22 mm), power = (1.5 × SE) + 1. Average eye (22–25 mm), power = (1.4 × SE) + 1. Long eye (>25 mm), power = (1.3 × SE) + 1.
  - Residual myopia. Short eye (<22 mm), power = (1.5 × SE) − 1.

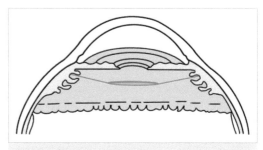

Fig. 20.8 Illustration of 360 sulcus PCIOL within the eye without any capsular support.

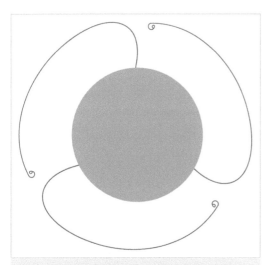

Fig. 20.7 Four-piece 360 sulcus PCIOL piggyback intraocular lens with an option of eyelets for scleral fixation when needed.

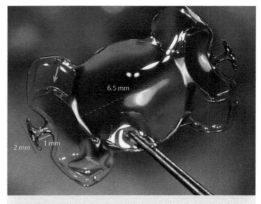

Fig. 20.9 The Carlevale sutureless sulcus PCIOL. Used from Mularoni et al,[16] with permission from Wolters Kluwer Health, Inc.

Average eye (22–25 mm), power = (1.4 × SE) – 1. Long eye (>25 mm), power = (1.3 × SE) – 1.

- Abulafia-Hill calculation.[18]
  - Hyperopic refractive error with SE <+7.00 D and Ks in a normal range: The piggyback IOL power = SE × 1.50 will give a plano outcome at the spectacle plane.
  - Myopic refractive error with SE <−7.00 D and Ks in a normal range: The piggyback IOL power = SE × 1.3 will give a plano outcome at spectacle plane.
- Barrett Rx formula at www.apacrs.org
  - This formula is more versatile with more parameters, hyperopic versus myopic refractive errors, 7.00 D or greater, unusual Ks, or if the refractive target is not plano. The Barrett Rx formula can also be used for IOL exchange and toric IOL rotation calculations.

20.6 How Do We Determine the IOL Power in a Very High Hyperope When a Single IOL Power Is Not Enough?

This is the most compelling indication for piggyback IOLs or polypseudophakia. First, we need to find out what total power is needed if a single in-the-bag lens were to be used. Then determine how to split the power between these two lenses. Logically, we want to have a higher power IOL in the bag and leave the rest to the sulcus piggyback lens. Because a ciliary sulcus-placed lens is more anteriorly located (closer to the principal plane of the cornea), an IOL at the level of the ciliary sulcus will have a greater effective power than if were located at the level of the capsular bag. For this reason, the residual IOL power originally calculated for placement in the capsular bag will need to be adjusted. If we do not make this adjustment, the final outcome can be widely off target. The amount of adjustment will depend on the power of the piggyback IOL. The best resource with a sample case and step-by-step instructions is from Warren Hill's instruction at his website https://www.doctor-hill.com/iol-main/polypseudophakia_calculations.html.[19]

The good news is that we can get very high power, up to 60 D, IOLs from HumanOptics (Erlangen, Germany).[20] For those very short eyes, choosing a single IOL is preferred to a piggyback

to avoid associated side effects discussed in this chapter. HumanOptics has −20.0 to +60.0 D in 1.0 D steps, +10.0 to +30.0 D in 0.5 D steps for the monofocal version, both clear and yellow IOLs. Toric IOLs also have the same extended diopter range. They also have multifocal, trifocal, and toric IOLs. Three-piece monofocal IOLs are also available (+10.0 D to +30.0 D only). The inconvenience is the fact that they are not FDA approved. They can be only imported under compassionate use via the FDA Access program if applicable.

20.7 Is White-to-White Measurement Accurately Correlated with the Ciliary Sulcus Diameter?

An early cadaver study[21] by Werner and Apple and their associates demonstrated that sulcus size is not proportional to white to white. A positive correlation was found between the white-to-white measurements and the anterior chamber diameter in the 10 eyes studied at the 6 o'clock to 12 o'clock meridian but not at the 3 o'clock to 9 o'clock meridian. The latter is the meridian frequently used by surgeons to perform white-to-white measurements and thus choose the overall size of the intraocular lens to be implanted. No correlation was found between the white-to-white measurements and the ciliary sulcus diameter in these two meridians. However, modern anterior segment OCT can accurately measure ocular structures. This is likely the future for choosing and placement of piggyback IOLs.

20.8 What Are our Recommended Enhancement Principles When You Have a Refractive Surprise?

- Do not rush to make the piggyback use decision. In general, wait a few weeks until the refractive status is more stabilized, unless there is a case of an obviously wrong IOL power or toric misalignment or rotation. This is especially important for patients with a history of radial keratotomy. Two to three months are needed to let the cornea return to a stable condition in these patients.

- Make sure there is no other major ocular pathology contributing to unhappiness, such as dry eye, epiretinal membrane, etc.
- If not sure, consider a trial of glasses or contact lenses first.
- Cylinder problem:
  - If the spherical equivalent is close to plano, less than ±0.50 D and the residual astigmatism is 1 D or less, LRI may be the first thing to consider, since this is not going to affect the spherical equivalent.
  - If the cylinder is over 1 D, laser vision correction will be better than an LRI.
- Sphere problem:
  - Piggyback.
  - IOL exchange.
  - Laser vision correction (LVC) can be very good for small degrees of error.
    - Photorefractive keratectomy (PRK).
    - Laser in situ keratomileusis (LASIK). These work better for myopic enhancement, which is more predictable and more forgiving than hyperopic enhancement. Avoid in eyes with loose epithelium and/or a thin cornea.
- If there are both cylindrical and spherical equivalent errors with a toric IOL, this is best managed by laser vision correction if the error is small (<1 D) and there is a myopic SE. If there is a hyperopic SE or large degree of myopic SE, IOL exchange and rotation to the ideal axis is preferred.

References

[1] Masket S, Fram NR, Cho A, Park I, Pham D. Surgical management of negative dysphotopsia. J Cataract Refract Surg. 2018; 44(1):6–16

[2] Masket S, Fram NR. Pseudophakic dysphotopsia: review of incidence, cause, and treatment of positive and negative dysphotopsia. Ophthalmology. 2020:S0161–6420(20) 30787–9

[3] Werner L, Mamalis N, Stevens S, Hunter B, Chew JJ, Vargas LG. Interlenticular opacification: dual-optic versus piggyback intraocular lenses. J Cataract Refract Surg. 2006; 32 (4):655–661

[4] Intraocular lenses, OVDs & accessories. Product guide. Johnson & Johnson Vision; 2017

[5] Karakelle M. The science behind the AcrySof IQ. Cataract & Refractive Surgery Today. Published May 2018. Accessed April 8, 2021. https://crstoday.com/articles/the-blueprint-for-exceptional-image-quality/the-science-behind-the-acrysof-iq-iol/#:~:text=The%20AcrySof%20IQ%20IOL%20(Alcon,lens%20to%20patients%20with%20cataracts.

&text=The%20design%20of%20the%20AcrySof,versus%20the%20prior%20spherical%20control

[6] Findl O. Intraocular lens materials and design. In: Colvard M, ed. Achieving excellence in cataract surgery: a step-by-step approach. Self-published; 2009

[7] Chang WH, Werner L, Fry LL, Johnson JT, Kamae K, Mamalis N. Pigmentary dispersion syndrome with a secondary piggyback 3-piece hydrophobic acrylic lens. Case report with clinicopathological correlation. J Cataract Refract Surg. 2007; 33(6):1106–1109

[8] Kirk KR, Werner L, Jaber R, Strenk S, Strenk L, Mamalis N. Pathologic assessment of complications with asymmetric or sulcus fixation of square-edged hydrophobic acrylic intraocular lenses. Ophthalmology. 2012; 119(5):907–913

[9] Ollerton A, Werner L, Strenk S, et al. Pathologic comparison of asymmetric or sulcus fixation of 3-piece intraocular lenses with square versus round anterior optic edges. Ophthalmology. 2013; 120(8):1580–1587

[10] McIntyre JS, Werner L, Fuller SR, Kavoussi SC, Hill M, Mamalis N. Assessment of a single-piece hydrophilic acrylic IOL for piggyback sulcus fixation in pseudophakic cadaver eyes. J Cataract Refract Surg. 2012; 38(1):155–162

[11] Amon M. Early results from the new Sulcoflex trifocal. EuroTimes. 2019 suppl:2–3

[12] Reiter N, Werner L, Guan J, et al. Assessment of a new hydrophilic acrylic supplementary IOL for sulcus fixation in pseudophakic cadaver eyes. Eye (Lond). 2017; 31(5):802–809

[13] Tsaousis KT, Werner L, Trindade CLC, Guan J, Li J, Reiter N. Assessment of a novel pinhole supplementary implant for sulcus fixation in pseudophakic cadaver eyes. Eye (Lond). 2018; 32(3):637–645

[14] Trindade BLC, Trindade FC, Werner L, Trindade CLC. Long-term safety of in-the-bag implantation of a supplementary intraocular pinhole. J Cataract Refract Surg. 2020; 46(6): 888–892

[15] Trindade BLC, Trindade FC, Trindade CLC. Bilateral implantation of a supplementary intraocular pinhole. [Published online ahead of print, 2020 Nov 12]. J Cataract Refract Surg. 2021; 47(5):627–633

[16] Mularoni A, Imburgia A, Forlini M, Rania L, Possati GL. In vivo evaluation of a 1-piece foldable sutureless intrascleral fixation intraocular lens using ultrasound biomicroscopy and anterior segment OCT. J Cataract Refract Surg. 2021; 47 (3):316–322

[17] Holladay JT, Gills JP, Grabow H. Piggyback intraocular lenses. Ann Ophthalmol. 1998; 30(4):203–206

[18] Abulafia A, Hill WE. Enhancement with piggyback or intraocular lens exchanges. In: Hovanesian JA, ed. Refractive cataract surgery. 2nd ed. Slack. 2017:225–232

[19] Piggyback IOL intraocular lens power calculations primary polypseudophakia eye cataract surgery eyes. doctor-hill.com IOL Power Calculations. Accessed April 15, 2021. https://www.doctor-hill.com/iol-main/polypseudophakia_-calculations.html

[20] Monofocal platform. HumanOptics. Accessed June 17, 2021. https://www.humanoptics.com/en/physicians/intraocular-lenses/monofocal-1p-aspira/

[21] Werner L, Izak AM, Pandey SK, Apple DJ, Trivedi RH, Schmidbauer JM. Correlation between different measurements within the eye relative to phakic intraocular lens implantation. J Cataract Refract Surg. 2004; 30(9):1982–1988

21 Refractive Lens Exchange

Fuxiang Zhang, Alan Sugar, and Lisa Brothers Arbisser

Abstract

This book is about refractive cataract surgery for beginners, but most beginners will not consider refractive lens exchange (RLE) due to the high cost for the patient, the risk-benefit ratio given vision still correctable to 20/20 with glasses, and significantly higher patient expectations. Then why do we still include this chapter? As technology advances with more and more new premium intraocular lenses (IOLs), the fear of loss of accommodation for prospective younger patients undergoing RLE has drastically reduced as good functional vision across all distances can be achieved. A refractive cataract surgeon will sooner or later encounter younger patients who want RLE. Patients with high degrees of myopia, hyperopia, and astigmatism may not always be the best candidates for keratorefractive surgery. The added advantage of not developing a cataract in the future and having to undergo a second surgical procedure makes RLE an attractive alternative. For those patients who are intent on less dependence on glasses and who seek laser-assisted in situ keratomileusis (LASIK) but are well into the presbyopic age range with a dysfunctional lens, RLE is an alternative without the vagaries of soon having to choose an IOL in the presence of a surgically altered cornea. This chapter discusses some of the fundamental principles and challenges of RLE. We will also discuss the major differences between RLE and regular cataract surgery before, during, and after surgery. Main indications and contraindications will be reviewed. There are several surgical modalities for RLE; the pros and cons of monofocal IOLs versus multifocal diffractive optic IOLs will be considered.

Keywords: refractive lens exchange, clear lens exchange, refractive cataract surgery, pseudophakic monovision, Symfony IOL, EDOF, multifocal IOLs, trifocal IOLs, PanOptix

21.1 Introduction

Refractive lens exchange (RLE), in this case refractive lens extraction, was performed in Europe as early as the 19th century. Over 3,000 patients with high myopia underwent surgery in Europe before the 20th century.[1] At the beginning of the 20th century, it was realized that retinal detachment, at the time untreatable, occurred as a late complication in many cases. As a consequence, RLE was gradually abandoned in the following decades.[1]

Over half of Americans over the age of 40 have ametropia of sufficient magnitude to require refractive correction.[2] About 36 million people in the United States used contact lenses in 2005.[3] RLE, also called clear lens exchange, seems to have become more popular with the advancements in new technologies, including intraocular lenses (IOLs), IOL formulas, preoperative biometry and other measurements, intraoperative devices, efficacy of off-label intracameral antibiotics, etc.

Laser vision correction is the mainstay for the surgical management of refractive error for the young generations. When presbyopia (now often defined as early dysfunctional lens syndrome) is present in addition to significant refractive error, RLE is another alternative. For the presbyopia-aged population, especially if one has already started to have early cataracts, RLE may be better than laser-assisted in situ keratomileusis (LASIK), small incision lenticule extraction (SMILE), corneal inlays, phakic IOL, and other options, since it offers a single one-stop-shopping surgery. The cornea will remain relatively unchanged in contour with no significant extra aberrations, although some patients may have significant against-the-rule (ATR) astigmatism drift down the road. Another advantage of RLE is that it simultaneously eliminates the need for cataract surgery in the future. The goal of RLE is to eliminate or significantly decrease the need for using contact lenses and glasses for the remainder of the patient's postoperative life.

A survey was presented at the 2020 virtual ASCRS meeting ($n = 204$) regarding the prevalence of RLE for presbyopia among ophthalmologists and to assess the willingness of these ophthalmologists to recommend RLE to immediate family members.[4] Eighty-nine percent (89%) of surveyed surgeons were currently performing RLE. The survey showed that 23% of responders would undergo lens replacement for presbyopia correction in the absence of a cataract; 32% reported that they have recommended RLE to immediate family members; and 19% reported immediate family members have had RLE.

Based on an RLE cohort from a private eye clinic ($n = 675$) and a cataract cohort from the outcomes of the Swedish National Cataract Register,[5] RLE patients were younger (52.1 ± 7.7 vs. 73.8 ± 9.3 years) with a smaller percentage of women (45.28% vs. 60.46%; $p < 0.001$, fewer females than males) and were more often myopic than the cataract patients. Our limited experience suggests, however, more females than males are exploring RLE.

21.2 Why Should a Beginner Need to Know RLE?

Often RLE is not suitable for early beginners due to the nature of self-payment with high cost (an average of cost up to about $4,000–4,500/eye[6,7]) and higher expectations in this relatively young active patient population. Once you engage in refractive cataract surgery and if you are doing well with a good reputation, you will have patients coming to you for RLE. This chapter is to discuss some of the basic but fundamentally important principles to consider when an RLE candidate walks into your office.

21.3 What Are the Indications for Refractive Lens Exchange?

- Presbyopia, with normal ocular anatomy and clear lens or early cataract, but demanding independence from presbyopic glasses, with or without high refractive errors, such as myopia or hyperopia. Generally speaking, corneal refractive surgery cannot correct presbyopia unless monovision is offered, but not everyone desires or is a good candidate for monovision. The ideal candidates of RLE are hyperopic, presbyopic patients, contact lens intolerant, aged 50 to 55, with or without astigmatism, and with mild incipient cataracts. If we do keratorefractive surgery on these patients, they will be happy immediately, but the happiness may not last long as the cataract gets cloudier. They often, as we have witnessed, blame the corneal refractive surgery.

- High refractive errors with clear lens and abnormal ocular anatomy, in patients who are not good candidates for keratorefractive surgery or phakic IOL implantation, with or without presbyopia. Patients with higher degrees of myopia, hyperopia, and astigmatism are not the best candidates for keratorefractive procedures. RLE is a viable option in younger patients where the anterior chamber is too shallow and excludes the use of a phakic IOL in high hyperopia individuals.[8] If a myopic patient is to be considered for RLE, the presence of a spontaneous complete posterior vitreous detachment makes them lower risk candidates as this may reduce the otherwise increased risk of retinal detachment. As technology advances with more and more types of premium IOLs, the fear of loss of accommodation for younger populations undergoing RLE has drastically reduced and good functional vision across all distances can be achieved. The added advantage of not developing a cataract in their future and having to undergo a second surgical procedure makes RLE a very attractive alternative.[9]

- The dysfunctional lens syndrome is another way to view the dynamic and progressive pathophysiology of lens dysfunction and RLE. Dysfunctional lens syndrome is described in three stages[8,10]:
  - A dynamic process of loss of accommodation beginning roughly at age 40.
  - Increase in light scatter and decrease in contrast sensitivity from age 50.
  - Early opacification of the crystalline lens at 65 years or older.

Based on the concept of dysfunctional lens syndrome, there is an objective way of evaluating candidates for RLE.[8] Devices, such as iTrace (Tracey Technologies, Houston, TX), can be used to generate an objective parameter termed dysfunctional lens index (DLI) with the measurement of internal higher order aberrations, contrast sensitivity, and dynamic pupil size. A poor DLI score is represented by a blurred and distorted "E" which becomes well defined and clear as the DLI score improves. Poor DLI is an indicator of dysfunctional lenses. RLE in such cases may help in improving symptoms.[8] There are patients who complain of reduced visual quality despite having normal visual acuity quantitatively, and a bright-light acuity test (BAT) may not necessarily confirm much decrease in vision per se; but these patients really complain of not seeing well. Possible etiologies include increased internal higher order aberrations and decreased contrast sensitivity with greater light scatter due to a dysfunctional lens.

When we make a decision to do cataract surgery for our usual patients, we typically follow the vision criteria set by each State. Sometimes, however, we still agree to do the cataract surgery on those patients whose Snellen visual acuity does not meet such criteria, even with the BAT test scores. The legitimate reasons are that we believe visual acuity is not the only factor affecting visual function and that we do expect the surgery will significantly improve quality of life for these patients.

21.4 What Are Contraindications and Relative Contraindications?

The following is the list of contraindications and relative contraindications based on the 2017 Preferred Practice Pattern (PPP) from the American Academy of Ophthalmology for refractive lens exchange.[11]

Contraindications:
- Unstable refraction.
- Corneal endothelial disease, including Fuchs dystrophy.
- Uncontrolled glaucoma.
- Uncontrolled external disease.
- Active or recently active uveitis, or uveitis that requires ongoing treatment or is recurrent in nature.
- Uncontrolled autoimmune or other immune-mediated disease.
- Unrealistic patient expectations.

Relative contraindications[11]:
- Significant eyelid, tear film, or ocular surface abnormalities related to keratoconjunctivitis sicca, blepharoconjunctivitis, acne rosacea, conjunctival cicatrization, corneal exposure, neurotrophic keratitis, or other corneal abnormalities.
- Inflammation of the anterior segment.
- Presence of a filtering bleb.
- Pseudoexfoliation.

- Functional monocularity.
- History of uveitis.
- Autoimmune or other immune-mediated disease.
- Diabetes mellitus.
- Pregnancy or lactation.

Our advice in terms of RLE contraindications/relative contraindications for beginners is that surgeons should not consider a patient for RLE if:
- Unable to expect a good quality of vision, such as central corneal haze, epiretinal membrane.
- Good vison is not maintainable, such as active diabetic retinopathy.
- Unable to provide spectacle freedom to meet the patient's desired activities, such as s/p radial keratotomy with significant irregular astigmatism/spherical aberration/coma.
- Of note, the PPP did not include younger patients (40 years old and younger) in the above list; but we believe another surgical modality, such as a keratorefractive procedure, might be preferred to RLE for these patients to preserve their accommodation unless their cornea or ocular anatomy is not suitable for corneal refractive surgery.
- High myopes without a posterior vitreous detachment (PVD) who might be better served by phakic lenses.

21.5 Is RLE FDA Approved? Will Everyone Need Cataract Surgery if S/he Lives to the Average Lifespan in the United States?

The FDA has not approved use of pseudophakic IOLs for the sole purpose of correcting refractive error in the absence of visually significant cataract.[11,12] This should be explained to the patient and documented in the medical record.

Everyone will develop a cataract if they live long enough, but based on 2010 data from the National Eye Institute, only about 30% to 40% of white Americans will actually require cataract surgery by 70 years of age.[13] By age 75, half of white Americans have a cataract when defined as "A cataract is a clouding of the lens in the eye that affects vision" (▶ Fig. 21.1). By age 80, 70 percent

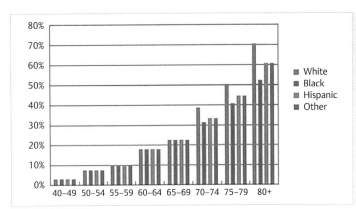

Fig. 21.1 2010 data on US prevalence rates for cataract by age and race.[13] Courtesy of National Eye Institute, National Institutes of Health (NEI/NIH).

of whites have cataract compared with 53 percent of blacks and 61 percent of Hispanic Americans.[13] The average lifespan of Americans is 78.7 years, based on 2018 CDC data.[14] For younger patients, postoperative retinal detachment and cystoid macular edema risks are also higher than for older patients because the prevalence of posterior vitreous detachment in older population is much higher.[15]

21.6 What Percentage of Presbyopic Patients Are RLE versus Conventional Cataract Cases?

Based on the 2019 ASCRS clinical survey, 4% of cataract surgeries are RLE[16] (▶ Fig. 21.2). It seems to be higher in Europe than in the United States (▶ Fig. 21.3).

21.7 What Are the Biggest Challenges for RLE?

From a patient's perspective, the biggest challenge for RLE may be the cost. For surgeons, we believe it is how to make our patients happy and cause no complications. For pseudophakic monovision, we typically do not use a preoperative contact lens trial for the average cataract patient, but for RLE, we recommend a preoperative contact lens trial unless these patients have had a history of contact lens or corneal laser-induced monovision. If the patient chooses to have a diffractive lens-based procedure, including multifocal IOLs (MFIOLs), trifocal IOLs, or extended depth-of-focus (EDOF) lenses, they need to have a thorough preoperative understanding and explanation. Pictures, or, even better, videos, to show candidates how nighttime dysphotopsia looks are highly recommended; simple verbal explanation is usually not sufficient. Remember that the cataract patient, having gradually lost vision, will be amazed by the improvement, while the clear lens patient is comparing postoperatively to the quality of vision they were enjoying while spectacle or contact lens corrected. Missing refractive targets can be managed with other surgical modalities, but subjective complaints are harder to manage. Neuroadaptation does not always develop and the patient can remain unhappy for the rest of their life. The key preoperative point for RLE is not to explain how much they can see without any spectacles or contact lenses, but how much relevant downside they may expect to have for the rest of their lives.

21.8 What Are the Major Differences between Refractive Lens Exchange and Regular Cataract Surgery?

21.8.1 Preoperatively

You really need to know your patient very well, his/her job, hobbies, needs and desires, etc. As we explained earlier, having the patient really

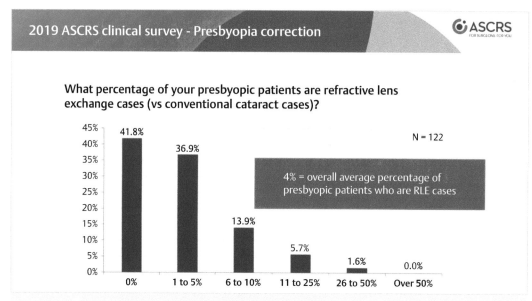

Fig. 21.2 2019 ASCRS clinical survey.[16] Used with permission from ASCRS.

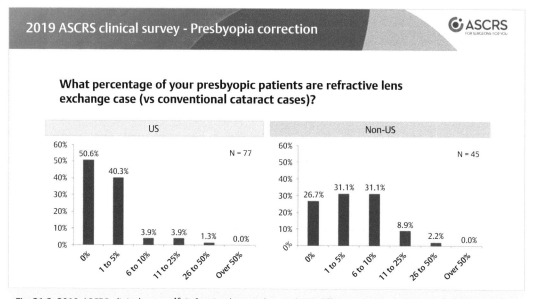

Fig. 21.3 2019 ASCRS clinical survey.[16] Refractive lens exchange (RLE) difference between Europe and the United States. Used with permission from ASCRS.

understand the disadvantages related to a specific IOL is the most important part of the consultation. If you are to consider MFIOL, EDOF, or trifocal, you should not miss the aberration profile, pupil size, angle alpha, and angle kappa evaluations.

Considering the generally younger age of this group of patients, it is reasonable to avoid IOLs prone to development of glistenings, although, to our knowledge, there is, as of yet, no conclusion that they impact visual acuity. That we cannot definitely confirm the inferiority with current technology does not mean it does not exist. When there are hundreds or thousands of imperfect glistening dots in the optic a few years after surgery, it should be a concern. There are ample studies suggesting the impact of glistenings on visual quality, such as straylight,[17] light scatter,[18] spherical aberration, and contrast sensitivity.[19]

Very highly myopic patients should have a retinal examination by a retina specialist prior to the procedure to document and manage any possible predisposing factors for retinal detachment and for documentation of the status of PVD.

21.8.2 Intraoperatively

From the phacoemulsification perspective, RLE is usually easier than most routine cases, because this is a younger group and sometimes irrigation/aspiration will be enough to aspirate the soft crystalline lens without the need for phacoemulsification. Hydrodelineation can be most beneficial in dysfunctional lenses to facilitate easy removal of the slightly denser endonucleus.

In long highly myopic eyes, anterior chamber depth and fluctuation can be a challenge. Sudden deepening of the anterior chamber should be avoided by gentle insertion of the phaco needle in foot position zero in an ophthalmic viscosurgical devices (OVD) controlled chamber with low bottle height, and upward tenting of the pupillary rim by a second instrument upon initial irrigation (▶ Video 21.1). Volumetric changes in the vitreous occurring intraoperatively due to changes in intraocular pressure (IOP), which may result in traction or vitreous degeneration, are believed to be the iatrogenic etiology of high rate of retinal detachment.[8]

There are some challenges associated with operating on short eyes in high hyperopia, such as shallow anterior chamber, vulnerability for uveal effusion, and expulsive choroidal hemorrhage. Increasing bottle height to oppose positive

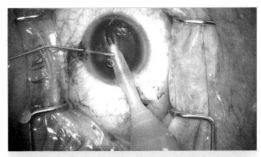

Fig. 21.4 Adding dispersive OVD to coat the back side of cornea before one starts the "quadrant removal" phaco section.

vitreous pressure and good incisional integrity to minimalize leaking can be beneficial. Never allowing the chamber to shallow in these patients can be very beneficial (see Chapter 23, "Surgical Pearls"). Dilating these patients with intracameral epinephrine-lidocaine on the table may also have merits, rather than risking preop dilation that can cause them to come to the surgery a relative pupillary block. Also, these patients benefit hugely from bolus IV push mannitol ¼ g/kg 20 minutes prior to surgery, as well as the use of Healon GV as the cohesive part of the Arshinoff OVD soft shell instead of Provisc or Healon. A small paracentesis incision (about 0.5 mm preferred) is very important to avoid overleaking which can make the anterior chamber shallower. Try to avoid overhydrodissection which can also make the anterior chamber shallower. Effectively coating the endothelium of the cornea just prior to quadrant nuclear removal is especially important in these short eyes. A pearl we recommend is to inject the coating dispersive OVD over the phaco needle to facilitate creating a layer of OVD to cover the central cornea (▶ Fig. 21.4; ▶ Video 21.2).

21.8.3 Postoperatively

Close follow-up is necessary, especially for those patients who are not perfectly happy (see Chapter 22). If a patient receives a piggyback IOL for high hyperopia, diligent visits are warranted to make sure there is no interlenticular opacification and iris chafing. For high myopia patients, retinal detachment rate can be as high as 8%[11] to 10%.[20] A large review noted that the higher the level of myopia, the higher the incidence of rhegmatogenous

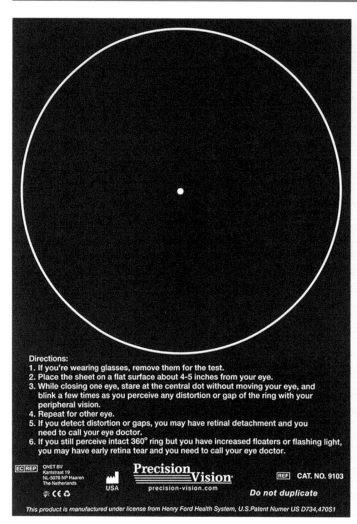

Fig. 21.5 Zhang Ring Test for retinal detachment.

Directions:
1. If you're wearing glasses, remove them for the test.
2. Place the sheet on a flat surface about 4-5 inches from your eye.
3. While closing one eye, stare at the central dot without moving your eye, and blink a few times as you perceive any distortion or gap of the ring with your peripheral vision.
4. Repeat for other eye.
5. If you detect distortion or gaps, you may have retinal detachment and you need to call your eye doctor.
6. If you still perceive intact 360° ring but you have increased floaters or flashing light, you may have early retina tear and you need to call your eye doctor.

EC REP ONET BV
Kantstraat 19
NL-5076 NP Haaren
The Netherlands

Precision═══**Vision**
precision-vision.com

USA

REF CAT. NO. 9103

Do not duplicate

This product is manufactured under license from Henry Ford Health System, U.S.Patent Numer US D734,470S1

retinal detachment.[21] The Zhang Ring Test (▶ Fig. 21.5) is recommended for these high-risk patients for self-monitoring purposes.

21.9 When a Patient Suspects Something Is Wrong with His/ Her Vision, How Should They Check It?

The correct way is to check each eye separately. Surprisingly, not every patient knows that. In November 2019, a 62-year-old male experienced a bright flash of light in his right eye with a little blurriness; he rubbed the eye hoping the problem would disappear. Three months later, he happened to cover his left eye and he became alarmed that he was unable to see out of his right eye. The patient came to see me in 2020. The diagnosis was rhegmatogenous retinal detachment with macula off. The patient cried in the exam room upon learning the diagnosis. I asked the patient if he had known to cover each eye prior to the visit to identify if the problem was occurring in only one eye or both eyes and he said no. Because of this case, we designed a vision survey research project for public education. Our preliminary survey data as indicates that, among more than 2,000 surveyed patients (we plan to survey 5,000 patients), about 50% of the surveyed (18 years and older and cognitively capable of understanding the survey question at fz office since October 2020) do not know they should test each eye monocularly or understand how to check peripheral vision by maintaining stable central fixation. The Zhang Ring Test requires the patient to test each eye individually.

21.9.1 Zhang Ring Test Instructions

- If you are wearing glasses, remove them for the test.
- Place the sheet on a flat surface about 4 to 5 inches from your eye.
- While closing one eye, stare at the central dot without moving your eye and blink a few times to see if you perceive any distortion or gap of the ring with your peripheral vision.
- Repeat for the other eye.
- If you detect distortion or gaps, you may have a retinal detachment and you need to call your eye doctor.
- If you still perceive an intact 360-degree ring but you have increased floaters or flashing lights, you may have an early retinal tear but no retinal detachment yet, so you still need to see your eye doctor.
- If you want to see what the distorted/missing ring image looks like with a retinal detachment eye, you can Google "Zhang Ring Test," which will lead you to the Precision Vision web.

21.10 What Is the Role of the Light Adjustable Lens (LAL, RxSight, CA) in Refractive Lens Exchange?

The typical RLE patient asks for at least two things: to not have to wear thick glasses and/or contact lenses and to see well. These patients usually listen to our recommendations, although occasionally they know what they want, based on their own research and/or recommendation from their family/friends. No doubt, diffractive optic IOLs, such as traditional multifocal IOLs, Symfony EDOF (Johnson & Johnson), and trifocal PanOptix (Alcon), are doing well in most of our patients, but there are a percentage of patients who are not happy due to nighttime dysphotopsia, especially when additionally missing the refractive target.

With the arrival of the light adjustable lens (LAL; Light Adjustable Lens, RxSight Aliso Viejo, California), we have a new modality for RLE, although monofocal pseudophakic monovision has been used and doing well in the management of cataract and presbyopia for decades. Our deidentified survey of our 10-year monofocal IOL monovision patients indicated satisfaction to be 97%[22] (68.6% really like it and 28.4% like it). It is well known that when asked what IOL they would want for their own eyes, monofocal IOLs with some level of monovision are chosen by most practicing ophthalmologists.[23,24] As indicated by the 2019 ASCRS clinical survey, minimonovision (15% <1.0 D myopic defocus) and "true" monovision (12% 1.0 D or higher) together represented 27% of cataract surgery, while only about 8% had presbyopia-correcting IOLs in the United States.[16] The cost, vision quality, patient satisfaction, etc., may be the reasons behind these numbers.

- What the light adjustable lens adds is the capability of obtaining best vision possible to 20/15 and determining how much myopic defocus is desired for the near eye at a series of postoperative adjustment visits. (See more detailed discussion in Chapter 13) Of course, it is clear that neither the patient nor the surgeon will have the stress and pressure regarding how much anisometropia to plan prior to the surgery any more. In terms of vision quality, we do not need to worry about halo and glare either. The LAL has the highest premium IOL rate of uncorrected vision of 20/20 with outstanding patient satisfaction.[25] A press release from RxSight at the time of the FDA approval stated that patients with the LAL, compared to the control group, were twice as likely to achieve 20/20 or better without correction at 6 months postoperative.[25] It is even more impressive, with 20/15 in around 50%.[26] With this IOL we have the ability to operate on both eyes without delaying the second eye to assess refractive outcome in the first, which actually helps with customization. We cautiously predict that monofocal IOLs will still dominate in the future due to vision quality, especially when Refractive Index Shaping becomes available.

21.11 Should We Always Try to Make Our RLE Patients Completely Spectacle Free?

That is not always the case. The goal is to make the patient satisfied, not necessarily 100% glasses/contact lens independent. To provide what the patient wants and needs is the core of RLE. Review the preoperative survey and listen to the patient's feedback. Making a prospective RLE patient happy may be more art than science in the spectrum of all the premium IOLs and IOL monovision. For example, if a patient is quite happy for digital reading (dashboard, GPS, computer, and cell phone) after the first eye with a Symfony EDOF, UDVA 20/25, and UNVA J2, but wishes to have sharper UDVA and no additional photic phenomena, and willing to have readers for small print reading, then offering a monofocal of the same company's Tecnis ZCBOO (Johnson & Johnson Vision) for the fellow eye aiming at plano regardless of dominance may be a better approach than using another Symfony or trifocal for the fellow eye, especially if the patient is relatively young and outdoors-oriented.

21.12 Why Is a Pair of Backup Readers Easier than Dealing with Nighttime Dysphotopsia?

Our anecdotal experience suggests that there is no easy solution if a patient is not happy with diffractive optic-related dysphotopsia, even if they agreed and signed the consent form prior to the surgery. On the other hand, for a patient with minimonovision (anisometropia <1.0 D) or moderate monovision (anisometropia 1.0–1.5 D), a pair of over-the-counter readers can always solve the problem. The typical difference is that the former may not be very happy but the latter is satisfied. Neuroadaptation does not always occur and it is not always predictable. To preserve binocular summation and stereoacuity, mini mono and moderate monovision have become more popular than traditional full monovision (anisometropia between −1.75 to −2.50 D) in the last decade. As a consequence, these patients may often need readers for small print or actual full progressive glasses for challenging nighttime driving and extended pleasure reading. A full progressive glasses prescription allows each eye to see its best with full binocularity for occasional use, though not all will feel it necessary to fill the prescription.

An interesting study[27] in the Journal of Refractive Surgery by Schallhorn and his colleagues compared visual outcomes and patient satisfaction between two groups based on 3-month postoperative data: LASIK monovision versus EDOF Symfony (Johnson & Johnson Vision) for refractive lens exchange patients (LASIK monovision had 608 patients and Symfony group had 590 patients). There were four subgroups based on preoperative refractive status: plano, hyperopia, low myopia, and moderate-to-high myopia. There was a statistically significant difference in patient satisfaction in favor of monovision LASIK for moderate-to-high myopia (94.3% for monovision LASIK vs. 79.1% for refractive lens exchange, $p < 0.01$). For all other refractive categories, there was no significant difference in patient satisfaction. All myopic patients with refractive lens exchange experienced more postoperative visual phenomena than patients with monovision LASIK. Based on this paper, we are unable to say that IOL monovision does better than EDOF Symfony because LASIK monovision was used rather than IOL monovision in this study. We do have a head-to-head prospective study which showed statistically significantly better patient satisfaction in monofocal IOL monovision patients than in a multifocal IOL group.[28]

21.13 If IOL Power Calculation Suggests a Zero Diopter Lens, Can I Maintain Aphakia or Should I Place a Plano IOL in the Bag?

IOL power can be either very low or very high for RLE. A plano IOL is still better for the patient than leaving aphakia. The IOL can serve as a barrier between vitreous and anterior chamber in case future Nd:YAG laser is needed for posterior capsular opacification. Since the incidence of RD increases with Nd:YAG over that from the surgery itself, posterior optic capture may be the best choice once mastered. Down the road, when we have the Refractive Index Shaping technology, the presence of this IOL will let us make changes as indicated.

References

[1] Alio JL, Grzybowski A, El Aswad A, Romaniuk D. Refractive lens exchange. Surv Ophthalmol. 2014; 59(6):579–598

[2] Vitale S, Ellwein L, Cotch MF, Ferris FL, III, Sperduto R. Prevalence of refractive error in the United States, 1999–2004. Arch Ophthalmol. 2008; 126(8):1111–1119

[3] Barr JT. Contact lenses 2005. Contact lens spectrum. Published January 1, 2006. https://www.clspectrum.com/issues/2006/january-2006/contact-lens-2005. Accessed June 25, 2021

[4] Hura A, Kezirian G. Prevalance of refractive lens exchange in ophthalmologists who perform refractive surgery. Presented at ASCRS Virtual Annual Meeting. May 2020. https://ascrs.org/clinical-education/presbyopia/2020-pod-sps-107-63366-prevalence-of-refractive-lens-exchange-in-ophthalmologists-who-perf

[5] Westin O, Koskela T, Behndig A. Epidemiology and outcomes in refractive lens exchange surgery. Acta Ophthalmol. 2015; 93(1):41–45

[6] McIntire L. Refractive lens exchange (LASIK alternative). Heart of Texas Eye Institute. Published January 8, 2020. https://www.heartoftexaseye.com/blog/refractive-lens-exchange-surgery/. Accessed June 25, 2021

[7] Evans D. Better vision guide. https://www.bettervisionguide.com/refractive-iols-rle/. Accessed June 25, 2021

[8] Kaweri L, Wavikar C, James E, Pandit P, Bhuta N. Review of current status of refractive lens exchange and role of dysfunctional lens index as its new indication. Indian J Ophthalmol. 2020; 68(12):2797–2803

[9] Alió JL, Grzybowski A, Romaniuk D. Refractive lens exchange in modern practice: when and when not to do it? Eye Vis (Lond). 2014; 1:10

[10] Fernández J, Rodríguez-Vallejo M, Martínez J, Tauste A, Piñero DP. From presbyopia to cataracts: a critical review on dysfunctional lens syndrome. J Ophthalmol. 2018; 2018:4318405

[11] Chuck RS, Jacobs DS, Lee JK, et al. American Academy of Ophthalmology Preferred Practice Pattern Refractive Management/Intervention Panel. Refractive errors & refractive surgery preferred practice pattern. Ophthalmology. 2018; 125(1):P1–P104

[12] Hamill MB, ed. Intraocular refractive surgery. 2017–2018 Basic and Clinical Science Course (BCSC), Section 13: Refractive Surgery. Volume 13. American Academy of Ophthlamology;147

[13] Cataract Data and Statistics. National Eye Institute. Updated July 17, 2019. https://www.nei.nih.gov/learn-about-eye-health/resources-for-health-educators/eye-health-data-and-statistics/cataract-data-and-statistics. Accessed June 25, 2021

[14] Xu J, Murphy SL, Kockanek KD, Arias E. Mortality in the United States, 2018. NCHS Data Brief. 2020(355):1–8

[15] Reinstein DZ. Laser treatment options yield safer, better outcomes. What is the future of presbyopic correction in patients younger than 65 years old? Ocular Surgery News. 2018:11

[16] ASCRS. 2019 Clinical Survey. ASCRS Database

[17] Łabuz G, Knebel D, Auffarth GU, et al. Glistening formation and light scattering in six hydrophobic-acrylic intraocular lenses. Am J Ophthalmol. 2018; 196:112–120

[18] Henriksen BS, Kinard K, Olson RJ. Effect of intraocular lens glistening size on visual quality. J Cataract Refract Surg. 2015; 41(6):1190–1198

[19] Luo F, Bao X, Qin Y, Hou M, Wu M. Subjective visual performance and objective optical quality with intraocular lens glistening and surface light scattering. J Refract Surg. 2018; 34(6):372–378

[20] Passut J. Age, degree of correction determine surgery choice for myopes. EyeWorld. 2011; 16(9):50

[21] Ullrich M, Zwickl H, Findl O. Incidence of rhegmatogenous retinal detachment in myopic phakic eyes. J Cataract Refract Surg. 2021; 47(4):533–541

[22] Zhang F, Sugar A, Barrett GD, eds. Pseudophakic monovision. A clinical guide. Thieme Publishers; 2018

[23] Gossman M. What intraocular lens would you want in your eyes. EyeWorld. 2016; 21(7):34–36

[24] Logothetis HD, Feder RS. Which intraocular lens would ophthalmologists choose for themselves? Eye (Lond). 2019; 33(10):1635–1641

[25] Hillman L. Insights on the light adjustable lens. EyeWorld. 2020; 25(7):28–29

[26] Berdahl J. Light adjustable IOL. Our refractive IOL armamentarium, more choices than ever. 20/Happy in 20 webinar. August 29, 2020

[27] Schallhorn SC, Teenan D, Venter JA, et al. Monovision LASIK versus presbyopia-correcting IOLs: comparison of clinical and patient-reported outcomes. J Refract Surg. 2017; 33 (11):749–758

[28] Zhang F, Sugar A, Jacobsen G, Collins M. Visual function and patient satisfaction: comparison between bilateral diffractive multifocal intraocular lenses and monovision pseudophakia. J Cataract Refract Surg. 2011; 37(3):446–453

22 Management of the Unhappy Refractive Cataract Surgery Patient

Samuel Masket

Abstract

Dissatisfaction following "premium" intraocular lens (IOL) cataract surgery is often associated with missed diagnoses prior to surgery, with emphasis on ocular surface disease and occult maculopathy. Moreover, patient expectations may exceed available technology. A realistic view of the patient's optical and physical conditions in combination with a careful discussion of surgical options prior to surgery will benefit surgeon and patient alike. True spectacle independence is a very desirable surgical goal but may be difficult to achieve for some patients and impossible for others.

Assuming no meaningful surgical complications occur, patient dissatisfaction postoperatively is most often associated with induced or worsened ocular surface disease, ametropia, and pseudophakic dysphotopsia. Contemporary cataract surgery is commonly associated with induction of or worsening of preexisting dry eye disease, resulting in foreign body sensation and fluctuation of vision. The latter may be quite problematic with respect to diffractive optic IOLs that tend to reduce contrast sensitivity function. Despite ever improving IOL power calculation formulae, roughly 80% of cases can be expected to fall within 0.5 D of the desired optical outcome. Negative, positive, and diffractive optic dysphotopsia may occur individually or cumulatively after surgery.

All of these concerns should be known to the patient prior to surgery, so that unhappy surprises after surgery are minimized. The doctor–patient relationship is best established preoperatively and, should problems occur afterward, the patient and doctor can approach them as a "team."

Keywords: ocular surface disease, ametropia, occult maculopathy, premium IOL, refractive cataract surgery, pseudophakic dysphotopsia, patient dissatisfaction, diffractive optic IOL

22.1 Introduction

In reality, all cataract surgery in the developed nations is to be considered as refractive whether or not a "premium" intraocular lens (IOL) is implanted. For the purposes of this section a "premium" IOL is one for which the patient has an additional out-of-pocket fee, irrespective of whether the device is diffractive, toric, or another form of advanced technology IOL. While the patient who pays added fees for a given lens may develop a sense of entitlement, in practical experience virtually all patients have expectations of reduced spectacle dependence, even those who opt to wear eyeglasses as part of their "daily costume." However, one distinction between premium and standard cataract/IOL surgery is that premium IOLs require a more thorough preoperative evaluation and a more diligent intraoperative management for optimal visual outcomes. As an example, diffractive optic multifocal (MFIOL) or extended depth-of-focus (EDOF) IOLs require that the macular region be free of any significant abnormality for best performance, and a recent investigation uncovered a roughly 25% incidence of macular abnormalities when routine cataract patients were screened by optical coherence tomography (OCT) prior to surgery.[1] An important consideration is that it is best to avoid creating an unhappy patient after surgery by knowing what comorbidities exist and avoiding diffractive IOLs in those conditions. Those conditions include: Keratopathy (anterior and posterior), Zonulopathy, Pupillopathy, Optic Neuropathy, and Maculopathy. Moreover, certain personality disorders may also be a hindrance to favorable outcomes with MFIOLs. Similarly, with regard to any form of toric IOL, the surgeon must be diligent in determining the appropriate cylinder axis and must also implant the lens in the correct position.

For what reasons would a patient be dissatisfied with the surgical outcome and what measures can be taken to assuage those concerns? We can consider patient complaints as falling into two chief categories: Visual or physical symptoms; and, certainly they may coexist. With regard to the former, uncorrected optical error and undesired optical effects of surgery are the most likely, whereas for the latter, foreign body sensation is the most often encountered chief complaint. Moreover, while visual and physical symptoms may create dissatisfaction, the manner with which the surgeon approaches the problem(s) can have a marked impact on their resolution.

Let's consider the patient–physician relationship at the outset. As I see it, among the chief responsibilities of the cataract surgeon is to educate the patient about what cataract surgery is, what are the limitations of the technology, what are the options for optical outcomes, what is the accuracy of the IOL power formulae, what are the possible side effects and complications of surgery, what can be done to fix potential problems, what are realistic goals, etc. With that information the patient can make an informed decision regarding IOL choices and surgical "upgrades" regarding use of the femtosecond laser, intraoperative aberrometry, etc. Should the patient request a "premium" IOL or optional technology, cost will be added to the situation and the patient automatically becomes a consumer. The surgeon must anticipate that consumerism brings with it a potential need for added time, explaining the benefits of the added technology prior to surgery. That said, the more time spent prior to surgery, the less time will be necessary explaining any less than expected results after surgery. There is a potential bias to over promise an unattainable goal prior to surgery ("You can throw away your glasses after surgery, etc."). However, should the patient perceive (accurately or not) less than their desired outcome, it will be easier to manage their disappointment if they were under- rather than overpromised. In addition, patients must be made aware of their comorbidities prior to surgery as they may impact the outcome. One way to consider this issue is that if the patient was aware of a problem prior to surgery (dry eye as an example), it is their problem. On the other hand, if they only become apprised of the condition after surgery, it is your problem. It can be noted that many of the causes for patient dissatisfaction after surgery stem from preexisting conditions or patient's misunderstanding of what to expect after surgery.

In this chapter we will consider those conditions that may have negative consequences after uncomplicated cataract surgery, how to evaluate and manage them prior to surgery, and how to deal with the unhappy patient following surgery; illustrative cases will be considered.

22.2 Ocular Surface Diseases

Ocular surface conditions, most typically dry eye disease (DED) and epithelial basement membrane dystrophy (EBMD), may impact surgery in two ways: they can interfere with biometry resulting in an unexpected optical outcome and they can lead to physical discomfort, manifesting as dry eye or epithelial breakdown after surgery. As corneal power readings are essential for accurate biometry, both with regard to IOL power and cylinder, the surface needs to be near pristine for accuracy. Among the best ways to evaluate the corneal surface is Placido disc imaging. At the slit lamp, physical signs (whorls, map dots, etc.) and negative fluorescein staining provide evidence for EBMD and punctate staining along with rapid tear film breakup time suggest DED (▶ Fig. 22.1). In evaluating a patient for surgery and in deciding on lens type and power, the surgeon should employ corneal topography or similar technology. Let's consider the following case:

A 70-year-old woman was referred by her cataract surgeon for management of a malpositioned toric lens implant (▶ Fig. 22.2). At initial and uncomplicated cataract surgery, a toric IOL was implanted. However, following surgery the patient was noted

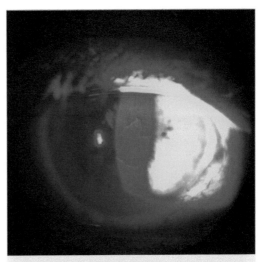

Fig. 22.1 Characteristic "negative" fluorescein staining in a case with paracentral epithelial basement membrane dystrophy (EBMD).

to have significant residual astigmatism and the surgeon believed that the IOL was off axis and planned surgery to rotate it. Unfortunately, the second surgery resulted in zonulysis and rupture of the posterior capsule and the patient was referred for management of the dislocated toric IOL.

At initial examination, slit lamp findings, corneal surface analysis by keratoscopy, and automated keratography revealed irregular astigmatism, consistent with EBMD (▶ Fig. 22.3). A careful and tactful discussion was held with the patient and the tests shared with her. Subsequent superficial keratectomy was well tolerated and 7 weeks later repeated corneal surface analysis appeared "pristine" and surgery to remove and replace the IOL was planned (▶ Fig. 22.4). One can note that the normalized cornea revealed less than 0.70 D of with the rule (WTR) anterior corneal cylinder, indicating that a toric IOL was not necessary. The offending IOL was exchanged for a scleral fixated monofocal IOL resulting in a happy patient.

The take-away message in this case is that the referring surgeon failed to evaluate the corneal surface prior to selecting the IOL. EBMD, obvious on testing and by slit lamp examination, was missed and the surgeon was "fooled" into selecting an unnecessary toric IOL. Worse, attempted IOL rotation resulted in surgical complications. However, a tactful, nonincriminating educational patient conversation, in combination with recognition and amelioration of the problem, resulted in a favorable outcome and happy patient.

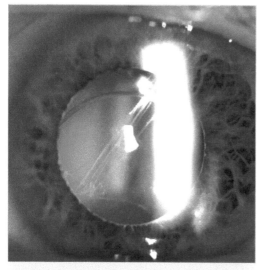

Fig. 22.2 Malpositioned intraocular lens (IOL) left eye (LE); note torn posterior capsule and dehiscence of superonasal zonular fibers.

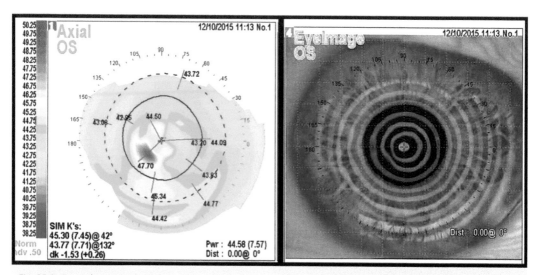

Fig. 22.3 Corneal topography (left) and Placido disc image (right) reveal obvious irregular astigmatism and corresponding characteristic surface distortion consistent with epithelial basement membrane dystrophy (EBMD).

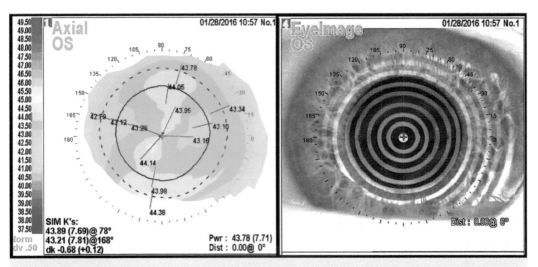

Fig. 22.4 Same eye as in ▶ Fig. 22.2 seven weeks after superficial keratectomy. Note marked improvement in the Placido image and topography.

Another concern regarding EBMD is breakdown of the corneal epithelium in the immediate or early postoperative period; this creates marked discomfort and reduced vision if the defect is central or paracentral. That combination creates unhappy patients. However, a well-informed patient will be more tolerant of the problem. Moreover, the ocular surface can be carefully "babied" during surgery to help prevent damage to the intercellular desmosomes that help keep the epithelium intact:

1. If using preoperative drops in advance of surgery, prescribe nonpreserved agents where possible and continue nonpreserved agents after surgery. There is an understandable and progressive interest in "drop-free" cataract surgery.
2. Do not use tetracaine on the corneal surface as it promotes epithelial breakdown; it can be swabbed with a cellulose sponge on the limbal conjunctiva and cul-de-sacs after applying proparacaine which is much kinder to the corneal epithelium.
3. Apply 2% hydroxypropyl methylcellulose (HPMC) ophthalmic vicosurgical device (OVD) to the cornea repeatedly during surgery; it protects and lubricates the cornea and enhances the view.[2] Avoid allowing the surface to dry.
4. Apply a bandage contact lens at the close of surgery and remove it at the first postoperative visit (▶ Video 22.1).

Dry eye disease (DED) is a very common ocular surface disorder that impacts many cataract age patients, women in particular, prior to and after surgery. The literature varies significantly regarding the incidence of DED after surgery; however, most reports place it above 35%, a rather sobering number.[3] Postoperatively, it manifests as a burning or foreign body sensation and may induce fluctuation of vision, the latter particularly if there is rapid evaporation of the tear film with each blink. DED may be due to aqueous tear deficiency, Meibomian gland dysfunction (MGD) with evaporative DED, chronic blepharitis, or a combination of these issues. As a result, postoperative patients with DED may be unhappy with regard to both physical discomfort and reduced vision; the latter is likely to be more evident with diffractive IOLs. Management of DED has become a near major industry and perhaps a subspecialty of its own. There are evolving diagnostics to help identify those patients who could manifest symptoms following surgery.[4,5] Although DED is not rare prior to surgery, there are a number of other factors associated with cataract surgery that can make it worsen or become manifest. They include: Interruption of corneal nerves in similar, but less extensive, fashion as with laser-assisted in situ keratomileusis (LASIK) flaps, toxic effect of (nonpreserved) eye drops and povidone iodine, intraoperative drying and anesthetics, microscope light phototoxicity, physical injury to the corneal surface, etc.

As postoperative patients may be quite unhappy with symptoms of DED, one key is to identify problem eyes prior to surgery; however, nearly 20% of asymptomatic cases preop will develop DED postoperative, owing to a "frail" ocular surface.[6] But, there are a plethora of diagnostic tests and therapeutic regimens that have evolved to identify and manage both aqueous deficiency and MGD.[5,6] Moreover, certain physical conditions should alert the surgeon to the potential for DED. Those include, but are not limited to blepharitis, prior blepharoplasty or other causes for poor lid closure, autoimmune disorders, and use of systemic medications that have a proclivity to induce mucous membrane drying. Physical examination at the slit lamp can often establish the diagnosis; however, as in the case of EBMD, the Placido disc image and surface topography can be very beneficial. When reviewing biometry for IOL selection, it is essential to inspect the topographic images for evidence of dry spots or "bleeding" of the edges of the colored images. If the findings suggest that DED is present, consideration should be given to postpone surgery until the ocular surface can be properly managed and improved. With good counseling, patients are likely to be understanding of this plan and cooperative in carrying it out.

Intraoperative management of the patient with DED is quite similar to the regimen for those with EBMD. In addition, and where possible, avoid astigmatic keratotomy, reduce surgical and microscope time, exercise particular caution when placing the lid speculum, consider **not** using the femtosecond laser as it requires additional time, added surface anesthetic, extra trauma to the ocular surface, etc. Postsurgery, it is best to use nonpreserved drops, lubricate aggressively, and be judicious with the use of topical NSAIDs as they can impact surface healing in this background, even more so in dry eye patients with autoimmune disorders.[7] Moreover, and based on findings and symptoms, consideration can be given to the use of punctal plugs and/or topical cyclosporine or lifitegrast. One comment on the use of punctal plugs prior to cataract surgery: While some DED patients may benefit from their use, it has been my policy to remove them shortly before surgery as they may harbor mucus and provide a biofilm for microbes. They can be replaced shortly after surgery as indicated.

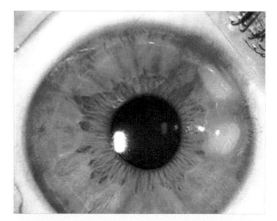

Fig. 22.5 Salzmann nodular degeneration right eye (RE) seen classically as two white elevated lesions nasally and superonasally.

Less common, but potentially as troubling with regard to a poor visual outcome if missed prior to surgery is Salzmann nodular degeneration (▶ Fig. 22.5). While this condition most often affects the periphery and midperiphery of the cornea, it can have a major impact on corneal topography and, in turn, biometry with a resultant improper IOL power. The condition is readily treated with superficial keratectomy and peeling of the nodule(s). ▶ Fig. 22.6 and ▶ Fig. 22.7 demonstrate the impact of Salzmann degeneration on corneal topography and biometry for IOL power calculations. Had the surgeon not viewed the topography and looked only at the biometry for IOL selection, a large error could have eventuated as the pretreatment biometry suggested that a high toric IOL was appropriate. However, following treatment, topography appeared normal and there was only 0.5 D of regular corneal astigmatism. The important message is that corneal topography is an essential element of cataract evaluation and surgical planning.

The posterior corneal surface (endothelium and Descemet membrane) may harbor preexisting conditions that, when missed preoperatively, can also result in less than desirable surgical outcomes. The most common is Fuchs endothelial corneal dystrophy (FECD) with central guttae that induce light scatter, glare, and reduced contrast sensitivity (▶ Fig. 22.8).[8] This can result in poor nighttime visual function, especially with diffractive optic IOLs. It is apparent that the surgeon

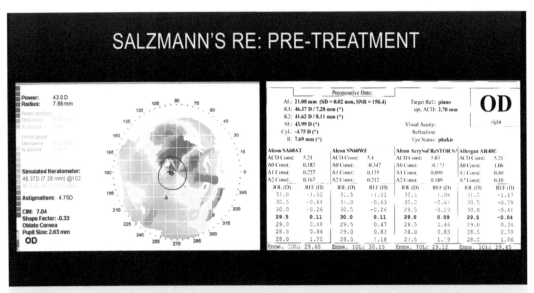

Fig. 22.6 Corneal topography (left) and biometry (right) in a case with Salzmann nodular degeneration (RE). Note marked irregular astigmatism, high degree of measured astigmatism and biometry suggesting a 30 D high toric intraocular lens (IOL).

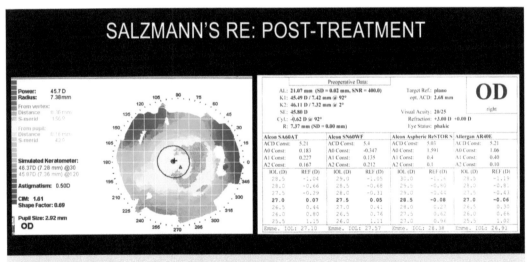

Fig. 22.7 Corneal topography (left) and biometry (right) following treatment for Salzmann nodular degeneration (RE). Note marked improvement in topography and reduction in astigmatism as compared with ▶ Fig. 22.5. Also note that biometry suggests a 27.5 D nontoric intraocular lens (IOL).

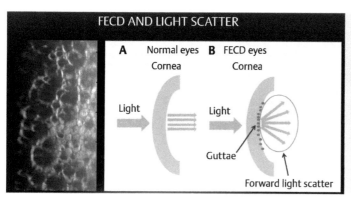

Fig. 22.8 Fuchs endothelial corneal dystrophy (FECD), noted on the left with specular microscopy can induce light scatter and reduce visual function (noted schematically on the right), particularly with diffractive optic intraocular lens (IOLs) at night time.

must carefully evaluate both anterior and posterior corneal surfaces prior to cataract surgery, consider those findings, and, in light of pathology, involve the patient in the IOL decision-making process, as the risk for postoperative dissatisfaction increases greatly if an abnormal corneal condition is ignored prior to surgery. In general, it is best to avoid diffractive optic IOLs in patients with FECD, as the latter is likely to progress.

22.3 Unexpected Optical Outcomes of Surgery

As discussed above, missed preexisting OSD is a chief cause for dissatisfaction following cataract surgery. However, equally as important are residual optical error and undesired optical imagery, the latter referred to as dysphotopsia. In fact, according to Tester et al, dysphotopsia is the chief cause for dissatisfaction after otherwise uncomplicated cataract surgery.[9]

With regard to residual optical error, surgeon and patient alike must appreciate the limitations of preoperative biometry and intraoperative aberrometry in predicting the correct IOL power to achieve the planned outcome. At present, under best case circumstances, approximately 80% of eyes will fall within 0.5 D of the intended optical outcome.[10] As a result, one in five cases will fall outside of that "goalpost." When other factors are taken into consideration, short or long axial lengths, steep or flat corneas, and prior refractive surgery, the percentage eyes within that range goes down.[10] Furthermore, while intraoperative aberrometry may be beneficial under some circumstances, in general it is not helpful in reducing

the overall percentage of eyes that fall outside of desired range.[11,12,13] For all IOL power predictive methods this is chiefly due to the fact that it is impossible to know with certainty where the IOL will sit in relationship to fixed ocular structures, or the final physical lens position (PLP). That point of fixation (PLP), when combined with certain attributes of the IOL, determines the effective lens position (ELP), and IOL power prediction formulae engage a variety of parameters to **predict** it. The higher the IOL power, the more critical is the estimated ELP. As a result, short hyperopic eyes are very prone to inaccuracies in refractive outcomes. Highly myopic eyes are also prone to optical error after surgery, but more likely due to biometric inaccuracy, rather than ELP issues. Formulae continue to emerge and artificial intelligence is also becoming a valuable tool for IOL power prediction.[14] Nevertheless, as ELP will always be an estimate, some patients will experience an undesired refractive outcome. On a positive note, however, technology now exists to allow for nonsurgical postoperative IOL power adjustment, a potential game changer.[15]

Unfortunately, even under the best of circumstances with routine eyes, a considerable number of patients will not be satisfied with their refractive outcome. When use of premium IOLs, for which the patients pay out of pocket, is added to the situation, the surgeon must have a clear plan for dealing with the optical error. The first order of business is to determine, if possible, the source of the error, while explaining the nature of the "detective work" to the patient:

1. Perform an accurate refraction.
2. Confirm that the intended IOL was placed by comparing the preoperative planning to the

actual IOL used by inspecting the stickers supplied with the IOL, etc. This is one situation where human error may be responsible for wrong IOL power. It's good practice for the surgeon to have a written plan for each patient's surgery and to double check the IOL selection at the outset of the procedure.

3. Review the original readings and repeat corneal topography and biometry—perhaps the original biometry was performed with a contact lens in place; typically, soft contact lenses have flat anterior powers. Or, perhaps the contact lenses were removed just prior to biometry, rather than allowing adequate time for the cornea to return to its normal curvature.

4. Be certain that the IOL is in the intended anatomic position and that the anterior chamber is not excessively shallow (wound leak, aqueous misdirection, capsule block syndrome), inducing myopia, or unexpectedly deep, owing to (iatrogenic?) diffuse zonulopathy, causing a hyperopic error.

An improperly planned or selected IOL, a human error, or an anatomic abnormality should be uncovered with this algorithm. There is only a **very** remote chance that all of the above will fail to uncover the problem and that an improperly marked and boxed IOL could have been inserted. However, given the heavily controlled IOL manufacturing process, this is the least likely possibility. Once the problem is discovered, a plan can be made to correct the error. All during this process, the patient must be involved in the discussion and decision making. It is far better that the patient is made aware of the situation from the surgeon, rather than a nearby competitor. What are the options for dealing with the unexpected optical outcome? For some corrective strategies the source of the error is irrelevant, as the management method does not require that information. In addition, before any corrective surgery, where possible, a contact lens trial should be done to be certain that the patient will be satisfied with the new optical plan. Moving from least expensive and least risky, the following algorithm can be considered:

1. If the error is small and well tolerated, perhaps no correction is needed. An example would be a small degree of unplanned myopia with a monofocal IOL; enhanced intermediate vision would ensue and potentially benefit the patient. However, in the case of a diffractive MFIOL or EDOF IOL, ametropia is generally not well tolerated.

2. Spectacles can be considered; however, refractive cataract surgery patients have already expressed their desire, and perhaps paid out of pocket, to eliminate or reduce spectacle dependence.

3. Contact lens wear: Similar to spectacle wear, patients are not likely to accept CLs unless they have a long history of comfort with them. Those unfamiliar with their use are unlikely to accept them. Moreover, they should not be used for several weeks after surgery, allowing for incision healing.

4. Laser refractive surgery: This may be a good option for those patients who have had prior LASIK or similar procedures, particularly if there is no added personal expense. However, the prolonged healing time and initial discomfort associated with surface ablation (PRK) may not be desirable for an already dissatisfied patient. Therefore, LASIK and SMILE, in my view, are better options but require a healing period after cataract surgery and the eye must be otherwise suited for such a procedure. This is a very good option for those with MFIOLs or EDOF IOLs as small degrees of uncorrected ametropia can hinder performance of these IOLs. ▸ Fig. 22.9 demonstrates a chart of five cases with diffractive IOLs and moderate residual mixed astigmatic errors and poor VA. Custom wavefront laser vision correction improved all cases to excellent visual acuity and satisfactory outcomes.

5. "Piggy Back" or ciliary sulcus add on IOL: While this option can create rapid improvement, it does engender expense and the added risk of secondary intraocular surgery. Moreover, in the US market there are fewer IOLs available for this option than in other countries. In addition, this procedure should only be considered if the initial IOL is fully confined to capsule bag, if there is complete zonular integrity, and if there is adequate space in the posterior chamber. There are also concerns about late IOL decentration and iris chafe with this method.

6. Toric IOL realignment: Toric IOLs should be carefully aligned on the correct axis for best performance as each degree of off-axis rotation

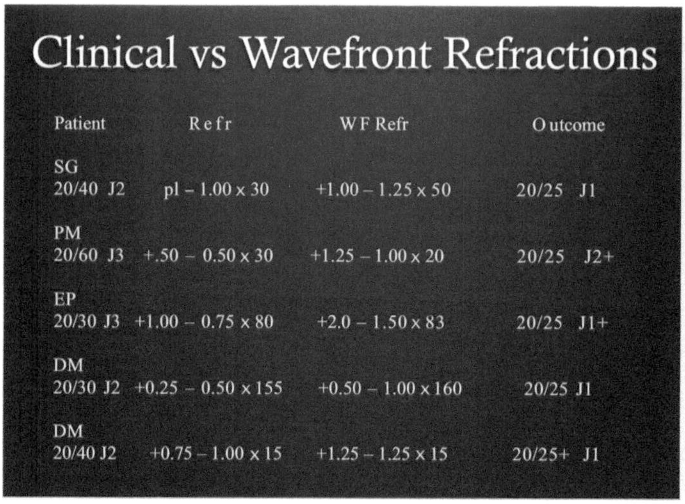

Clinical vs Wavefront Refractions

Patient	Refr	WF Refr	Outcome
SG 20/40 J2	pl − 1.00 × 30	+1.00 − 1.25 × 50	20/25 J1
PM 20/60 J3	+.50 − 0.50 × 30	+1.25 − 1.00 × 20	20/25 J2+
EP 20/30 J3	+1.00 − 0.75 × 80	+2.0 − 1.50 × 83	20/25 J1+
DM 20/30 J2	+0.25 − 0.50 × 155	+0.50 − 1.00 × 160	20/25 J1
DM 20/40 J2	+0.75 − 1.00 × 15	+1.25 − 1.25 × 15	20/25+ J1

Fig. 22.9 Chart reveals five patients with less than satisfactory vision with diffractive multifocal intraocular lens (IOLs) and mixed astigmatism. Clinical refractions uncovered smaller degrees of ametropia than did wavefront refraction in each case. All cases were treated with custom wavefront-guided laser-assisted in situ keratomileusis (LASIK) resulting in excellent visual outcomes and satisfied patients.

is associated with a 3% loss of toric function; therefore, just a 10-degree malalignment will result in nearly a one-third reduction of toric correction. Proper use of toric IOLs requires attention to anterior and posterior corneal astigmatism for determining axis and amount of correction, accurate axis marking and IOL positioning during surgery, and rotational stability of the IOL after surgery.[16] Manufacturers of toric IOLs often supply nomograms to determine best power and axis for each given case and the printed forms should accompany the patient chart at surgery to prevent human error. There is an increasing number of imaging devices to help measure, mark, and align toric IOLs at surgery. Should a lens be off-axis it is best repositioned between 2 and 6 weeks after surgery. An excellent guide to determine the correct axis for rotated toric IOLs is the website astigmatismfix.com.[17]

7. IOL exchange: This is the most physiologic, albeit most invasive, expensive and riskiest procedure. However, it leaves the eye in the original and intended state. The surgeon should have comfort with IOL exchange at various times following initial surgery. One consideration for this method, unlike the other options where the cause of the error is irrelevant, one must be certain that the incorrect IOL power is the culprit. Otherwise, there is a risk that an exchange may not yield the desired outcome.

Let's consider some case examples and the decision-making process:

A 55-year-old-woman was referred for difficulty with nighttime driving after cataract surgery with implantation of a Crystalens (B&L). Her history revealed that 10 years prior she had myopic LASIK followed a year later by additional "touch-up" ablation. She was satisfied with her vision until a cataract ensued. Although cataract surgery was uneventful and the IOL perfectly centered, the patient had a residual myopic and astigmatic refractive error. In addition, her mesopic pupil was larger than the size of the optic and evaluation of axial corneal topography revealed a centrally flat cornea with modest nasal decentration of the ablation profile (▶ Fig. 22.10 and ▶ Fig. 22.11).

Given two prior laser vision correction (LVC) procedures and a premium IOL at cataract surgery, neither spectacles nor contact lenses would be well-accepted options for this patient. In addition, attempted miotic therapy with brimonidine (0.15%) and dilute pilocarpine (0.5%) was not tolerated but could be useful for other patients. Moreover, the post-LASIK status of the cornea suggests that additional LVC would require surface ablation that could be unreliable with an already decentered ablation. IOL exchange is potentially difficult with the Crystalens even early after surgery owing to the "moustache" haptics. In all, the best option for this patient was a "piggy-back" IOL combined with peripheral corneal relaxing incisions for the residual astigmatism. At surgery (▶ Video 22.2) a −1.0 D

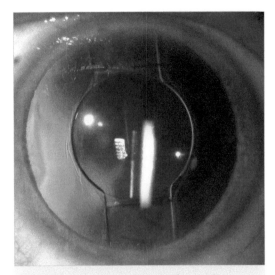

Fig. 22.10 Post cataract surgery with Crystalens (Bausch & Lomb) intraocular lens (IOL). Note large corneal diameter with well centered but relatively small IOL diameter.

6.3-mm silicone three-piece IOL (AQ5010V, Staar Surgical) was implanted in the ciliary sulcus without difficulty. Unfortunately, that IOL is no longer available. Improving the optical result of surgery and having a larger anterior IOL succeeded in correcting the patient's nighttime difficulties (▶ Fig. 22.12). Given that the Staar AQ5010V IOL is no longer manufactured, current alternative add-on IOLs in the US market would include the Sensar AR 40 M or Z 9002 (both from J&J), the MA60BM (Alcon), or the LI 61 series (B&L).

For the case described above, consideration was given for all of the methods for managing post-operative ametropia. Although the patient did well, she will require long-term observation as there is a possibility of iris chafe and IOL dislocation. This case also illustrates that the presurgical planning for the cataract surgery was flawed, in that the surgeon did not consider a disparity between pupil and IOL diameters in selection of the implant. Moreover, IOL power selection was

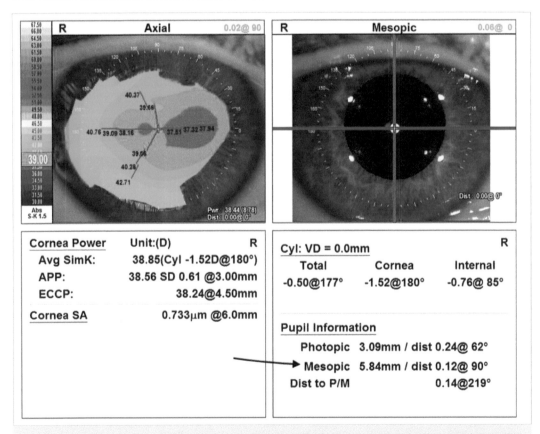

Fig. 22.11 Corneal topography (left) reveals results of prior laser-assisted in situ keratomileusis (LASIK) with central flattening and nasally decentered ablation. Image on right demonstrates a mesopic pupil size of 5.84 mm (*arrow*).

inaccurate, but given two prior LVC procedures, that outcome is understandable.

A 51-year-old highly myopic female contact lens wearer sought a second opinion following uncomplicated cataract surgery for the RE. She noted difficulty seeing within 10 feet for the operated eye, problems balancing between the two eyes, and positive dysphotopsia. Her examination revealed the results of excellent cataract surgery; however, there was a +0.75 D hyperopic refractive error that was intolerable, given previous high myopia and the low-powered (+3.0 D Tecnis, J&J), acrylic, IOL-

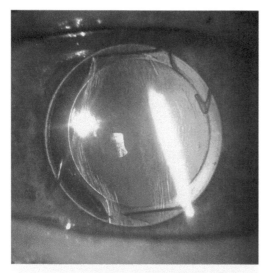

Fig. 22.12 Postoperative view after sulcus "piggy-back" implant. Note the greater size of the secondary intraocular lens (IOL).

induced dysphotopsia. After contact lens trials, the patient preferred a plano outcome for the RE and low myopia for the LE. Given the combination of ametropia and dysphotopsia the best option was IOL exchange. At surgery (▶ Video 22.3), the existing IOL was bisected and removed, and a lower Index of Refraction +4.0 D silicone IOL was placed in the capsule bag. Subsequent cataract surgery for the LE resulted in planned −1.0 D minimonovision and a gratified patient.

This case illustrates that IOL power calculation in patients with high myopia often results in an undesirable hyperopic error unless special formulae are applied. I have had excellent results with the Wang-Koch formula and the Barrett Universal II formulae.[18],[19] In addition, low-powered, high index of refraction acrylic IOLs are prone to induce positive dysphotopsia.

A 64-year-old woman was referred for realignment of a toric IOL (SN6AT9, Alcon) for the LE about 6 months following cataract surgery. She had radial and astigmatic keratotomy surgery bilaterally approximately 25 years earlier. She complained of poor vision. Both eyes revealed evidence of 4-cut RK and AK in the vertical meridian. Corneal topography (▶ Fig. 22.13) suggested a degree of irregular astigmatism and there is question whether a toric IOL was the best course of action. It is unclear if the surgeon chose the incorrect axis or the IOL rotated postoperative. However, overrefraction yielded marked improvement in VA and when the data was entered to the astigmatismfix.com website (▶ Fig. 22.14), I was encouraged that rotation to the correct axis would be beneficial.[17] At surgery (▶ Video 22.4) it

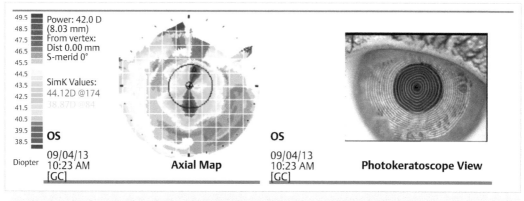

Fig. 22.13 Corneal topography indicates a high degree of "against-the-rule" astigmatism that is somewhat irregular as indicated by the Placido images and the nonorthogonal "hourglass" topo image.

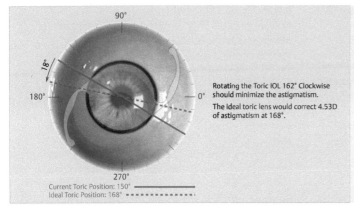

90°

18°

180° ——————————— 0°

Rotating the Toric IOL 162° Clockwise should minimize the astigmatism.
The ideal toric lens would correct 4.53D of astigmatism at 168°.

270°

Current Toric Position: 150° ————————
Ideal Toric Position: 168° ▪▪▪▪▪▪▪▪▪▪▪▪▪

Fig. 22.14 Printout from astigmatismfix.com website suggests that an 18-degree counterclockwise rotation would correct the optical condition.

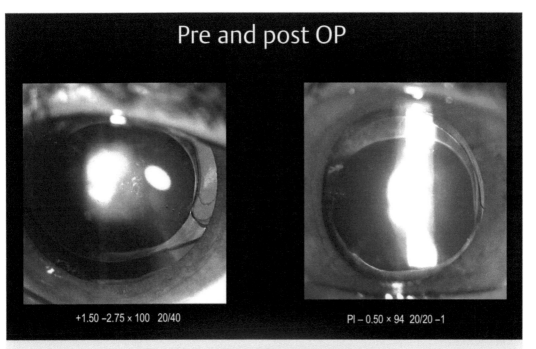

Pre and post OP

+1.50 −2.75 × 100   20/40

PI − 0.50 × 94   20/20 −1

Fig. 22.15 Intraocular lens (IOL) rotation resulted in a markedly improved best corrected visual acuity (BCVA) and reduction of residual optical error.

was necessary to free the tenacious adhesions of the haptics to the peripheral capsule, remove the IOL from the bag, reopen the bag for 360 degrees, reposit the IOL, place it on correct axis, remove the OVD, and perform intraoperative aberrometry to assure the proper axis. This resulted in improved objective and subjective vision (▶ Fig. 22.15).

There is always a risk when using high-powered toric IOLs in post-RK eyes unless astigmatism is regular and reproducible over several methods for determining corneal power (topography, tomography, keratometry, Lenstar, or IOL Master). In this case a T9 (Alcon) (4.1 D toric power at the corneal plane) caused markedly poor vision when rotated just 18 degrees off axis. More currently, for this case, other forms of treatment could be considered in lieu of toric rotation; they include inducing a small pupil by miotics, suture pupilloplasty, or implantation of a small pupil aperture (Trindade XtraFocus Morcher) add-on sulcus implant (off-label in the United States).[20,21]

22.4 Dysphotopsia—Undesired Optical Side Effects of Surgery

Dysphotopsia represents undesired optical imagery that is associated with otherwise uncomplicated lens-based (cataract or clear crystalline lens replacement) surgery; as such, the condition disturbs the view of the desired object of regard or the visual field. Dysphotopsia is an exclusionary diagnosis and a full examination must be done to assure that there is no pathology that could account for the symptoms, including significant refractive error and posterior capsule opacification (PCO). Dysphotopsia may be classified into three general types: positive dysphotopsia (PD) is reported as light streaks, light flashes, light arcs, starbursts, etc., that are induced by an external light source, typically one of oblique incidence.[22,23] It may also be stimulated by nearly incident light under certain circumstances.[24] This condition must be distinguished from entoptic phenomena that are associated with vitreoretinal traction and noted without an external light source. Negative dysphotopsia (ND) is generally noted as a temporal dark shadow that simulates the effect of "horse blinders."[25] It too is stimulated by a temporally incident light source. Diffractive optic dysphotopsia (DD) consists of halos, rings, spiderwebs, etc., that surround point sources of light, most typically at night. These occur specifically from the diffractive rings associated with multifocal (MFIOLs) or diffractive extended depth-of-focus (EDOF) IOLs. Each of the dysphotopsias has unique causes, courses, and solutions. As they are different entities they may coexist in the same patient. Given that patients may be quite symptomatic and concerned, despite uncomplicated surgery, they may require support and should be managed with compassionate assurance. All too often patients' dysphotopic symptoms are dismissed by the surgeon.

The incidence of PD has not been well studied; however, the literature suggests that somewhere between 20 and 50% of patients will note dysphotopsia of some type after surgery.[9] There are no laboratory testing devices that can record or plot the symptoms of PD. There appears to be little neuroadaptation to PD and those patients who cannot tolerate it may benefit nonsurgically from the use of miotics, such as brimonidine 0.15% or dilute pilocarpine (0.5%). Should that strategy fail, IOL exchange may be offered. Square-edged design of the optic and surface reflectivity owing to high index of refraction is the chief cause of PD. There are no round-edge foldable IOLs on the market in the United States. While some manufacturers have modified the anterior portions of the edge of IOLs in an attempt to reduce PD, the posterior portion of all foldable IOL edges is squared and contributes to PD. A recent investigation regarding surgical management of PD suggests that using an IOL of lower index of refraction as the replacement IOL brings an 85 to 90% chance for success.[26] This is particularly true if the inciting IOL was made of acrylic material and replaced by silicone with lower I/R and reflectivity.[24]

ND is reported by patients as a blockage of the temporal field of view, most typically inferotemporally.[25] Unlike PD, there are fewer apparent causes for ND and the subject remains somewhat controversial as there is seemingly a discrepancy between clinical findings and optical laboratory bench testing.[27,28,29] The incidence of ND has been reasonably well studied and indicates that when specifically asked, between 15 and 20% of cases will report ND early after surgery; the incidence falls to about 3% at one year.[30,31] The reduction in ND symptoms over time appears to be due to neuroadaptation. Also, unlike PD, an ND "scotoma" can be plotted with Goldmann peripheral kinetic visual field testing.[32,33,34] Until recently, it was perplexing to note that some ND patients could be highly symptomatic despite a relatively small VF defect plotted on monocular Goldmann testing; however, binocular VF studies have shown that the ND scotoma is markedly larger with both eyes open than with the fellow eye occluded (▶ Fig. 22.16).[34] Although the mechanism for this phenomenon is presently unexplained, it suggests that the central nervous system (CNS) contributes to ND in some fashion. Also, the binocular VF changes add to our understanding of, and the intensity of, some patients' symptoms. Curiously, ND is more likely to occur in females than males, more so in left than in right eyes, and often in only one eye of the same patient even if the anatomy appears identical between the two eyes.[28] These observations also suggest CNS modulation of ND.

Although initial theories regarding the etiology of ND incriminated high I/R, square-edged IOLs as causal, it is now recognized that ND can and does occur with "in-the-bag" IOLs of any material and design.[27,28,29] Unlike PD, ND appears to be more related to IOL position relative to the capsule bag,

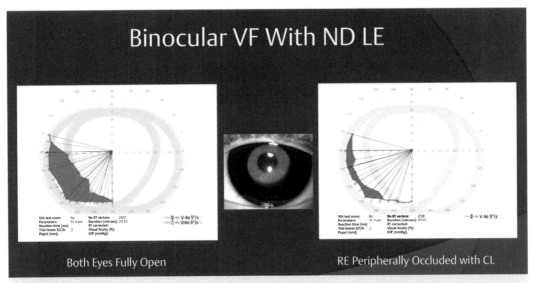

Fig. 22.16 Negative dysphotopsia "scotoma" for left eye (LE) under binocular Goldmann visual field testing. On the left, both eyes are fully open. On the right, the "scotoma" is markedly smaller after placing a peripherally opaque contact lens (center) on the fellow right eye (RE). (Used with permission from Masket et al 2020.)[34]

rather than features of the specific IOL, as the same IOL in a given patient with ND will "cure" the condition if that IOL is elevated with the optic placed in front of the anterior capsule edge either by placing the IOL in the sulcus or elevating the optic portion, leaving the haptics in the bag (reverse optic capture).[27,28,29] In fact, ND has not been reported with ACIOLs, sulcus-placed IOLs, or scleral fixated posterior chamber IOLs. The clinical findings indicate that reverse optic capture is nearly always successful in preventing or improving ND symptoms.[28]

ND may be managed nonsurgically by occluding temporally incident light with spectacle frames or peripherally opaque contact lenses. ND is not benefitted by pharmacologic miosis, but conversely it can be helped by pupil dilation, though the induced glare is not a worthwhile trade-off. Should ND persist chronically and be intolerable, secondary surgery can be performed with a high degree of success. Varying with the size and position of the existing anterior capsulotomy and the nature of the IOL, secondary reverse optic capture or sulcus placement (with IOL exchange if needed) will bring nearly universal success, as will primary reverse optic capture for the second eye of symptomatic cases.[27,28,29] As a general rule of thumb, optic over capsule will prevent or cure existing

ND, but in-the-bag IOL exchange for a lens of different design or material is generally unsuccessful.[27,35] In addition, using an Nd:YAG laser to amputate the overlying nasal capsule has been reported as successful in reducing ND symptoms.[36,37]

A 58-year-old woman was referred by her cataract surgeon for evaluation and management of positive and negative dysphotopsia 3 months following uneventful cataract surgery with placement of toric IOL (SN6AT3, Alcon). Her exam was unremarkable and the patient was counseled with regard to her condition. She was made aware that the surgery was without flaw and she was asked to wait a few additional months in the hope that her symptoms would improve. Owing to a family medical problem the patient was unable to return for a full year; however, symptoms were unchanged and she requested corrective surgery. At surgery the toric IOL was removed from the bag; one haptic was challenging to remove and a capsular tension ring (CTR) was placed owing to stress on the inferior zonule. A three-piece silicone IOL was placed with the haptics in the bag and the optic then elevated into a reverse optic capture position (▶ Video 22.5). Peripheral corneal relaxing incisions were made to correct astigmatism, as the original IOL was toric. Both forms

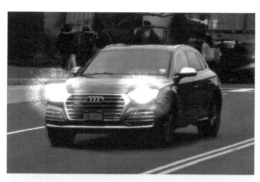

of dysphotopsia were resolved and patient was very grateful. A year later cataract surgery was performed for the fellow eye, employing reverse optic capture. Both eyes are free from dysphotopsia or any type.

By nature of their design, diffractive optic MFIOLs and diffractive EDFIOLs produce undesired optical imagery that is manifest as concentric circles, "star bursts," or "spiderweb" patterns around point sources of light in addition to glare and halos (▶ Fig. 22.17). As a result, the symptoms of DD tend to be exaggerated by headlights and streetlamps during nighttime driving. While the majority of patients with diffractive optic IOLs will note these optical effects, over time most find the side effects tolerable and an acceptable "trade-off" for reduced spectacle dependence; moreover, there appears to be a gradual improvement in tolerance, suggesting neuroadaptation. Bear in mind that the effects of diffractive optic dysphotopsia may be superimposed on PD, ND, or both.

Newer, lower add, and trifocal design IOLs seem to be better tolerated than the original series. With regard to the US FDA trials of the original Alcon ReStor +4.0 D add bifocal IOLs, 93% of patients indicated that they would have the same IOL implanted again, despite the fact that the patients were all "best case."[A] Contrast that with the more recent investigation of the Alcon trifocal Panoptix where 99% of patients indicated that they would have the same IOL again.[B] On a similar

note, with respect to the original Johnson and Johnson (J&J) +4.0 D add Tecnis MFIOL, 87% indicated that they would have the same IOL implanted again, whereas 96% would have the more recently designed +2.75 D add J&J Tecnis MFIOL in repeated surgery.[C] Both the Alcon and J&J examples indicate that trifocal and lower add MFIOLs are better tolerated than the original higher add power designs. In addition, much has been learned regarding patient selection for presbyopic IOLs with regard to ocular surface disease, maculopathy, preexisting higher order optical aberrations (HOAs), etc., allowing greater success with these devices. All of that notwithstanding, and despite the best information and improved IOL technology, a small but given percentage of patients will be unhappy with the outcome of surgery and require help.

Managing patients who are doing poorly with diffractive optic IOLs generally requires careful evaluation and treatment of the ocular surface and precorneal tear film, examination of the macula region with OCT to rule out cystoid macular edema, as well as correcting any meaningful residual optical error. Ametropia is not well tolerated with diffractive optics. Patients may improve over time and should be given 3 months or so to allow for neuroadaptation. However, should visual dissatisfaction exist once those items have been adequately attended to and time given, IOL exchange must be considered for a monofocal optic.[38] In my experience in dealing with patients referred for dissatisfaction with multifocal or EDOF lenses, those patients with chronic comorbidities have little chance for successful management, whereas those free from other conditions have a better likelihood for success, with attention paid to residual optical error, ocular surface disease, etc. The surgeon must be prepared to offer IOL exchange along with encouragement to those in need. Moreover, patients may be comforted to know that even under the best of circumstances somewhere between 5 and 8% of cases would not opt for the same IOL again, even though the need for reading glasses is markedly reduced. Once again, they need to be reassured that there is not a problem with them or with the surgery, but that the technology doesn't match well with their visual system and that this could not have been known prior to surgery. Let's consider a case management example:

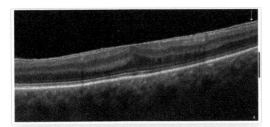

Fig. 22.18 Macular epiretinal membrane with thickening and loss of foveal depression but no cystoid edema.

A 63-year-old woman was referred for poor vision following implantation of a three-piece diffractive optic (Tecnis, J&J) IOL. Her examination revealed a BCVA of 20/40 and she was noted to have a residual astigmatic refractive error and an epiretinal membrane without macular edema (▶ Fig. 22.18). She was given a trial contact lens to manage the astigmatic error but was still unhappy with her vision quality. She requested an IOL exchange. At surgery (▶ Video 22.6) the multifocal IOL was exchanged for a monofocal toric and BCVA improved to 20/20-, resulting in a happy outcome.

This case illustrates the importance of careful patient selection (epiretinal membrane) and stepwise management of the issues, first correcting the residual optical error with a trial contact lens. Should the latter have satisfied her vision complaints, laser vision correction would have been the appropriate option. However, in this case the best option was to exchange the diffractive optic for a monofocal (toric, in this situation).

22.5 Conclusion

In this chapter we have considered only those problems that are related to **uncomplicated** cataract surgery. Complications can and will occur, but they are the subjects of other chapters. What should be apparent is that dealing with the potentially unhappy (refractive) cataract surgery patient begins **before** surgery with careful evaluation of the patient's needs, lifestyle, and prior method for dealing with presbyopia. Those factors, in association with a comprehensive ocular examination to uncover comorbidities, ocular surface disease, and maculopathy in particular can help guide the surgeon, and in turn the

patient, to the best strategy for success after surgery. That said, there are real potentials for refractive errors and undesired optical imagery (dysphotopsia) that may accompany the best of surgery. The surgeon and patient should form a "partnership" to first determine the source of the problem and then how best to manage it. All too often surgeons are reluctant to appreciate patients' complaints after what appears to be anatomically perfect surgery. But, by making the patient an ally rather than an "enemy," most problems can be overcome. Moreover, should it seem appropriate, seeking a second opinion for the patient can also lead to a satisfactory outcome.

References

[1] Weill Y, Hanhart J, Zadok D, Smadja D, Gelman E, Abulafia A. Patient management modifications in cataract surgery candidates following incorporation of routine preoperative macular optical coherence tomography. J Cataract Refract Surg. 2021; 47(1):78–82

[2] He Y, Li J, Zhu J, Jie Y, Wang N, Wang J. The improvement of dry eye after cataract surgery by intraoperative using ophthalmic viscosurgical devices on the surface of cornea: The results of a consort-compliant randomized controlled trial. Medicine (Baltimore). 2017; 96(50):e8940

[3] Naderi K, Gormley J, O'Brart D. Cataract surgery and dry eye disease: a review. Eur J Ophthalmol. 2020; 30(5):840–855

[4] Gupta PK, Drinkwater OJ, VanDusen KW, Brissette AR, Starr CE. Prevalence of ocular surface dysfunction in patients presenting for cataract surgery evaluation. J Cataract Refract Surg. 2018; 44(9):1090–1096

[5] Starr CE, Gupta PK, Farid M, et al. ASCRS Cornea Clinical Committee. An algorithm for the preoperative diagnosis and treatment of ocular surface disorders. J Cataract Refract Surg. 2019; 45(5):669–684

[6] Villani E, Marelli L, Bonsignore F, et al. The Ocular Surface Frailty Index as a predictor of ocular surface symptom onset after cataract surgery. Ophthalmology. 2020; 127(7):866–873

[7] Ting DSJ, Ghosh S. Acute corneal perforation 1 week following uncomplicated cataract surgery: the implication of undiagnosed dry eye disease and topical NSAIDs. Ther Adv Ophthalmol. 2019; 11:2515841419869508

[8] Watanabe S, Oie Y, Fujimoto H, et al. Relationship between corneal guttae and quality of vision in patients with mild Fuchs' endothelial corneal dystrophy. Ophthalmology. 2015; 122(10):2103–2109

[9] Tester R, Pace NL, Samore M, Olson RJ. Dysphotopsia in phakic and pseudophakic patients: incidence and relation to intraocular lens type(2). J Cataract Refract Surg. 2000; 26(6):810–816

[10] Melles RB, Holladay JT, Chang WJ. Accuracy of intraocular lens calculation formulas. Ophthalmology. 2018; 125(2):169–178

[11] Sudhakar S, Hill DC, King TS, et al. Intraoperative aberrometry versus preoperative biometry for intraocular lens power selection in short eyes. J Cataract Refract Surg. 2019; 45(6):719–724

[12] Hill DC, Sudhakar S, Hill CS, et al. Intraoperative aberrometry versus preoperative biometry for intraocular lens power selection in axial myopia. J Cataract Refract Surg. 2017; 43 (4):505–510

[13] Kane JX, Chang DF. Intraocular lens power formulas, biometry, and intraoperative aberrometry: a review. Ophthalmology. 2020; 13:S0161–6420(20)30789–2

[14] Carmona González D, Palomino Bautista C. Accuracy of a new intraocular lens power calculation method based on artificial intelligence. Eye (Lond). 2021; 35(2):517–522

[15] Chang DF. Disruptive innovation and refractive IOLs: how the game will change with adjustable IOLs. Asia Pac J Ophthalmol (Phila). 2019; 8(6):432–435

[16] Abulafia A, Barrett GD, Kleinmann G, et al. Prediction of refractive outcomes with toric intraocular lens implantation. J Cataract Refract Surg. 2015; 41(5):936–944

[17] Potvin R, Kramer BA, Hardten DR, Berdahl JP. Toric intraocular lens orientation and residual refractive astigmatism: an analysis. Clin Ophthalmol. 2016; 10:1829–1836

[18] Wang L, Shirayama M, Ma XJ, Kohnen T, Koch DD. Optimizing intraocular lens power calculations in eyes with axial lengths above 25.0 mm. J Cataract Refract Surg. 2011; 37 (11):2018–2027

[19] Zhou D, Sun Z, Deng G. Accuracy of the refractive prediction determined by intraocular lens power calculation formulas in high myopia. Indian J Ophthalmol. 2019; 67(4):484–489

[20] Narang P, Agarwal A, Ashok Kumar D. Single-pass four-throw pupilloplasty for Urrets-Zavalia syndrome. Eur J Ophthalmol. 2018; 28(5):552–558

[21] Dick HB. Small-aperture strategies for the correction of presbyopia. Curr Opin Ophthalmol. 2019; 30(4):236–242

[22] Masket S, Geraghty E, Crandall AS, et al. Undesired light images associated with ovoid intraocular lenses. J Cataract Refract Surg. 1993; 19(6):690–694

[23] Holladay JT, Lang A, Portney V. Analysis of edge glare phenomena in intraocular lens edge designs. J Cataract Refract Surg. 1999; 25(6):748–752

[24] Erie JC, Bandhauer MH, McLaren JW. Analysis of postoperative glare and intraocular lens design. J Cataract Refract Surg. 2001; 27(4):614–621

[25] Davison JA. Positive and negative dysphotopsia in patients with acrylic intraocular lenses. J Cataract Refract Surg. 2000; 26(9):1346–1355

[26] Masket S, Rupnick Z, Fram NR, Kwong S, McLachlan J. Surgical management of positive dysphotopsia: U.S. perspective. J Cataract Refract Surg. 2020; 46(11):1474–1479

[27] Masket S, Fram NR. Pseudophakic negative dysphotopsia: surgical management and new theory of etiology. J Cataract Refract Surg. 2011; 37(7):1199–1207

[28] Masket S, Fram NR, Cho A, Park I, Pham D. Surgical management of negative dysphotopsia. J Cataract Refract Surg. 2018; 44(1):6–16

[29] Masket S, Fram NR. Pseudophakic dysphotopsia: review of incidence, cause, and treatment of positive and negative dysphotopsia. Ophthalmology. 2020; 12:S0161–6420(20)30787–9

[30] Osher RH. Negative dysphotopsia: long-term study and possible explanation for transient symptoms. J Cataract Refract Surg. 2008; 34(10):1699–1707

[31] Makhotkina NY, Nijkamp MD, Berendschot TTJM, van den Borne B, Nuijts RMMA. Effect of active evaluation on the detection of negative dysphotopsia after sequential cataract surgery: discrepancy between incidences of unsolicited and solicited complaints. Acta Ophthalmol. 2018; 96(1):81–87

[32] Makhotkina NY, Berendschot TT, Nuijts RM. Objective evaluation of negative dysphotopsia with Goldmann kinetic perimetry. J Cataract Refract Surg. 2016; 42(11):1626–1633

[33] Masket S, Rupnik Z, Fram NR. Neuroadaptive changes in negative dysphotopsia during contralateral eye occlusion. J Cataract Refract Surg. 2019; 45(2):242–243

[34] Masket S, Magdolna Rupnik Z, Fram NR, Vikesland RJ. Binocular Goldmann visual field testing of negative dysphotopsia. J Cataract Refract Surg. 2020; 46(1):147–148

[35] Vámosi P, Csákány B, Németh J. Intraocular lens exchange in patients with negative dysphotopsia symptoms. J Cataract Refract Surg. 2010; 36(3):418–424

[36] Folden DV. Neodymium:YAG laser anterior capsulectomy: surgical option in the management of negative dysphotopsia. J Cataract Refract Surg. 2013; 39(7):1110–1115

[37] Cooke DL, Kasko S, Platt LO. Resolution of negative dysphotopsia after laser anterior capsulotomy. J Cataract Refract Surg. 2013; 39(7):1107–1109

[38] Braga-Mele R, Chang D, Dewey S, et al. ASCRS Cataract Clinical Committee. Multifocal intraocular lenses: relative indications and contraindications for implantation. J Cataract Refract Surg. 2014; 40(2):313–322

Other Cited Material

A, B—Data on file, Alcon Labs (Ft. Worth, TX).

C—Data on file, Johnson and Johnson (Santa Ana, CA).

23 Surgical Pearls

Lisa Brothers Arbisser, Fuxiang Zhang, and Alan Sugar

Abstract

To be a refractive cataract surgeon, first be a great cataract surgeon. I (FZ) am very grateful for this chapter written by my coauthor *Lisa Brothers Arbisser*. I continue learning tips and pearls from Lisa since we met in 1998. This chapter details maneuvers to sharpen our surgical skills for each intraoperative step. She also covers many seemingly "minor," yet important items needing the attention of beginners, such as preoperative preparation, anesthesia, and surgical draping. Efficiency and speed are important for all cataract surgeons, but a great refractive surgery seeks to optimize each step.

Keywords: rhexis rescue, biaxial vitrectomy, vocal local, optic capture, primary posterior capsulorhexis, circumferential disassembly

23.1 Introduction

Refractive surgery success requires surgeon competence, consistency, and empathy. Efficiency demands meticulous attention to detail more than speed. This chapter shares pearls gleaned from three decades of both high-volume refractive and challenging complex cataract cases of one of the authors (LBA). Every surgery and each patient deserves our highest level of skill. With the exception of monocular patients, the stakes are rarely higher than for those who elect spectacle independence. They expect perfect uncorrected acuity, rapid recovery, comfort, and predictable outcomes. Day one postop should be both celebratory and the basis for surgical planning for the second eye.

23.2 Scheduling

I recommend scheduling refractive cataract patients early in the day, saving more unpredictable complex cases for later. It is difficult to apply your best surgical skills when pressured.

23.3 Customizing

Customize your routine preop and postop protocols for individual patient's eyes and comorbidities.

Consider ordering ocular antihypertensives upon discharge for any patient at risk for postoperative pressure spikes. These comorbidities include glaucoma, ocular hypertension, pseudoexfoliation, very dense cataract, narrow angle or shallow anterior chamber (AC), complicated cases, and patients who had a significant postoperative pressure rise after fellow eye surgery. I use an acetazolamide sequel for nonsulfa-allergic patients given once upon discharge. One study found alfentanil also works well.[1]

All of my patients since 2007 have received intracameral moxifloxacin off label. Its use is particularly essential in complicated cases and for same-day sequential bilateral cataract surgery.[2,3]

I order capsular tension rings (CTR) and three-piece implants (along with the standard one piece) for back up for pseudoexfoliation patients. I may choose to optic capture a three-piece lens from the sulcus along with a CTR in the bag as a best option in severe zonulopathy for long-term stability if it won't foil my refractive plans. Beware of patients with asymmetric AC depths unexplained by axial length disparity, as this may signal zonulopathy. Consider intracameral dilation augmentation for small pupils and intraoperative floppy iris syndrome (IFIS) cases. Options include Shugarcane,[4] preservative-free epinephrine, Omidria in the balanced salt solution (BSS) bottle, and topical scopolamine added to the typical dilating regimen of mydriacyl and phenylephrine to help with "staying power," though it won't provide added dilation. Don't hesitate to use Malyugin rings or other pupil devices. Do not stretch IFIS irises and enlarge the pupil only to the size of the circular capsulorhexis (CCC) to avoid damaging the iris sphincter muscle.

Pediatric cataracts and shallow chambered eyes get Healon GV in addition to my usual Duovisc ophthalmic viscosurgical device (OVD) strategy. I reserve Healon 5 (viscoadaptive) for intumescent lenses, providing the most control of the anterior capsule shape to prevent rhexis runout. All patients with intralenticular or posterior pressure benefit from a bolus of intravenous Mannitol 0.25 g/kg pushed 20 minutes prior to incision. It cannot be simply added to the IV but must be pushed as a bolus to achieve the desired osmotic effect. When properly timed, it can make a world of difference in the efficacy and safety of the procedure. Administered too early, the patient may need to void on the table (always have a bedpan or urinal available). Preorder Trypan blue dye for visualization to avoid delays in getting it to the table.

Reinforce anti-inflammatory treatment for patients with uveitis, diabetic retinopathy, macular edema (especially fellow eye cystoid macular edema (CME)), or even just those requiring iris manipulation such as a Malyugin ring. Though off label, I instill 0.1 mL of triamcinolone acetonide (Triessence by Alcon) diluted 1:10 with BSS into the AC at the completion of the case for these individuals. Conceptually we "hide" the inflammatory event from the immune system which will deliver consistently quiet eyes and has not been linked to a steroid response pressure rise. For chronic uveitis, treat as needed to quiet the eye. In all but severe diabetics, consider adding 60 mg of prednisone PO Q AM beginning 2 days preoperative through 4 days postop, an effective regimen requiring no taper.

Thinking ahead about a particular patient's needs will reduce omissions and improve facility efficiency.

23.4 Communication

We depend on patient cooperation for best results. Our active communication quells fear and fills knowledge gaps. Consider consciously practicing psychiatric ophthalmology. Most cases receive topical and intracameral anesthetic without airway control. Even a dedicated and experienced anesthetist can't afford to cause slumber for fear of unconscious (and even combative) patient movement. Make sure the patient understands what is and will happen. "Vocal local" allows sparing use of the anxiolytic and amnestic properties of systemic drugs without resorting to doses or compounds that induced hypnotic sleep. Good intraoperative rapport also promotes patient compliance with postoperative medications and appointments.

We prepare hard of hearing patients preoperatively to expect their hearing aid to be temporarily replaced intraoperatively on the ipsilateral side for a device that allows me to speak directly into their ear with a microphone clipped to my surgical mask. This prevents the draped hearing aid

from squealing and greatly facilitates communication, reducing the need for anesthesia. For those with more profound hearing loss, if I can communicate well with an intelligent patient and a signing interpreter, I offer communication by touch, making topical anesthesia possible, similar to Fuxiang Zhang's described "touch language."[5]

I offer patients' families the opportunity to hear and watch the live televised surgeon's view in a remote room. This provides all an appreciation of the skill and complexity involved in restoring vision.

I select every word for its psychological impact on the patient and to signal efficient progress to my staff (▶ Video 23.1). I've had patients call their experience "fun," and artists have drawn the explosion of colors and images they experienced with interest rather than fear.

23.5 Anesthesia

Office assessment precedes scheduling surgery. Consider peribulbar block for patients unable to fixate on a light or uncooperative for the indirect ophthalmic exam due to blepharospasm, photophobia, or lack of gaze control; they never improve on the table. Reliance on systemic medication for compliance leads to unnecessary complications. If you anticipate sewing iris, requiring large incisions or scleral fixating a lens, peribulbar block is optimal. General anesthesia is reserved for young or uncooperative patients and other rare situations.

Identify and discuss claustrophobia in the office. We have a device which blows air and elevates the drape off the face which need only adhere on the operative side. It, however, occludes the view of the fellow eye so the patient doesn't accidentally perceive and follow movement in the room. Claustrophobic patients can have the drape taped up entirely off the face before starting surgery (except for the part that must stick to the operative periocular area) reducing the closed-in sensation. We ask them to keep the fellow eye closed as much as tolerated. I reassure them by demonstrating this in the office but still ask them to remain NPO for surgery so they can be safely converted to general PRN. I have never needed to convert.

I learned (and taught my anesthesiologist) a single inferior peribulbar injection technique as taught by Howard Gimbel's anesthesiologist Roy Hamilton.[6] We virtually never supplement with a second injection as, even when incomplete, given my expertise with topical, we only need to take the punch out of the squeeze and movement. I've had no complications in over 30 years with this technique (avoiding it in anticoagulated patients). Still, there is no anesthetic as safe as "vocal local."

I employ Propofol only for the moment of peribulbar block. Use Versed (short-acting anxiolytic) and Alfenta (short-acting analgesic less likely to cause nausea than fentanyl) for topical patients. We have a saline lock IV to facilitate this and any emergency measures in all patients.

In routine cases, one might consider a newer cost effective and safe protocol consisting of sublingual Midazolam, Ketamine, Ondansetron (MKO) melt avoiding the need for an IV.[7]

Anesthesia Protocol for Topical Anesthesia for Cataract Surgery for Dr. Lisa Brothers Arbisser:
1. All patients have saline lock.
2. In OR, after monitor hookup, majority of patients receive 1 mg Versed (range 0.5–2 mg).
3. During prep and drape, if patient is tense and squeezes lids then give 125 mg Alfenta and 10 mg Diprivan (Propofol).
   (Alfenta is diluted eight times so final concentration is 2 mL = 125 mg or else volume is too small to push without having to follow with saline.)
4. Intraop, if patient feels pressure or at surgeon's request give 125 µg Alfenta which may be repeated ×1. If patient is still uncomfortable add 10 mg Diprivan (Propofol) with the Alfenta in same syringe ("pinacolada").

Thanks to Dr. Sang Sapthevie (permission obtained).

23.6 Preparedness

When precision is measured in microns nothing replaces muscle memory gained from practice. I strongly recommend the use of eye models such as the SimulEye for practicing every step of cataract surgery. Experience can be gained rapidly and without consequence to patients. By following a routine, I attempt to make each eye behave the same as the last no matter how they differ, resulting in fewer complications. Keeping your focus on a repetitive process also empowers you to see any complication or deviation from routine at its inception, resulting in timely and effective intervention for best outcomes.

23.7 Get Ready for Draping

Once topical anesthetic is instilled, patients should be encouraged to close their eyes as much as possible due to a reduction in blink frequency. If OR protocol has the patient draped with speculum placed by the assistant ahead of the surgeon's presence, a wet cellulose sponge placed on the cornea with an occasional drop of BSS instilled protects the epithelium until surgery actually begins. The sponge aids the patient's adjustment to the microscope light when moved into place by the surgeon.

It is efficient to either schedule ipsilateral eyes consecutively or arrange the machinery in a fashion that doesn't require frequent rearranging when switching sides. This wasn't an issue when we operated superiorly.

Despite preop review of charts, post critical information in full view. Never allow any but the patient's IOLs into the surgical suite. The rest of the day's lenses stay outside, awaiting their intended recipient's entry into the OR.

Presbyopic scrub assistants deserve the clever little autoclavable Osher Magnifier HD (Storz), offering them the acuity for reliable orientation of your irrigating sleeve, accurate loading of IOLs, and detail verification.

When attaching the OVD cannula to the syringe, always fill the hub with BSS first. The small amount of ambient air in the hub cannot be expressed by the OVD in the way it would with a liquid. As a consequence, a bubble will appear unpredictably, often at the most exasperating time, while instilling OVD. This is totally eliminated by having your scrub tech develop this consistent habit.

My draping protocol creates double protection to isolate the lashes and lid margins where the majority of infective organisms reside. A small Tegaderm sheet is cut in half and placed prior to the main drape. The topical anesthesia patient is asked to look down as a cotton tipped applicator is placed superior to the upper tarsus, just under the brow, parallel to the lid margin and rolled or twirled upward allowing friction to do the work of opening the palpebral fissure without any pressure on the globe. This everts the lashes, making them easy to capture with the first half of the Tegaderm. Once the superior lashes are draped, the same maneuver in up gaze twirling in the downward direction everts the lower lid sequestering inferior lashes. This gentle maneuver without downward pressure does not cause the patient to squeeze and doesn't milk the Meibomian glands avoiding debris in the tear film. After the lashes are isolated with the Tegaderm, the standard drape is placed with adequate space to slit it open with a blunt lower jawed scissor. The drape edges are folded backward into the fornix with the speculum, thereby, in effect, double draping the lid margins.

I have tested many specula. Use one that locks into position to prevent the patient compressing it with a squeeze. In addition, it must accommodate variations in anatomy from proptotic to enophthalmic, ideally without putting pressure on the globe. It must not restrict our temporal maneuvers. I have a strong preference for the Koch-Cionni adjustable speculum (Duckworth and Kent). The ubiquitous wire speculum is truly inferior.

A small pearl regarding the oily debris which can sometimes disturb the surgeon's view: Though this is vanishingly rare when one doesn't press on the lid margin while draping, this meibum is impossible to wash away no matter how vigorously it's irrigated. One quick rinse with warmed BSS however makes it instantly disappear, leaving a cleaner surface and a clear view. We keep a 5 mL bottle of BSS handy in the blanket warmer to address this uncommon but disturbing problem.

Communication in the OR begins, but does not end, with patient communication. I believe an important tool for efficiency is that everyone, from the circulator to the scrub tech and anesthesiologist, be on the same page at all times. The staff becomes attentive and finds my consistent and routine "patter" very helpful as it lets them know exactly where I am in the case. In the event of a complication, I simply say "timing." Everyone knows to get the "vit kit" and suspend draping in the other room waiting for further calm direction.

23.8 Epithelial Protection

The integrity of the epithelium is recognized as a critical factor for making preoperative measurements but is often poorly maintained perioperatively. Because preserved topical medications are necessary (unless a "dropless" routine is employed) we only offer nonpreserved tears. I encourage their use as frequently as every hour or

2; just not within 10 minutes of the medicine so they don't cause dilution.

I strongly prefer to coat the cornea with dispersive viscoelastic or Ocucoat just after incision and chamber stabilization. A one-time application of a few drops of BSS smooths it, assuring a uniform view for the entire case. I tell the patient they'll see a kaleidoscope of colors while this is being done and explain we're protecting the eye since they cannot blink. This maneuver prevents the need to irrigate the cornea throughout the case, which is tough on the epithelium and can cause flinching. Poorly timed irrigation, entirely dependent on the judgment and attentiveness of the assistant, can interfere with the surgeon's view during critical moments.

23.9 Incisions

Every step of the cataract procedure impacts the quality of what follows. A properly constructed incision avoids a possible cascade of complications from iris prolapse to endophthalmitis.

Although the historic standard paracentesis incision size is 1 mm, I feel it is essential that, unless we have a chopper or cannula that plugs that incision, we instead aim for a 0.5 mm paracentesis. My average case requires only 50 to 75 mL of BSS in total. It has been shown that up to 22 mL/min can flow through a 1 mm paracentesis when the internal valve is interrupted; say with a chopper. There is no reason to be chasing fragments to the leaking paracentesis. We cannot afford this loss of closed chamber and threat to endothelial integrity. The Centurion (Alcon) has active fluid dynamics which may mitigate this issue to some extent.

I fashion my paracentesis 90 degrees away from my main clear corneal incision (CCI). Although the effect may be minimal, at least I will be canceling out my surgically induced astigmatism (SIA) rather than creating an entirely unpredictable vector between the two. Although we have come to understand that the use of the centroid for toric calculations is superior to the SIA value, I still feel this is justified. This configuration also provides an excellent angle with which to apply mechanical forces and separate nuclear fragments.

The size of the CCI should be snug but not tight, permitting insertion of silicone-sleeved instruments with minimal leak. An oversized, leaking incision results in greater fluid turbulence, an unstable environment, and excess BSS flowing through the AC. An undersized incision restricts irrigation inflow, causing more occlusion surge and the potential for wound burn. A too small stretched incision may also compromise internal Descemet valve integrity, requiring more hydration for closure and providing a less secure barrier to inflow in the early postoperative period—a risk for endophthalmitis.

Remember the stroma is elastic, and Descemet membrane is not. This is why stretched wounds become incompetent, requiring copious stromal hydration and a high intraocular pressure to appear closed. As intraocular pressure rapidly falls to normal and stromal hydration resolves over just a few hours, such incisions can "suck" or leak, leading to severe complications.

Our goal is to approximate a square incision; this is shown to be strongest. If the blade enters too early, the tunnel may not be long enough to resist deformation or may lead to iris prolapse. A too long tunnel causes an awkward angle for our instruments, with oar-locking producing view-disturbing striae. We never want to encroach on the visual axis for fear of lasting, if subtle, irregular astigmatism. Although inherent scleral rigidity varies, the biggest factor in our control is intraocular pressure. We must establish a consistent intraocular pressure with our instillation of OVD right after the paracentesis and before we perform the CCI. When the eye is overpressurized, the tunnel will end up too short, when underpressurized, too long. Getting comfortable and consistent with this maneuver will allow a more consistently shaped and secure incision and better outcomes overall.

My preferred scalpel is a diamond trapezoidal blade (Arbisser-Fine Triamond blade from Mastel; no financial interest). This thin precision blade is capable of making any size incision from 0.3 to any size needed as defined by a dedicated marker (► Fig. 23.1) (► Video 23.2). Despite the choice of blade, Howard Fine described remaining in one intrastromal plane that follows the shape of the cornea and then dips slightly to enter Descemet in a straight line parallel to the Iris. This is my preference.[8]

Never instrument the incision, but rather use OVD to open it anytime that might prove necessary. When introducing anything through the main temporal CCI, I use a cannula or sweep through the side port for countertraction and stability.

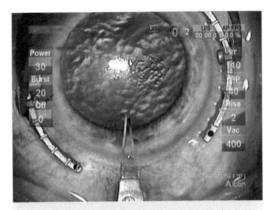

Fig. 23.1 Arbisser-Fine Triamond diamond blade incision (Mastel Precision Surgical Instruments. No financial interest for LBA).

I buck the trend for wound closure by not primarily depending on lateral stromal hydration. I irrigate the tunnel to clear debris from between the lips of the internal Descemet membrane valve and tunnel. Then I stromal hydrate the roof of the incision sufficiently for floor and ceiling to meet effecting wound closure. Although this may require modest lateral hydration in some cases, the key is an OVD and fragment-free tunnel and a thickened incisional roof meeting incisional floor. This will achieve a solid closure of a properly constructed and unstretched CCI confirmed by a dry gutter at normal pressure. The technique also reveals any errant and hidden lens fragments (► Video 23.3). Adjust the pressure to normal through the paracentesis which is treated in a similar fashion to the main CCI (one can use an intraoperative tonometer until experience allows just touch for assessment) and confirm the dry gutter with a cellulose sponge. One can use a fluorescein strip for confirmation, but I find this unnecessary. Once closed, only pinpoint pressure on the posterior lip will threaten incision integrity. Even if the eye becomes hypotensive, the incision will not "suck." If, for any reason, the incision will not close under these circumstances, I will not hydrate further but choose to supplement with a suture or glue.

23.10 Endothelial Protection

In refractive cataract surgery there is no tolerance for corneal edema. Critical to RCS is the status of the cornea not only at one month, but at one day postop. Beyond huge attention to all the parameters in the prevention of toxic anterior segment syndrome (TASS), more subtle methods of promoting endothelial integrity must be practiced.[9]

In phacoemulsification we use a microscopic jackhammer between two delicate membranes. To address this, Dr. Steven Arshinoff gave us the wonderful technique of "soft shell" using a dispersive viscoelastic under the cornea, ironed into place by a cohesive viscoelastic posterior to it.[10] I find Duovisc (Alcon) cost effective for routine cases offering me both OVDs.

In longer, denser cases, if sensing a loss of protection, reinstill dispersive viscoelastic through the paracentesis with the phaco tip held steadily in place in foot position zero. The goal is to fill the AC completely with the dispersive OVD so it fills into itself, eliminating visibility issues. Be absolutely certain to establish flow in foot position 2 before engaging foot position 3 to avoid wound burn.

If you protect the cornea, it will be clear the next day—even if you're dealing with 5 + brunescent lenses. Reducing turbulence and ultrasound time with a noncontinuous phaco strategy along with torsional ultrasound to improve followability and reduce chatter is another protective factor detailed below. There are many ways to harm the cornea: wasted ultrasound power, ultrasound too near the endothelium rather than at the iris plane, ricocheting lens particles, chamber bounce, and excessive flow of BSS through the eye associated with leaky incisions. Most of these can be mitigated by technique.

I always record my cumulative dispersed energy (CDE) (Alcon) or effective phaco time (EPT) (J&J) as well as the density of the nucleus for two reasons. One is medicolegal, but the other is for my continuous learning curve. You can track the efficiency and consistency of your ultrasound use and find ways to predictably reduce it if you try. One also learns to be consistent in judging density which helps to set the ultrasound parameters for efficiency. Reviewing your videoed cases improves your technique.

23.11 Visualization

Staying in focus helps surgeons know where the phaco tip is vertically located. Neophyte surgeons' fear of breaking the capsule causes unconscious raising of the phaco tip closer to the cornea, endangering endothelium. Maintaining the microscope in centered and focused position throughout the case will make a world of difference. We cannot control what we cannot see.

Staining poorly visualized anterior capsule assists our efficiency and reduces complications. There are many uses for the dye: the white or brunescent cataract, corneal scars or haze obstructing the view, absent red reflex due to posterior segment anomalies, questionable anterior capsule integrity, non-free-floating post femtolaser capsulotomy and to reduce capsule elasticity. Not all are likely to be refractive cataract cases but, whenever IOL fixation and centration are dependable, even in complex situations, toric- or even presbyopia-correcting strategies can be considered. The refractive cataract surgeon must be prepared for all contingencies. We know Trypan Blue dye can stiffen elastic pediatric cataract capsule by permanently changing its molecular structure without knowledge of the long-term consequences. In these cases, I use a retentive OVD such as Healon GV, change the vector to a more centripetal direction, and proceed cautiously.

Commercially available Trypan blue is nontoxic to the corneal endothelium, but higher concentrations demonstrate toxicity. Low concentrations have been used to identify endothelial cells in eye banking. Trypan blue was introduced to be used under an air bubble, but air is actually toxic. Some surgeons fill the AC with the dye and then exchange it for OVD. I believe the best way to apply Trypan blue is to first place the OVD soft shell, controlling the chamber but leaving the eye a little soft. Then irrigate the Trypan through an Osher dye cannula (Storz), one with a hole on the underside rather than at the tip. This facilitates "painting" a layer of dye onto the surface of the lens underneath the OVD. I wait at least one minute (by the clock, as it can seem like an hour) for adequate uptake and then move it out of the way with more OVD from distal to proximal essentially evacuating the dye. This won't create an extremely deep stain but achieves adequate visualization. One can place a copious amount or leave it in place longer and the stain will be more robust.

Soon Phaik Chee has shown that when a discrete cortical opacity in the path of a rhexis obscures the view, dye is unnecessary. The opacity is not anchored in place within the cortical layer and can be "milked" to the periphery with a sweep placed flatly on the intact anterior capsule. A sweeping motion, surprisingly, provides a clear view of the capsulorhexis progression, obviating the need for dye in these unusual cases.[11]

23.12 Continuous Circular Capsulorhexis (CCC)

A symmetric CCC, appropriately sized to the lens optic, promotes lens centration and a stable and predictable refractive error. Although these benefits extend to every IOL, they are critical for toric implant stability. Covering the IOL's truncated edge may improve long-term dysphotopsia risk as well as reduce posterior capsule opacification. An incomplete CCC dramatically increases the risk of a cascade of intraoperative complications. A CCC just smaller than the size of the optic is an essential safety net for IOL stability in the face of posterior capsule complications, allowing optic capture techniques.

Centering the CCC and, ultimately, the IOL is important, especially for multifocal IOLs. Understand the Purkinje images and your microscope and take advantage of the patient's ability to fixate under topical anesthesia. Although femtolaser assisted cataract surgery (FLACS) usually results in a capsulotomy that covers the edges of a centered IOL, this is not always the result. Since centration is done during docking and not by patient gaze or images, we have little control over this result. One technology that deserves consideration is the Zepto precision pulse capsulotomy device (Centricity Vision; author is a minor stockholder). The surgeon centers the device on the patient's line of sight creating a reproducibly sized and round capsulotomy with an even stronger edge than a manual rhexis. CapsuLaser is another automated device with fixation centration, though not FDA approved.

By the time we create the rhexis, we have a feel for the patient's ability to cooperate. Although I routinely use a partial ring fixation device for the incisions, it's rare to need manual fixation for the CCC. I usually just communicate the critical moment of CCC to the patient saying: "hold steady just as you've been doing, especially for the next minute or so." As long as you regrasp whenever the vector is no longer optimal, unpredicted movement will result in a too small rhexis (easily fixed) and not tear out.

Because of variations in white-to-white diameter and pupil dilation, an independent reference must be used to size the rhexis. I prefer not to mark the cornea as many do with an RK marker; pristine epithelium recovers faster. Perhaps you have a system with a reticule in the microscope for reference but I simply hover above the cornea with calipers centered on the pupil set to 5 mm for a 6 mm optic and 6 mm for a Crystalens. Although there is some trivial inaccuracy due to parallax, in a second, I've noticed how far the edge of the rhexis will need to be from the edge of this particular patient's dilated pupil. My mind's eye "sees" the goal.

I puncture the capsule with a sharp bent cystotome. In the same fluid movement, with a superficial forward pushing motion, I raise a flap of capsule in a curvilinear manner, and then manage the flap with forceps. When the initial opening is curvilinear rather than radial, if there is any intralenticular or posterior pressure potentially causing the tear to spontaneously progress, it will tear inward rather than outward.

Some surgeons prefer to make a needle rhexis without forceps, but they switch to forceps whenever faced with a truly challenging capsulorhexis. I prefer to use the most controllable method in every case as one doesn't always know when one might be challenged.

I initiate the tear along the nasal border of the CCC (distal to my temporal incision) and progress in a counterclockwise direction. I believe we have the least control over the vector subincisionally and prefer to establish the vector with the best view and most comfortable hand position.

Attend to the actual radius of the capsule flap, always constant. Don't assume one can easily gauge the actual diameter of the circle being created. I am further guided by my mental image of how closely to approach the pupil margin from the caliper placement a moment before. Once I establish this first quadrant radius, and assuming a symmetrically dilated pupil, I can follow the pupil edge for completion. With an asymmetric pupil, stay focused on the symmetry of the radius for each quadrant and not on the capsulotomy edge. One can recheck with the external caliper as you go or use a laser-marked CCC forceps like the one I developed for ASICO in the 1990s (no financial interest).

With topical anesthesia, I enlist the patient's help to stay central and planar with the microscope by asking them to "stand your ground and don't be dragged away from the light of the microscope."

Regrasp every time the vector is not optimal (about once per quadrant on average). If the patient suddenly moves, the rhexis ends up prematurely small instead of tearing out into the periphery. I always err on the small side as it is easy to enlarge the CCC with a tangential cut and a spiraling forceps motion once the lens is implanted to perfect the shape and size of the capsulorhexis with the optic under it as a template (▸ Video 23.4).

Concentrate your attention during CCC enabling you to recognize within a degree or two the vector going awry. At the first sign of an unpredictable tear direction, not corrected by regrasping, immediately withdraw and instill OVD over the capsule periphery at the crux of the errant portion of the flap and not centrally (▸ Video 23.5). Do not redeepen the AC by placing OVD in the center. Ideally this will halt the tear and allow what has become known as the "Little rhexis rescue maneuver," pulling the flap in the opposite or backward direction in the plane of the capsule to reestablish the correct vector completing the CCC.[12]

Correct an errant rhexis before it reaches the pupil edge; however, use an Iris hook for visualization. If needed, paint the capsule at the crux of the tear with a small amount of Trypan blue with the Osher cannula under the OVD. Wait a minute then move the blue cloud out of the way with more OVD. This reduces the elasticity of the capsule making it more responsive to the "Little maneuver" and also, of course, improving visualization of the actual edge of the tear (▸ Video 23.6).

If a tear has progressed into the equatorial zonular network it cannot be safely recovered. Approach instead from the other direction. Create a new flap, if necessary, to initiate the now clockwise progression of rhexis to finish just outside of the defect for continuity. If the capsulotomy is no longer continuous, all subsequent maneuvers must accommodate this suboptimal condition.

Zonular laxity, recognized by striae created upon attempts to puncture the capsule for rhexis initiation, can cause the tear to proceed unpredictably often requiring more frequent regrasping.

Beware of anteriorly inserting zonules (most commonly seen in myopic eyes) which can hinder the progression of the tear.

Knowledge of OVD rheology helps in their selection. Shallow chambered eyes deserve a more retentive cohesive OVD such as Healon GV to achieve space under conditions of low shear during the CCC. Intumescent cataracts, with intralenticular pressure, benefit most from the use of the viscoadaptive Healon 5 flattening the shape of the anterior capsule most effectively. These cohesives replace the standard Provisc for the soft shell under the ubiquitous dispersive OVD protecting the endothelium just for the CCC. I don't aspirate lens milk after puncturing the intumescent capsule as the intralenticular pressure may be loculated. I prefer to move it aside with dispersive OVD to facilitate visualization as the tear progresses in order to keep the chamber constantly controlled. I've never experienced an Argentinian flag sign (where the tear extends spontaneously to the equator in two directions) in my career using these techniques (▸ Video 23.7).

For these more challenging cases, patience is rewarded. Investing time in your rhexis avoids more time devoted to subsequent complications.

Just a word regarding femtosecond laser capsulotomy flap removal. This automation creates a perfectly round capsulotomy, but not with 100% assurance of a free-floating flap. In cases with potential remaining tags, my central dimple-down maneuver is safe and effective. Immediately following a small paracentesis, instill OVD to first control the chamber. Then use its cannula to press down centrally on the capsule flap to dislodge any attachment. This in effect creates a 360-degree "Little maneuver." We do not know where the tag is attached, and therefore in what direction to pull centripetally for safe completion. Pushing downward centrally will bring any tag in the right direction. My paper coauthor Burkhard Dick, who has done many more FLACS than I, never had a tear-out after employing the dimple-down technique[13] (▸ Video 23.8).

23.13 Hydrodissection and Hydrodelineation

Hydrodissection frees lens contents from the capsular bag mobilizing the nucleus, avoiding stress on the zonules. Freeing the nucleus is essential for most phaco disassembly techniques as well as for clean cortical removal. Hydrodissection is often taught as simple irrigation with a cannula through the CCI. Emphasis is appropriately on the tip's placement under the anterior capsular rim, and all ophthalmologists are taught to watch the fluid wave cross the nucleus' midline and exit peripherally. Hydrodissection should be understood as a more complexly nuanced maneuver beyond simple irrigation.

23.14 LBA's Seesaw Hydrodissection Technique

My technique for hydrodissection always involves a subtle seesaw ballottement of the nucleus using the posterior incision lip as the fulcrum during BSS injection. This avoids fluid entrapment tamponade causing either capsule blow out or iris prolapse. Once the cannula tip is correctly placed under the distal CCC rim, a slight downward movement of the cannula tip (once it is seated in the correct plane) pushes the nucleus slightly posteriorly, thereby "burping" the capsular bag and encouraging the fluid to dissect around the equator rather than building posterior pressure risking blowout. Alternate this downward movement with an equally subtle lifting of the cannula tip applying slight downward pressure on the posterior lip of the CCI burping the AC to avoid anterior pressure risking iris prolapse.

Posterior capsular blowout causes ruptures in a split second (pun intended). It is often not recognized until the tear extends as the eye is pressurized by insertion of the phaco tip, and the nucleus is lost to the posterior segment. Large dense lenses or hyperopic shallow segments face the most risk.

Seesaw hydrodissection slightly opens the internal valve of the CCI and allows controlled egress of irrigated fluid, avoiding explosive pressure change. Iris prolapse, particularly in eyes with intraoperative floppy iris syndrome, can cause pigment loss and atonicity of the stroma, leading to intraoperative difficulties as well as postoperative visual aberrations.

I employ a McCool flat 25-gauge cannula (Storz) on a 5-mL syringe for hydrodissection. This cannula's flattened irrigating tip creates a broad stream of fluid that is easy to place in the desired plane. All solutions are irrigated through micropore filters in my OR.

My goal is to free the nucleus and epinucleus separately (hydrodelineation) when the cataract is immature and together when the cataract is dense and there is no clear endonuclear plane.

Howard Fine described an efficient way of evacuating cortex during phaco called cortical-cleaving hydrodissection. He placed the hydrodissection cannula tip directly under the capsule.[14] I prefer to use I&A routinely, as his technique often leaves behind thin wisps of cortex which cannot adequately occlude the standard 0.3-mm opening of the I/A port required to build peristaltic vacuum. Residual sticky wisps must be forcefully irrigated off the capsule or manually removed under OVD with a 26- gauge cannula. This can be more time-consuming and riskier in my hands. If one prefers cleaving, consider a 0.2-mm I/A port.

After standard hydrodissection, nuclear and epinuclear evacuation with the phaco tip leaves more substantial amounts of residual cortex. This facilitates optimal cortex removal with the I/A handpiece. Always engage the anterior edge of cortex to facilitate clean stripping. Initiating removal from the posterior edge of a cortical remnant often leaves behind wisps. Although a radial vector for removal is tempting, a more tangential direction of pull is easier on zonules and allows a hurricane-like action which is highly efficient.[15]

Hydrodelineation is essential for soft, immature cataracts (or clear lens exchange) and posterior polar cataracts. Our goal is to create a "golden ring" signaling separation of endonucleus and epinucleus. This is achieved by digging into the central anterior cortex with our hydrodissection cannula to define that natural plane and irrigate BSS somewhat forcefully. "Inside out hydrodelineation" as described by Abhay Vasavada is a foolproof method to achieve this goal but I generally find it unnecessary.[16] Hydrodelineation facilitates chop techniques without any need for sculpting. For immature lenses, vacuum alone will remove the nucleus once dissected. Phaco chop, sometimes thought useful only in dense lenses, is actually highly efficient and effective in soft lenses prepared with hydrodelineation. The remaining epinucleus acts like a bandage avoiding posterior capsule rupture by the ultimate capsular-cortical adhesion (the posterior polar defect) which can then be peeled away in a safe manner.

Hydrodissection's goal is to mobilize the nucleus. Beware if it is difficult to achieve an adequate fluid wave or the nucleus isn't subsequently easily rotated. This signals significant peripheral cortical-capsular adhesion or poor zonular integrity. Never force rotation. Several options exist. First, try multidirectional hydrodissection by using a Binkhorst-hooked cannula, left and right (Storz) to create the fluid wave from the subincisional direction. If this doesn't loosen the nucleus, then a two-handed approach to rotation may be gently attempted. If the lens cannot be easily rotated, it is prudent to use an in situ vertical chop technique. Hemisections are created. Next a distal quadrant is chopped and removed leaving room to push the proximal quadrant distally in the bag without rotation to complete nuclear removal. One can also consider placing capsule suspension hooks along the CCC edge to support the lens and make any intralenticular movement totally independent of the zonular network.

23.15 Anterior Chamber Stability

AC stability is underrated. Trampolining of the chamber and associated movement of the vitreous body may increase the incidence of pseudophakic retinal detachment by stressing not only zonules but also the attachment of the vitreous base to the thinnest and most vulnerable part of the retina. Chamber collapse, and aggressive reexpansion, stresses zonules and may detach the Wiegert ligament allowing misdirection of fluid and increasing the propensity for complications.[17] Collapse of the chamber and aggressive redeepening as well as high fluidic parameters facilitate the ingress of potentially contaminated fluids from the ocular surface and the escape of lens particles into the Berger space. Maintenance of positive pressure discourages rock hard eye syndrome and choroidal effusion or hemorrhage, particularly in very short eyes. We have all learned to instill viscoelastic through the side port when there is a broken capsule before withdrawal of the phaco tip to avoid vitreous prolapse. I believe we should apply this principle, irrigating BSS not OVD, upon irrigating handpiece removal even in our routine cataract surgery cases.

Chamber collapse is common in distensible myopic eyes and in shallow chambered hyperopic eyes. It remains unpredictable in average eyes. Variations of incision integrity, posterior pressure, and scleral rigidity all play a role. The chamber is most likely to shallow upon removal of the phaco tip or the I/A tip from the eye and again, immediately following OVD removal after IOL placement.

Therefore, I would like to describe how I mitigate or eliminate AC collapse routinely.

Although this goal can be achieved with a chamber maintainer, this requires a second source of irrigation, an extra incision, and attention to when it must be turned on and off. I mimic a maintainer's effect with BSS in a 5-mL syringe with a 26-g cannula manually irrigated with my nondominant hand through the paracentesis whenever an irrigating instrument is removed threatening chamber collapse. These particular moments are further described below in detail. (I always attach a Millipore filter on any irrigation solution intended for the AC.)

At the conclusion of phaco, before withdrawing the tip from the incision, the scrub nurse (tech) exchanges my chopper for a BSS syringe. I irrigate fluid manually through the paracentesis as I withdraw the phaco (and similarly when finished with the I&A tip), cause the internal Descemet valve to seal, or, in some cases just continuously irrigating for chamber maintenance. This maintains positive pressure for the few seconds it takes to get the next irrigating handpiece or OVD in place through the main incision. This maintains physiologic chamber depth continuously throughout the case.

The syringe's cannula in the nondominant hand through the paracentesis doubles as an instrument like a sweep (when I'm not irrigating), permitting bimanual control of the globe during I/A. Similarly, I irrigate again upon withdrawing the I/A tip until OVD has been used through the main incision to secure the chamber prior to IOL insertion. The same syringe is then used to irrigate the main CCI free of debris prior to OVD removal after IOL insertion to prevent AC collapse and potential IOL-corneal touch in a widely dilated pupil.

Almost as important as preventing chamber collapse is preventing overdeepening of the AC, especially in the detachment-prone myope or the previously vitrectomized eye. Reverse pupillary block where the pupil edge contacts the anterior capsule flap for 360 degrees preventing fluid from distributing between the anterior and posterior chambers causing extreme chamber deepening. In the at-risk eye (pars plana vitrectomy, loose zonules, or myopia) I place a small space occupying bolus of dispersive OVD between the iris and the anterior capsule rim in 1 or 2 clock hours nasally when filling the chamber with OVD after hydrodissection and before entry with the phaco tip.

I lower the irrigation (or forced infusion) and enter the OVD-filled chamber on foot position 0. Prior to initiating irrigation, I insinuate the tip of the nondominant hand instrument (chopper) on its side between the pupil edge and the anterior capsule where the OVD allows me space. I slightly lift the iris away from the capsule with the chopper preventing reverse block occlusion in this small area, enough to eliminate deepening entirely. It is widely known that this maneuver of lifting the iris (or depressing the anterior capsule rim) can resolve the deepening once it occurs, but few surgeons prevent this very predictable event.

The moment foot position 1 is applied, the bottle or infusion is raised to the usual homeostatic level for the routine fluidic settings. One must take great care that foot position 2 (aspiration) is entered and flow established (it just takes a second or two) before going into foot position 3 (ultrasound) to prevent wound burn.

This prophylactic maneuver avoids the pain felt by the patient on sudden deepening, spares stress on zonules, and allows a normal and unchanging plane for the angle of the phaco tip. Complications occur when the artificially deep chamber necessitating a more acute phaco handpiece angle of attack suddenly and unpredictably shallows, exposing the posterior capsule to trauma (▶ Video 23.9).

23.16 Avoiding Iris Prolapse

Maintain normotension whenever possible. Hypotony is toxic to the eye. Although a high pressure can be tolerated, it poses risks both intraoperatively and postoperatively. Never allow the iris to fully prolapse through the incision but, rather, strive to identify it as it begins to enter the tunnel. This is the ideal time to lower the intraocular pressure by burping the side port but not the incision. If still required, reposit iris by sweeping from the paracentesis, not poking backward through the incision. Any breach of Descemet valve can cause further iris prolapse. If this happens early in the case, keep the previously prolapsed iris depressed and covered with dispersive OVD whenever instruments enter the incision. Never exit the incision on foot position 1 (irrigating) but only foot position 0. If the iris prolapses more than once, consider closing the incision and creating a new clear corneal incision remote from the damaged iris, perhaps with a longer tunnel.

Never fill the chamber in this situation with viscoelastic from distal to proximal promoting prolapse (▶ Video 23.10).

A homeostatic chamber depth lessens influx of surface debris, discourages misdirection of fluids, reduces iris damage, and stress on zonules, ciliary body, as well as the vitreous base. The described maneuvers lead to more comfortable patients intraoperatively. quieter eyes perioperatively, and fewer long-term retinal and corneal sequelae.

23.17 Fluidics

Do not "set it and forget it." You are the captain of the ship. Be intimately familiar with your phacoemulsification machine. It is beyond the scope of this chapter, but I highly recommend an excellent review article by L. Benjamin.[18] Efficiency and followability can be modulated without ultrahigh settings that overwhelm zonular attachments and push lens material into the Berger space. Understand the differences and benefits of peristaltic versus venturi pumps and when it might be good to toggle between the two. The nuances are endless but, knowing what to do, especially when things aren't going right, how to minimize surge and maximize followability are essential to becoming the expert cataract surgeon your patients deserve.

23.18 Phacoemulsification for Vertical Chop with Burst Mode

There are many techniques for phacoemulsification. Most surgeons employ the techniques they were trained in. This author (LBA) learned phaco while in practice, being trained in the intracapsular and extracapsular days. My technique, used on tens of thousands of cataracts, has worked well and is perhaps worth your consideration. It is effective for every lens density, even those that, with hydrodelineation, are so soft they simply suck up without ultrasound. The technique I will describe is especially helpful for the brunescent lens which causes so many surgeons to struggle.

Although there are other excellent phaco platforms and strategies, I'm most experienced with the Alcon machines. Vertical chop without any sculpting is my procedure of choice. Divide and conquer is energy inefficient, horizontal chop requires the second-hand chopper to leave the safe zone within the CCC traveling out to the equator outside the surgeon's view inviting complication.

23.18.1 Phaco Machine Settings

Ozil (torsional ultrasound) is ideal for sculpting as it makes a wider trough than longitudinal phaco; a true advantage for divide-and-conquer techniques. Ozil segment removal offers superior followability as it mitigates repulsive forces compared to traditional longitudinal phaco, making it ideal for fragment removal. For these same reasons Ozil is inefficient for the disassembly phase of chop techniques because it makes a wider hole and instantly "eats" whatever it touches, discouraging holdability.

Less used today, Burst Mode with longitudinal phaco remains best for the disassembly phase of vertical chop in lenses of all densities in my hands. In continuous Ozil the linearity in foot position 3 controls ultrasound power so you are only potentially clogging with too little power to be effective until you progress low enough into foot position 3 to get to the right power for the particular nucleus density. Worse, conversely, in a soft lens it is not difficult to go too far too fast into the nucleus toward the posterior capsule if you are heavy footed and end up with a complication. Regardless of lens density it is almost impossible not to travel just a fraction too long in foot position 3 and "eat" what you're trying to hold for the chop maneuver.

Chop is an energy-sparing technique, as ultrasound is never used continuously. Time in foot position 3 is only staccato and never constant. Ultrasound has two purposes in chop: to grab onto the nucleus, holding it steady for disassembly by the second-hand instrument and to assist aspiration flow avoiding clogging while removing lens fragments.

I do make full use of Ozil in all but brunescent lenses for the fragment removal phase of vertical chop (especially once IP was added where longitudinal is automatically thrown into the motion when a micro clog develops). In the standard density lens, while the nucleus is held steady by the imbedded phaco tip, the second-hand instrument applies mechanical forces dividing it through the posterior plate into four or more manageable sections that won't threaten the endothelium. To accomplish this hold on the nucleus, burst mode (with longitudinal phaco) allows a measured approach to diving into the lens at the right depth and then maintaining that hold. The burst interval rather than the ultrasound power percentage is under foot pedal linear control. At the top of foot position 3 the bursts are far enough apart to give the needed time to exquisitely control stopping the progress into the meat of the nucleus and also holding it there by easing off into foot position 2. Equally important, Burst Mode allows panel setting of the US power percentage appropriate to the nuclear density in available memory settings. Tailoring power to the cataract's density helps control the phaco tip travel down into the nucleus, facilitating occlusion for the chop. I record cataract density on the schedule. For example, if a 3+ nucleus is scheduled, the scrub chooses my memory 2 setting which I have preset with 40% ultrasound. Rarely is adjustment required. Having that appropriate power immediately upon engaging foot position 3 (ultrasound) saves cumulative use of phaco energy in dense lenses, and prevents inadvertent deep travel into a soft nucleus. I use memory 3 for brunescent nuclei where I've set a 70% phaco power as a good starting point. I have never used over 40 seconds of CDE in the most brunescent lens with my technique.

When operating on truly brunescent lenses, Ozil can prove superfluous. It requires extensive toggling between disassembly and removal, given that my technique of circumferential disassembly requires peeling sections out of the center of the dense nucleus and removing them repeatedly. Circumferential disassembly leaves the leathery posterior fibers intact to protect the bag until sufficiently thinned to fold in and be easily removed without threatening endothelial integrity. Ozil is less useful for very brunescent lenses also because IP automatically engages longitudinal phaco almost continuously to avoid clogging.

My version of vertical chop sometimes includes a cross action maneuver rather than the standard chop. This means that rather than lift the piece of nucleus held by the phaco tip (which requires constant vacuum in foot position 2) while pushing down and away on the section to be chopped with the chopper, I often place the chopper on the far side of where the phaco tip is embedded and push that hemisection-to-be away in an "X" pattern, all in the same plane. This is more forgiving of potentially losing suction by not staying perfectly in foot position 2 and accomplishes the division of the two sections anyway. There is less likelihood for lens tilt with this cross-action maneuver compared to the standard phaco chop version. This hard to describe maneuver is best appreciated in the linked video.

23.18.2 Circumferential Disassembly Technique

Brunescent lenses are best handled without chopping down through the posterior plate. Leathery endonuclear sections of brunescent fibers are debulked and stripped away, thinning the nucleus from the inside out during multiple rotations. Ultrasound is again only necessary to assist aspiration during fragment removal while the second hand guides the pieces to the phaco tip and "stuffs them in" (without of course allowing touch between instruments). The thinned brunescent "nucleofied" epinucleus remains to protect the posterior capsule and expand the bag, often associated with weak zonules, until the final moments when it folds in on itself and is removed at the iris plane.

In standard density lenses all disassembly is accomplished first, leaving sections to protect the posterior capsule and keep it expanded followed by the switch from burst to continuous Ozil—most efficient for removing all sections. Occasionally, toggling back and forth as the individual lens removal most naturally dictates, works better with removal of some fragments as they become available and then returning to Burst mode for further disassembly. This is accomplished seamlessly with the foot pedal side-kick enabled or can be done by the scrub at verbal request.

With experience, these techniques require very low CDE. A mature surgeon can predict the CDE based on the nuclear density and, conversely, predict what the lens density had been based on the CDE used. Consistency goes hand in hand with a low complication rate and clear corneas. These principles allowed 94% of day one postop patients to have sufficiently clear corneas to refract to 20/25 or better (assuming full visual potential of course) in this author's hands (LBA) and permitted us to refract patients on day one and begin to plan for the second eye if needed. Also, in general, my techs couldn't tell the difference between a brunescent lens and a 2+ at the slit lamp on day one postop: a goal worth striving for (▶ Video 23.11).

23.19 Irrigation and Aspiration

Thorough cortical removal leads to faster recovery, better centration, less cystoid macular edema, and a lower Nd-YAG capsulotomy rate. I prefer a 45-degree bent tip and a silicone sleeve that lets me take care of subincisional cortex without a bimanual approach. Confirm proper sleeve position relative to the I/A tip. A sleeve that is too far back causes irrigation into the tunnel, leading to wound hydration and chamber instability. If the sleeve is too far forward, it impedes cortical occlusion of the port. Use the irrigating cannula through the paracentesis as described above during irrigation and aspiration (IA) to stabilize the globe. Anytime we have two hands controlling the topically anesthetized eye, we are safer.

Always remove the subincisional cortex first while the bulk of the cortex expands the capsular fornix, making this ergonomically tougher area more accessible. Taking a sequential and systematic approach from subincisional then clockwise half-way to nasal and then subincisional counterclockwise back toward the nasal quadrant avoids missing any hidden sector of cortex.

Always engage cortex from the anterior edge of the remnant and not the posterior part attached to the capsule for cleaner stripping. Linear vacuum is helpful, though the capsule vacuum mode can be very useful to safely "fish" for nonvisualized residual wisps peripheral to the CCC edge. Once cortex is engaged, with vacuum building, one will hear the occlusion tone signaling it is time to immediately change to standard I/A vacuum to strip it away within the rhexis safe zone. Linear vacuum can be used for this maneuver rather than toggling back and forth between vacuum and full I/A setting but requires nuanced foot pedal control.

Don't hesitate to gently retract iris to visually confirm a clean bag. Very dense and white cataracts often look clean since there is no central cortex but retain the cortex in the periphery which should be removed to promote a quiet postoperative course (▶ Fig. 23.2).

Although bimanual I&A is ubiquitous outside the United States, coaxial became the standard here. I prefer to avoid the extra incision except in complicated cases with vitreous prolapse. Separating the irrigation from the aspiration keeps the higher pressure anteriorly while targeting residual cortex at any clock hour. Bimanual I/A can be

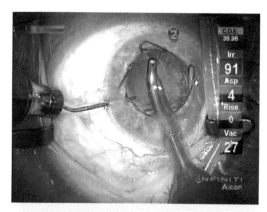

Fig. 23.2 Bent I/A tip finding hidden cortex in mature cataract.

helpful for stubborn subincisional cortex or in FLACS where the cortex is sometimes welded to the CCC edge.

23.20 Dealing with Complications

The only way to avoid complications of cataract surgery entirely is not to do cataract surgery. For most surgeons the entry into refractive cataract surgery means that one already has a significant volume under one's belt. The higher the volume, the less likely we are to have complications. As we apply skills for vitrectomy infrequently, we must be certain that our entire staff has in mind what's needed. I recommend practice by periodically calling a "code V." Ask your industry representative for one clean vitrectomy pack for practice. Be certain everyone knows how to attach it and what the ideal machine settings are. Also, rarely used additional instruments, medications, sutures, IOL styles, etc., which I loosely refer to as the "vit kit," must be sterilized and locatable.

Whatever your experience or preferred incisional approach for anterior vitrectomy, be it biaxial anterior incisions or, as I have taught for years, one port pars plana incision with irrigation anteriorly, establish a precise protocol prior to the moment of crisis.[19]

The earlier a complication is recognized and limited, the better the results. A torn posterior capsule with an intact anterior hyaloid, converted to a continuous posterior capsulorhexis, uniformly results in optimal outcomes. Rupture of the hyaloid membrane with prolapse of vitreous into the AC changes the risk of late complications because we now face posterior segment harm. We will forever deal with a one chambered eye. Once vitreous is lost through incisions, there's a greater likelihood of retinal tear or detachment and another set of actions is indicated to provide a stable intraocular environment. Depending on the timing, this may be associated with residual lens remnants which must be isolated from vitreous for removal or left for another surgery. An ounce of prevention is meaningfully worth a pound of cure.

Our anterior vitrectomy strategy must be based upon a set of cardinal principles that can't be violated. Avoid intraoperative and postoperative vitreous traction since the peripheral retina is 100 times thinner than posterior retina and prone to tears and detachment.[20] Maneuvering instruments and devices through vitreous, as well as improper settings, promotes traction. Although classically taught, using a sweep from the side port to drag entrapped vitreous out of the main incision actually increases traction through the pupil rather than efficiently freeing it from incarceration in the wound. This practice, and that of wicking entrapped vitreous strands with a cellulose sponge, should be replaced by amputating anterior–posterior prolapsed vitreous connections with the vitreous cutter. This amputation method can be clearly visualized when using particulate identification with triamcinolone acetonide. Once connection to the vitreous body is eliminated, such strands and sheets can be easily removed without consequence to the retina (▶ Video 23.12).

Maintenance of a normotensive globe is achieved through the use of tight fitting and closed incisions as well as proper management of inflow and outflow. Judicious use of OVDs are necessary to avoid hypotony and wide pressure swings. Acute pressure variations promote choroidal effusion and catastrophic suprachoroidal hemorrhage. Vitreous always follows along a high- to low-pressure gradient which is why strict prevention of AC collapse throughout the case is essential to prevent re-presentation of vitreous and avoid postoperative traction of vitreous strands left associated with AC structures. Strictly embracing proper technique generally avoids impaired visual outcomes, all-the-more important if there is a refractive goal.

A key part of our strategy must be to protect other tissues from collateral damage. Though we must deal with vitreous, there is no justification for losing much needed capsule support, chewing up iris, or causing corneal edema by failing to protect the endothelium. The anterior segment surgeon must leave a clean anterior segment with a stable implant whenever appropriate and a clear visual axis for rapid visual rehabilitation or for allowing further timely management if needed.

One-piece presbyopia correcting IOLs and toric implants should only be placed when there is assurance of stable and maintainable centration. Any time we can convert a tear to a continuous posterior rhexis we can optic capture below the posterior capsule with haptics in the bag. Our most commonly reliable back-up when the posterior capsule is breached is to reverse optic capture if the IOL is already in the bag at the time a break is noted. Alternatively, a capsular tuck implantation: placing the IOL in the sulcus and tucking both haptics into the bag is a safer approach to the same configuration.[21] Any time optic capture is accomplished, the lens cannot rotate or subluxate (assuming zonules are competent). The IOL power may change by about 0.50 D depending on the dioptric power. It is nice to have a chart (and IOLs) available in the OR to convert powers accurately.

Only a three-piece lens can be placed with haptics in the sulcus. The optic is captured through a continuous anterior or posterior capsulotomy (or both), or otherwise fixated to iris or sclera for reliable long-term centration. Few recognize that sulcus implantation is off-label in the United States. Sadly, no three-piece toric- or presbyopia-correcting lenses designed for the sulcus are available in the United States. An accommodating IOL (Crystalens) should not be placed in the setting of a broken posterior capsule. Refractive cataract surgeons should be prepared to include peripheral keratotomy as a substitute maneuver for toric lenses. Patients should be informed as part of consent that it may not be safe to implant the chosen technology in rare circumstances.

There are many details to successful complication management, both intraoperative and postoperative, which are beyond the scope of this chapter; the authors encourage you to read widely.

23.21 Capsule Polishing

Always strive to leave a clean visual axis. I avoid vacuuming the posterior capsule with the I/A tip and limit vacuum mode to the anterior capsule rim. The latter is firmly supported in the normal eye by the anterior and equatorial zonules unlike the more flaccid PC. Vacuuming the PC is zonule unfriendly. Although high velocity irrigation can succeed, I prefer using a Terry Squeegee (Alcon Laboratories, Inc., Fort Worth, TX). It is soft and tends not to have burrs like diamond-dusted instruments can develop. The cannula has a silicone sleeve over its barrel and can be attached to the viscoelastic syringe used for IOL placement. This arrangement avoids an extra entry into the eye. OVD is useful for achieving safe capsular polishing by "greasing" the capsule so friction won't catch it, causing a tear. I usually first inject a small amount of viscoelastic on the surface of the posterior capsule to put a little tension on the capsule before attempting to polish it. I then inject more as needed to maintain a taut capsule.

A PC fibrotic membrane can sometimes have the edge teased off the capsule allowing a peel with forceps. If this proves too risky, particularly in a posterior polar cataract, I consider a planned hyaloid-sparing posterior continuous capsulorhexis (PCCC). Absent capsule provides a clearer visual axis than the clearest intact capsule and, in adults, PCCC drastically reduces the risk of subsequent visual axis obscuration requiring Nd:YAG posterior capsulotomy. PCCC is a skill worth learning. It will help you in complex and complicated cases. Along with posterior optic capture into Berger space, PCCC could be the truest "premium surgery" as it is one and done[22] (▶ Video 23.13).

Leaving a refractive cataract patient with a visually significant posterior capsule opacity leads to frustration. It delays visual recovery and requires an early laser procedure with real risk, especially in the presence of any subclinical postoperative inflammation or significant myopia. It is especially problematic in the setting of multifocality where it becomes impossible to interpret the cause of patient dissatisfaction. Any subsequent lens exchange or even piggyback procedure, should the patient remain dissatisfied after opening the hazy capsule, increases the risk of vitreous presentation.

Although many surgeons now use curettes routinely to "scrape" residual cells off the anterior capsule there are pros and cons to this procedure. It reduces fibrosis of the anterior capsule. It also hastens or increases posterior capsule opacity by delaying the sandwich effect that closes the capsule around the square-edged implant preventing equatorial cells (which are never eliminated) from migrating to the visual axis.[23] We certainly want to prevent lens cells' fibrotic metaplasia but I'm not sure our goal should be to eliminate these epithelial cells entirely. They may play a significant role in the maintenance of lens capsule and zonular basement membrane integrity over time. We are experiencing an epidemic of late bag-lens subluxations even in patients without clinical pseudoexfoliation, often associated with phimosis. We also are beginning to rarely see dead bag syndrome where the lens is no longer adherent to the bag and the tissue is friable. Time will hopefully inform us about etiology and prevention.

23.22 Implant Insertion

Fill the bag with OVD, making certain the distal capsular fornix is well expanded to receive the IOL without risking proximal zonule stress. I have previously mentioned that I won't stretch an incision, and therefore I prefer to have the tip of the cartridge just inside the Descemet membrane internal incision rather than in the tunnel before pushing it down the barrel. I use a sweep in the paracentesis as countertraction to get to this point. Because I prefer control over speed, I use a two-handed screw-type inserter and I ask the patient to "…fight to look at the light while the lens goes inside. The light will brighten up. The lens is folded into this little tube and springy arms will open to keep it centered and secure." This patter empowers the patient to help me with counterpressure.

Rather than withdrawing the plunger immediately, I use it as a finger to immediately tuck the optic-haptic junction and haptic elbow underneath the anterior capsule so the trailing haptic cannot open out of the bag, threatening the endothelium. As it slowly unfolds, I position my I/A handpiece for final OVD removal. If the chamber has tended to be collapsible during the case, I irrigate the incision and hydrate the incision's roof before using the I/A to be sure the AC won't shallow upon I/A removal. With the I/A tip in the chamber and the bag open and controlled with OVD, nudge the IOL into the correct toric meridian and center it if needed.

In the rare event that the IOL doesn't open but has a haptic stuck to the optic, just deform the haptic slightly by gently squeezing it with forceps on either side of the stuck haptic; it will immediately unfold.

Now is the time to evaluate the size and conformation of the CCC relative to the optic. It is a simple maneuver to enlarge the rhexis or improve symmetry at this time with a tangential cut and spiraling motion with capsulorhexis forceps.

23.23 OVD Removal

The "rock-and-roll" technique of OVD removal often doesn't work. If we want to assure stability of the IOL position, especially for toric implants, we must fully remove OVD from the posterior chamber. This will also eliminate capsule distention syndrome and reduce the chances of postoperative pressure spikes. Since the posterior chamber and anterior chamber are expanded with OVD upon I/A insertion, it is safe and easy to remove the viscoelastic from the posterior chamber first. The I/A tip is insinuated under the edge of the optic, nudging it to the side if necessary, and lifting it up while in foot position 0 so there is no irrigation. Orient the port sideways so it is neither tamponaded by the optic nor, most importantly, able to engage the posterior capsule. Foot position 2 is then engaged directly from foot position 0, allowing all OVD to be evacuated from under the IOL. The lens is then allowed to fall backward into the bag. Now the AC is evacuated in the usual manner. This works in every case and for every model lens so long as the posterior capsule is intact to begin with. This is extremely safe and effective; I have never broken a capsule with this technique in tens of thousands of cases.

Before removing the I/A handpiece, nudge the IOL into the ideal position while the chamber is controlled with BSS in foot position 1. Center the lens on the visual axis and correct any toric misalignment. Then exit the incision abruptly, allowing it to snap shut. Always exit the eye on foot position 0 so that iris is not inclined to follow.

Immediately prepare your irrigation cannula to assure incision closure as discussed above.

23.24 Drape Removal

This seems like a minor detail easily delegated, but I highly recommend you do this yourself. Hold the skin as you remove the adhesive to minimize pulling lid skin upward, causing discomfort and potentially deforming the incision. Always avoid any possibility of pressure directly on the incision's posterior lip.

23.25 Conclusion

Attention to detail, attentive focus on the task, and the pursuit of perfection maximizes the likelihood of fulfilling the high-visual expectations of our refractive cataract patients.

References

[1] Hayashi K, Yoshida M, Sato T, Manabe SI. Effect of topical hypotensive medications for preventing intraocular pressure increase after cataract surgery in eyes with glaucoma. Am J Ophthalmol. 2019; 205:91–98

[2] Arbisser LB. Safety of intracameral moxifloxacin for prophylaxis of endophthalmitis after cataract surgery. J Cataract Refract Surg. 2008; 34(7):1114–1120

[3] Haripriya A, Chang DF, Ravindran RD. Endophthalmitis reduction with intracameral moxifloxacin prophylaxis: analysis of 600000 surgeries. Ophthalmology. 2017; 124(6): 768–775

[4] Myers WG, Shugar JK. Optimizing the intracameral dilation regimen for cataract surgery: prospective randomized comparison of 2 solutions. J Cataract Refract Surg. 2009; 35 (2):273–276

[5] Zhang F. Special communication for deaf patients during topical anesthesia cataract surgery. Am J Ophthalmol Case Rep. 2020; 20:100940

[6] Hamilton RC. Retrobulbar and peribulbar anesthesia for cataract surgery. In: Steinert RF, ed. Cataract surgery. 3rd ed. Elsevier; 2010

[7] Smith JC, Hamilton BK, VanDyke SA. Patient comfort during cataract surgery: a comparison of troche and intravenous sedation. AANA J. 2020; 88(6):429–435

[8] Fine IH, Hoffman RS, Packer M. Profile of clear corneal cataract incisions demonstrated by ocular coherence tomography. J Cataract Refract Surg. 2007; 33(1):94–97

[9] Chang DF, Mamalis N, Ophthalmic Instrument Cleaning and Sterilization Task Force. Guidelines for the cleaning and sterilization of intraocular surgical instruments. J Cataract Refract Surg. 2018; 44(6):765–773

[10] Arshinoff SA. Dispersive-cohesive viscoelastic soft shell technique. J Cataract Refract Surg. 1999; 25(2):167–173

[11] Chee SP, Chan NS. Capsule milking: Modification of capsulorhexis technique for intumescent cataract. J Cataract Refract Surg. 2017; 43(5):585–589

[12] Little BC, Smith JH, Packer M. Little capsulorhexis tear-out rescue. J Cataract Refract Surg. 2006; 32(9):1420–1422

[13] Arbisser LB, Schultz T, Dick HB. Central dimple-down maneuver for consistent continuous femtosecond laser capsulotomy. J Cataract Refract Surg. 2013; 39(12):1796–1797

[14] Fine IH. Cortical cleaving hydrodissection. J Cataract Refract Surg. 1992; 18(5):508–512

[15] Nakano CT, Motta AFP, Hida WT, et al. Hurricane cortical aspiration technique: one-step continuous circular aspiration maneuver. J Cataract Refract Surg. 2014; 40(4):514–516

[16] Vasavada AR, Raj SM. Inside-out delineation. J Cataract Refract Surg. 2004; 30(6):1167–1169

[17] Anisimova NS, Arbisser LB, Shilova NF, et al. Anterior vitreous detachment: risk factor for intraoperative complications during phacoemulsification. J Cataract Refract Surg. 2020; 46(1):55–62

[18] Benjamin L. Fluidics and rheology in phaco surgery: what matters and what is the hype? Eye (Lond). 2018; 32(2): 204–209

[19] Arbisser LB. Pars plana anterior vitrectomy. In: Fishkind WJ, ed. Phacoemulsification and intraocular lens implantation mastering techniques and complications in cataract surgery. 2nd ed. Thieme Publishers; 2017

[20] Wenner Y, Wismann S, Preising MN, Jäger M, Pons-Kühnemann J, Lorenz B. Normative values of peripheral retinal thickness measured with Spectralis OCT in healthy young adults. Graefes Arch Clin Exp Ophthalmol. 2014; 252 (8):1195–1205

[21] Gimbel HV, Marzouk HA. Haptic tuck for reverse optic capture of a single-piece acrylic toric or other single-piece acrylic intraocular lenses. J Cataract Refract Surg. 2019; 45 (2):125–129

[22] Menapace R. Posterior capsulorhexis combined with optic buttonholing: an alternative to standard in-the-bag implantation of sharp-edged intraocular lenses? A critical analysis of 1000 consecutive cases. Graefes Arch Clin Exp Ophthalmol. 2008; 246(6):787–801

[23] Menapace R, Wirtitsch M, Findl O, Buehl W, Kriechbaum K, Sacu S. Effect of anterior capsule polishing on posterior capsule opacification and neodymium:YAG capsulotomy rates: three-year randomized trial. J Cataract Refract Surg. 2005; 31(11):2067–2075

Index

Note: Page numbers set **bold** or *italic* indicate headings or figures, respectively.